PENGUIN CLASSICS

T0249359

ROOTS OF YOGA

JAMES MALLINSON is Senior Lecturer in Sanskrit and Classical Indian Civilization at SOAS, University of London. His research focuses on the yoga tradition, in particular the texts, techniques and practitioners of traditional *haṭhayoga*. He has edited and translated several texts on *haṭhayoga* from its formative period, the eleventh to fifteenth centuries CE, and published encyclopedia entries and journal articles on yoga's history. His primary research methods in addition to philology are ethnography and art history. He has spent several years living with traditional Hindu ascetics and yogis in India and was honoured with the title of 'mahant' by the Ramanandi Sampradaya at the 2013 Kumbh Mela festival. He is currently leading a five-year, six-person research project at SOAS on the history of *haṭhayoga*, funded by the European Research Council, whose outputs will include ten critical editions of key texts on *haṭhayoga*.

MARK SINGLETON is Senior Research Fellow in the department of Languages and Cultures of South Asia, SOAS, University of London, where he works with James Mallinson on the Indian and transnational history of *haṭhayoga*. He taught for six years at St John's College (Santa Fe, New Mexico), and was a Senior Long-Term Research Scholar at the American Institute of Indian Studies, based in Jodhpur (Rajasthan, India). He was a consultant and catalogue author for the 2013 exhibition 'Yoga: The Art of Transformation' at the Smithsonian Institute in Washington, DC, and has served as co-chair of the Yoga in Theory and Practice Group at the American Academy of Religions. He is a manager of the Modern Yoga Research website. His research focuses on the tensions between tradition and modernity in yoga, and the transformations that yoga has undergone in recent centuries in response to globalization. He has published book chapters, journal articles and encyclopedia entries on yoga, several edited volumes of scholarship, and a monograph entitled *Yoga Body: The Origins of Modern Posture Practice*. His current work involves the critical editing and translation of three Sanskrit texts of *haṭhayoga* and new research on the history of physical practices that were incorporated into or associated with yoga in pre-colonial India.

Roots of Yoga

Translated and Edited
with an Introduction by
JAMES MALLINSON *and* MARK SINGLETON

PENGUIN BOOKS

PENGUIN CLASSICS

UK | USA | Canada | Ireland | Australia
India | New Zealand | South Africa

Penguin Books is part of the Penguin Random House group of companies
whose addresses can be found at global.penguinrandomhouse.com.

Penguin
Random House
UK

This edition first published in Penguin Classics 2017

024

Set in 10.25/12.25 pt Adobe Sabon
Typeset by Jouve (UK), Milton Keynes
Printed and bound in Great Britain by Clays Ltd, Elcograf S.p.A.

ISBN: 978–0–241–25304–5

www.greenpenguin.co.uk

Contents

Note on the Reference System and Diacritics

The translated passages are numbered sequentially from the beginning to the end of the book, and are referred to in the introductions by these numbers, which are given in bold type. In cases where the chapter arrangement is entirely chronological, the first number indicates the chapter and the second the translation itself. So, for example, **3.4** denotes Chapter 3, translation 4. In cases where the chapters are arranged thematically, the first number indicates the chapter, the second the thematic section, and the third the translation. So, for example, **6.2.1** denotes Chapter 6, section 2, translation 1.

Historically, Sanskrit has been written using many different scripts. Since the advent of printing, the most common of these, especially in northern India, has been Devanāgarī (देवनागरी). It is important to understand, however, that these scripts are not Sanskrit itself but systems for representing its sounds. The Roman alphabet (used for writing English and other European languages) cannot represent the full range of sounds in Sanskrit, and so we must add diacritical marks to certain letters. In this book we follow the conventions of the International Alphabet of Sanskrit Transliteration (IAST), which allows for the lossless representation of the Sanskrit syllabary in Roman script.

Introduction[1]

Over the last three decades there has been an enormous increase in the popularity of yoga around the world. The United Nations' recent declaration of an International Day of Yoga[2] is symbolic of yoga's truly globalized status today. Along with this globalization, however, has come metamorphosis: yoga has adapted to social and cultural conditions often far removed from those of its birthplace, and in many regions has taken on a life of its own, independent of its Indian roots. The global diffusion of yoga began at least a century and a half ago, since which time yoga has continued to be refracted through many new cultural prisms, such as New Age religion, psychology, sports science, biomedicine, and so on.[3]

In spite of yoga's now global popularity (or perhaps, rather, because of it), a clear understanding of its historical contexts in South Asia, and the range of practices that it includes, is often lacking. This is at least partly due to limited access to textual material.[4] A small canon of texts, which includes the *Bhagavadgītā*, Patañjali's *Yogasūtra*s, the *Haṭhapradīpikā* and some Upaniṣads, may be studied within yoga teacher-training programmes, but by and large the wider textual sources are little known outside specialized scholarship. Along with the virtual hegemony of a small number of posture-oriented systems in the recent global transmission of yoga, this has reinforced a relatively narrow and monochromatic vision of what yoga is and does, especially when viewed against the wide spectrum of practices presented in pre-modern texts.

Of course, texts are not reflective of the totality of yoga's development – they merely provide windows on to particular traditions at particular times – and an absence of evidence for certain practices within texts is not evidence of their absence within yoga as a whole.[5] Conversely, the appearance of new practices in texts is itself often an indication of older innovations. Despite these limitations, however, texts remain a unique and dependable source of knowledge about yoga at particular moments in history, in contrast to often unverifiable retrospective self-accounts of particular lineages. In addition to texts, material sources, particularly sculpture and painting from the second millennium CE, provide invaluable data for the reconstruction of yoga's history. While we have not addressed such sources directly here, they have informed our analyses. Examples of our work with such sources can be found in Diamond 2013.

In some respects this book resembles a traditional Sanskrit *nibandha* (scholarly compilation) in that it gathers together a wide variety of texts on a single topic.[6] Unlike a *nibandha*, however, our approach does not have a sectarian religious orientation, and it will, we hope, be somewhat more accessible as a result. The material is drawn from more than a hundred texts, dating from about 1000 BCE to the nineteenth century, many of which are not well known. Although most of the passages translated here are from Sanskrit texts, there is also material from Tibetan, Arabic, Persian, Bengali, Tamil, Pali, Kashmiri, Old Marathi, Avadhi and Braj Bhasha (late-medieval precursors of Hindi) and English sources. This chronological and linguistic range reveals patterns and continuities that contribute to a better understanding of yoga's development within and across traditions (for example, between earlier Sanskrit sources and later vernacular or non-Indian texts which draw on them). Where possible, we have used the earliest available textual occurrence of a particular passage, rather than a later duplication. For this reason, perhaps better known but derivative texts, such as the later Yoga Upaniṣads,[7] are passed over in favour of the earlier texts from which they borrow. By and large we have not included material which is incidental to the mainstream of yoga theory and practice in South Asia, nor do we draw on non-textual sources popularly considered to be fundamental to yoga's history, but which have been discredited by scholarship.[8] Indeed, this collection benefits enormously from advances in historical and philological research in yoga traditions over the past three decades (see 'Yoga Scholarship' below, p. xxii).

The yoga whose roots we are identifying is that which prevailed in India on the eve of colonialism, i.e. the late eighteenth century. Although certainly not without its variations and exceptions, by this time there is a pervasive, trans-sectarian consensus throughout India as to what constitutes yoga in practice. One of the reasons for this is the rise to predominance of the techniques of *haṭhayoga*, which held a virtual hegemony across a wide spectrum of yoga-practising religious traditions, including the Brahmanical traditions, in the pre-colonial period.[9] The texts included in this collection reflect this historical development. As well as delimiting what would otherwise be an unmanageable amount of material, focusing on yoga as it was most commonly understood helps to reflect the actual practices of a majority of traditions in which yoga was undertaken. Such a focus can also help shed light on the immediate predecessors of the nineteenth- and twentieth-century yogis who helped disseminate yoga around the world.

The material represented here is largely practical in nature, not philosophical. In general, we do not include passages on metaphysics unless they are directly related to practice (e.g. meditation on the elements (*tattva*s)). Although traditional yoga rarely, if ever, occurs outside of particular religious and doctrinal contexts, these contexts vary considerably, while yoga itself retains essential theoretical and practical commonalities.[10] We therefore focus mainly on the practice of yoga and not on the philosophical systems that may underpin this practice in its specific sectarian settings. In addition, a distinction needs to be drawn between yoga as practice, as found across a wide range of Indian traditions, and Yoga as a doctrinal or philosophical system rooted in traditions of exegesis (i.e. textual interpretation) that developed from the *Pātañjalayogaśāstra*. Notwithstanding the popular notion that the *Pātañjalayogaśāstra* is the fundamental text of yoga, and fully recognizing its enormous impact on practical formulations of yoga throughout history (in particular *haṭhayoga*, with which it is sometimes identified in texts),[11] it is in fact a partisan text, representing an early Brahmanical appropriation of extra-Vedic, Śramaṇa techniques of yoga, such as those of early Buddhism (on which, see below p. xiii). Its long exegetical tradition is not one of practice but of philosophy. Although this exegesis is vital to understanding the development of metaphysical speculation in South Asia, particularly in orthodox contexts, it is not our focus here, in that it does not significantly contribute to a history of yoga practices. Those interested in the philosophical traditions associated with the *Pātañjalayogaśāstra* should consult Philipp Maas's forthcoming sourcebook of yoga's 'classical dualist philosophy'.

Finally, it is worth pointing out that this is not a manual of yoga practice. It is a work of scholarship documenting a wide range of yoga methods, a few of which may cause injury or illness, and some of which may even lead to physical and/or cognitive 'death', if practised successfully. The reader undertakes the practices described in this book entirely at his or her own risk.

HISTORICAL OVERVIEW

Yoga in Vedic-era Sources

Prior to about 500 BCE there is very little evidence within South Asian textual or archaeological sources that points to the existence of systematic, psychophysical techniques of the type which the word 'yoga' subsequently came to denote. Passages in the oldest Sanskrit text, the fifteenth- to twelfth-century BCE *Ṛg Veda* (the earliest of the four 'Vedas', the textual foundation of orthodox, 'Vedic' Hinduism) indicate the use of visionary meditation and its famous hymn to a long-haired sage (10.136) suggests a mystical ascetic tradition similar to those of later yogis.[12] The somewhat later *Atharva Veda* (*c.* 1000 BCE),[13] in its description of the Vrātya, who, like the long-haired sage, exists on the fringe of mainstream Vedic society, mentions practices which may be forerunners of later yogic techniques of posture and breath-retention (on the latter, see **4.1**), and the *Jaiminīya Upaniṣad Brāhmaṇa* (*c.* 800–600 BCE) teaches mantra-repetition, together with control of the breath. But it is entirely speculative to claim, as several popular writers on yoga have done,[14] that the Vedic corpus provides any evidence of systematic yoga practice.

Muddying the waters is the fact that later yoga texts composed in Brahmanical milieus incorporate Vedic motifs, such as the attainment of immortality. Similarly, the word *yoga* itself appears in the *Ṛg Veda*, but generally with reference to the chariot of war to which horses were yoked – 'yoke' being an English cognate of the Sanskrit *yoga*. This Vedic usage of the word is still in evidence a millennium later in the *Mahābhārata*, where dying heroes travel through the sun and onwards to heaven by means of their 'yoga chariot'.[15] Although the *Mahābhārata* also incorporates extensive instructions on yogic practice, and the Vedic image of yoking evolves into a metaphor of the soteriological method (i.e. a method which leads towards salvation or liberation), it would be wrong to read this backwards as proof of a similar understanding within the Vedas themselves. Similarly, the famous 'proto-Śiva' seals from the Indus Valley civilization (which developed from around 2800 BCE in modern-day Punjab and Sindh), in spite of their popular currency, offer no conclusive evidence of an ancient yogic culture.[16]

Śramaṇas

Around 500 BCE we see the rise of new groups of renunciant ascetics in India, sometimes collectively referred to as Śramaṇas ('strivers'), and identified by Johannes Bronkhorst as originating in the 'Greater Magadha' region, the area east of the confluence of the Ganges and Yamuna rivers in modern-day Allahabad in northern India.[17] These groups, which probably developed independently of the Brahmanical Vedic traditions, but were influenced by them to varying degrees, included Buddhists, Jains and the lesser-known Ājīvakas. They were concerned with finding ways to bring an end to the cycle of rebirth (*saṃsāra*) and the *karma*-driven suffering that characterizes human existence, and they developed techniques of meditation (*dhyāna*) to this end. The goal itself was known as *nirvāṇa* ('extinguishing') or *mokṣa* ('liberation'), and entailed the complete eradication of karmic traces, including the cessation of personal identity, in a kind of permanent ontological suicide (i.e. the irreversible destruction of one's very being). These ideas make their first appearance among the Śramaṇa traditions, and are only later incorporated into Vedic teachings.[18] The Śramaṇas did not refer to their practices as 'yoga' until later, and in fact the first mentions of *dhyānayoga* ('yoga [by means of] meditation' or 'the discipline of meditation') appear in the Brahmanical *Mahābhārata* (third century BCE to third century CE), with explicit reference to practices associated with Buddhism and Jainism.[19] Subsequently, the term *yoga* would become increasingly adopted among Buddhists themselves, and rather later among Jains, to indicate these meditational practices.

As well as meditational techniques, our early sources speak of ascetics within both the Śramaṇa and Vedic traditions engaged in arduous practices known as *tapas* (a singular noun which literally means 'heat', but which is translated in this book as 'austerities'). For the ascetics of the Vedic tradition, the aim of these austerities is usually to win a boon – often a protection or a special power – from the gods, while within the Śramaṇa traditions their purpose is said to be the stilling of the mind or the annihilation of past *karma*. In the *Mahābhārata* practitioners of *tapas* are referred to synonymously as *yogin*s, and their practices are frequently also termed *yoga*. Some scholars have attempted to draw a distinction between the early yoga of the non-Vedic Śramaṇas and the this-worldly, power-oriented *tapas* of the Vedic sages, asserting that even though the latter may be called *yoga*, it is not really yoga, because it is not concerned with liberation (*mokṣa*).[20] However, the texts of this period show that ascetics of all traditions engaged in austerities – the Buddha himself says that he tried various mortifying techniques (see **4.3**) – and that, in addition to liberation, the acquisition of supernatural powers, whether desirable or not, could result from these practices. It is clear that methods which might be differentiated as yoga and *tapas* were complementary parts of early ascetic practice, and this continues to be the case for Hindu ascetic yogis today.[21] *Tapas* is identified as a necessary preliminary for yoga practice in the *Pātañjalayogaśāstra* (see below and **1.2.2**)[22] and one of yoga's key practices, *prāṇāyāma* ('breath-control'), has long been identified as *tapas* (e.g. *Mānavadharmaśāstra* (**4.5**)). Textual teachings on extreme physical methods of *tapas* as practised by ascetics, such as the ancient *ūrdhvabāhu* ('raised arm') austerity, in which one or both arms are held up for years on end so that they atrophy, are not found, but the seals (*mudrā*s) and postures (*āsana*s) of *haṭhayoga*, which are first taught in texts from the beginning of the second millennium CE, appear to derive from some of the early Śramaṇa methods, and the word *haṭha* itself has overt connotations of asceticism, as we will see.[23] Many textual teachings on yoga can best be understood as attempts to instruct non-ascetics in techniques which emerged in ascetic milieus.

The Early Upaniṣads

The early Upaniṣads (*c.* seventh–first century BCE) are the first Brahmanical texts devoted to the teachings of ascetic renunciates.[24] The earliest known definition of yoga comes in the *c.* third-century BCE *Kaṭha Upaniṣad*, a dialogue between the boy Naciketas and Yama, the god of death (see 1.1.1). Drawing on an image familiar from the Vedic literature, but adapted to a soteriology of liberation, an analogy is drawn between living as a human being and riding a chariot. The body is the chariot itself, the self (*ātman*) is a rider in the chariot, the intellect (*buddhi*) is the charioteer, the mind (*manas*) is the reins, the senses (*indriya*) are the horses, and the sense objects (*viṣaya*) are the paths taken by the senses (3.3–4). If the senses are not brought under control, the result is rebirth. On the other hand, one who is able to control the senses by means of the mind, as a charioteer reins in his horses, is not reborn (3.7–8). He attains the highest state, which is identified as *puruṣa*, the indwelling person. The fourth, fifth and sixth chapters of the *Kaṭha Upaniṣad* are later than the first three. In the sixth chapter, the condition in which the senses are held still and one becomes undistracted is named *yoga* (6.11).

The *Kaṭha Upaniṣad*'s terms for the constituent elements of the human being are drawn from the ancient Indian dualistic philosophy known as Sāṃkhya. In the metaphysical narrative of Sāṃkhya, the material principle of existence, known as *prakṛti*, and the spiritual principle, called *puruṣa*, fall out of balance, resulting in a devolution into material existence. During the course of this process, *puruṣa* confuses itself with the twenty-four *tattvas* ('elements' or 'principles') of *prakṛti*, which include the senses, intellect and mind, as well as the grosser elements.[25] The human condition is therefore characterized by the delusory identification of the individual with the elements of *prakṛti*, the result of which is suffering and rebirth. As we shall see, this model provided a framework for much subsequent thinking about yoga, which developed as a practical solution to the ontological problem posed by Sāṃkhya.

Teachings on Yoga in the Mahābhārata, *including the* Bhagavadgītā

Teachings on Sāṃkhya and yoga are common in India's greatest epic the *Mahābhārata*, which had probably attained its current form by the end of the third century CE. They are especially common in a long section at the end of the twelfth book called the *Mokṣadharma*, several passages from which are included in this book. The *Mokṣadharma* contains probably the oldest systematization of yoga practice[26] and is thus a particularly important resource for information on the early practice of yoga. These extensive teachings have been utilized by a handful of scholars,[27] but remain little known outside of academia.

The *Bhagavadgītā* is part of the *Mahābhārata* and contains significant teachings on the practice of yoga, some of which are included in this book. As a text seeking to affirm Brahmanical religion, the *Bhagavadgītā* seeks to appropriate yoga from the renunciate milieu in which it originated, teaching that it is compatible with worldly activity carried out according to one's caste and life stage; it is only the fruits of one's actions that are to be renounced.

The Pātañjalayogaśāstra

The best-known early expression of yoga is the *Yogasūtra* of Patañjali, a series of one hundred and ninety-six short statements (*sūtra*s) concerning yogic techniques and states. Philipp Maas has shown that there is no manuscript transmission of these statements independent of their *bhāṣya* ('commentary'), which is commonly attributed to Vyāsa, and that the *sūtra*s and commentary are syntactically intertwined.[28] Maas convincingly argues that we should therefore consider the *sūtra*s and the commentary as the unified work of a single author who compiled the *sūtra* portion of the text from older sources some time between 325 and 425 CE.[29] He further suggests that the combined text should be called by the name by which it is referred to in the colophons of its manuscripts: the *Pātañjala-Yoga-Śāstra Sāṃkhya-Pravacana* ('the authoritative exposition of yoga that originates with Patañjali, the mandatory Sāṃkhya teaching'),[30] or the *Pātañjalayogaśāstra* as we will henceforth refer to it in this book. As this title would suggest, the metaphysical basis for the *Pātañjalayogaśāstra*'s teachings on yoga comes from Sāṃkhya, and the text describes practical means to escape the trap of existence characterized by suffering and rebirth. The influence of Buddhism is also evident in the text,[31] and the *Pātañjalayogaśāstra* represents a Brahmanical attempt to appropriate yoga from the Śramaṇa traditions.

Redactors subsequently divided the *Pātañjalayogaśāstra* into four chapters (*pāda*s) concerned, respectively, with the refined cognitive states known as *samādhi*; the practical methods to attain these states (*sādhana*, including the well-known yoga of eight 'limbs' or 'auxiliaries', *aṣṭāṅgayoga*, see 1.4.3); the special powers (*siddhi*, *vibhūti*; see Chapter 10) acquired through practice; and the final state of liberation (*kaivalya*, see Chapter 11). However, such a thematic division is not necessarily an accurate reflection of the contents of the chapters, which sometimes overlap with each other or include different themes from those their titles suggest. The *Pātañjalayogaśāstra* became an important reference for many – though by no means all – formulations of yoga which were to follow.[32] In about the twelfth century, yoga, with the *Pātañjalayogaśāstra* as its root text, is for the first time included in a list of philosophical systems (*darśana*s), both orthodox and heterodox, and it was subsequently included in a list of six orthodox *darśana*s that acquired canonical status.[33] Yoga's position as an orthodox *darśana* made the *Pātañjalayogaśāstra* of especial interest to early European scholars of Indian religion.[34] The many translations and studies that followed have ensured that the *Pātañjalayogaśāstra*, or at least the *sūtra* section of it, has enjoyed an enormous appeal globally both among scholars and in yoga-practitioner circles.

Yogācāra Buddhism

The two centuries prior to the composition of the *Pātañjalayogaśāstra* saw the beginnings of the Buddhist Yogācāra school, whose identifying feature was the practice of yoga. The Yogācāra textual corpus was considerably more extensive than that of the Pātañjala tradition and it influenced the text of the *Pātañjalayogaśāstra*. The importance of Yogācāra Buddhism for the understanding of yoga in India in the first millennium CE has been widely overlooked in scholarship for a variety of reasons, in particular the subsequent decline of Buddhism in India. We have drawn on its teachings only fleetingly in this book (see 1.1.4) because our aim is to trace the roots of yoga as it was practised in India on the eve of colonialism and Yogācāra and other early Buddhist yoga traditions do not pertain directly to this later development, other than in how they influenced the *Pātañjalayogaśāstra*. For an understanding of yoga's early history, however, the study of Yogācāra is essential.[35]

Tantra

Yoga was important in a range of traditions – predominantly Śaiva, Vaiṣṇava and Buddhist – that together constituted India's dominant 'religion' in the period from the sixth to the thirteenth century CE, and which has come to be known as 'tantra'.[36] The Sanskrit word *tantra* can refer to a text – many of the texts of the tantric traditions are called *tantra* – or 'a system of ritual or essential instructions', but in a more specific sense it indicates a body of soteriological knowledge, ritual and praxis regarded as distinct from, and more powerful than, Vedic revelation.[37] Usually associated with a deity or deities (even in doctrinally atheistic systems like Buddhism), the practices of tantra, which include ritual,[38] worship and mantra-repetition, as well as yoga, have as their aim either the attainment of supernatural powers (*siddhi*s) or the ascent of the practitioner through manifold stages of consciousness until he or she reaches either proximity to or non-differentiated union with the deity (the nature of the goal varies according to the many tantric traditions' different metaphysical systems).

An array of rituals and practices developed within the various tantric schools, sometimes (especially in the Śaiva systems known as Kaula) with a special emphasis on transgressive practices involving the ritual consumption of forbidden substances, sex rites and proximity to death. It is important to be aware, however, that tantric rituals are not themselves yoga (although they may contain yogic elements) and that in many tantric texts it is the section on ritual (*kriyāpāda*) – rather than the sections on yoga (*yogapāda*), knowledge (*vidyāpāda*) or rules (*caryāpāda*) – that is most important, while the other sections provide the conditions for the success of the ritual.[39]

Tantric yoga commonly involves complex visualizations of an ascent through the *tattva*s or elements taught in a particular system (tantric systems typically add eleven *tattva*s to the twenty-five of Sāṃkhya) until the yogi achieves dissolution (*laya*) in the supreme *tattva*, which is usually the deity of the system concerned. Tantric yogas may also include meditation on the body as the microcosm of the cosmos, with the *tattva*s aligned vertically along it (sometimes as characteristics of *cakra*s, on which see below), as well as the use of mantras, breath-control (*prāṇāyāma*) and other techniques.

In some tantric systems the body is conceived of as composed of a number of subtle channels (*nāḍīs*), which, when purified, conduct the vital energy of the body (*prāṇa*), which can then be manipulated and directed (see Chapter 5). The notion of a network of subtle channels can be traced back at least as far as the *Bṛhadāraṇyaka Upaniṣad* (2.1.19), but it increases in complexity and sophistication within the tantric tradition, beginning with the fifth-century CE *Niśvāsatattva-saṃhitā*. One of the most influential models of the tantric body is first described in the *c.* tenth-century *Kubjikāmatatantra*, which belongs to the Kaula tantric cult of the goddess Kubjikā, known as the 'Western Transmission' (*paścimāmnāya*). In this tradition a system of six power centres (*cakra*s, literally 'wheels') equivalent to six variant forms of Kubjikā and her consort are invested in the body of the yogi.[40] Although other such systems are found in tantric texts, it was the *cakra* system of Kubjikā that came to be accepted as the blueprint of the 'yogic body'. Another key feature of many later tantric yogas, which, in its developed form, is also first found in the *Kubjikāmatatantra*, is the goddess Kuṇḍalinī. Kuṇḍalinī resides at the base of the spine and, through practices that initially only included visualization, but subsequently, in the haṭhayogic traditions, acquired physical components, is made to rise up through the central channel (Suṣumnā)[41] to the crown of the head, where she is united with her male counterpart, Śiva. Kuṇḍalinī's ascent is a development from the earlier systems of sequential visualization of increasingly subtle elements mentioned above.

Haṭhayoga

At the end of the first millennium CE the first references to a method of yoga called *haṭha* appear in textual sources. Many of its principles and practices are taught for the first time in the *Amṛtasiddhi*, a *c.* eleventh-century tantric Buddhist work, but that text does not call its yoga *haṭha*. A formalized system of yoga called *haṭha* is taught for the first time in the *c.* thirteenth-century *Dattātreyayogaśāstra*, a Vaiṣṇava text. *Haṭhayoga*'s methods draw from those of Pātañjala and tantric yoga, but also include physical practices found in neither. These are cleansing techniques, non-seated postures (*āsana*s), complex methods of breath-control and physical means of manipulating the vital energy (*mudrā*s). Although these practices are taught for the first time in *haṭhayoga* texts, many of them, in particular the *āsana*s and *mudrā*s, bear a close similarity to ascetic practices first mentioned in the latter half of the first millennium BCE, shortly after the time of the Buddha. Indeed, the name *haṭha* ('force') is itself redolent of difficult austerities, and in the Tamil *Tirumandiram*, whose teachings on yoga are perhaps contemporaneous with or a little later than those of the *Dattātreyayogaśāstra*, *haṭhayoga* is called *tava-yoga*, *tava* being the Tamil form of the Sanskrit *tapas* ('austerity'). But the methods of *haṭhayoga* are not as extreme as many of the mortifications undertaken by Indian ascetics; only those techniques which might be used by more worldly yogis are taught. This adaptation of ascetic methods for a wider, non-ascetic audience is likely to be the reason for the composition of the texts on *haṭhayoga*.

In its first formalization, in the *Dattātreyayogaśāstra*, *haṭha-yoga* is taught as an alternative or supplement to a yoga consisting of the eight *aṅga*s taught in the *Pātañjalayogaśāstra*. In the middle of the second millennium CE the orthodox Brahmanical scholar Śivānanda Sarasvatī taught the methods of *haṭhayoga* alongside those of the *Pātañjalayogaśāstra* in his *Yogacintāmaṇi*, a lengthy compendium of passages on yoga. By the eighteenth century *haṭha* and Pātañjala yoga were seen as one and the same,[42] and *haṭha*'s rise to orthodox acceptance had been cemented by the compilation of a corpus of Upaniṣads (later referred to as the Yoga Upaniṣads) that borrowed wholesale from the texts of *haṭhayoga*.[43] *Haṭhayoga*'s rise to prominence spread to other traditions: from the eighteenth century onwards the revivalist Jain Terāpanthīs included its practice in their teachings.[44]

Modern Yoga

Although the most recent texts translated here date from the middle of the nineteenth century, it is worth mentioning that for about the past one hundred and fifty years yoga has been developing in new and important ways, inside and outside India, in response to the processes of globalization and modernization. Traditional Indian forms of yoga practice – in particular *haṭhayoga* – have undergone sometimes radical transformations and adaptations in the encounter with foreign ideas and practices, and 'diasporic' yogas have taken on a life of their own in many parts of the world. Adaptation and mutation have always been features of yoga's history, as competing and coexisting theories and practices exert their influence on one another, with some practices disappearing while others take on new, sophisticated forms. The texts represented in this book offer numerous examples of this, the seventeenth- and eighteenth-century proliferation of *āsana*s being one (Chapter 3), and the complex development of conceptions of the yogic body across the centuries another (Chapter 5). In the modern period similar processes are at work; however, the sheer range of new ideas and the speed with which they are transmitted within and between nations and cultures (for example, through travel, print and photography, and more lately via the internet) increase exponentially. Modern, global forms of yoga exist in a variety of complex and recursive relationships with 'traditional' yoga. Commonly, yoga in its global contexts has been interpreted by analogy with other concepts and practices that are more easily understood within the culture at hand. Thus, for example, over the past century yoga has been conceived variously as psychotherapy, philosophy, hypnotherapy and mesmerism, black magic, chiropractic bodywork, shamanism and sport (among other things). These analogical understandings have had a profoundly transformative effect on the way yoga is interpreted and practised in the world today.[45]

YOGA SCHOLARSHIP

One of the reasons we decided to embark on this project was to make available to a wide audience a range of primary sources that have not previously been used in scholarship on yoga (or at least not widely so), but are of key importance for understanding its history. Nevertheless, our work here is indebted to many scholars who have expanded our knowledge of yoga's history. In this section we review some of this scholarship in order to provide an overview of the scholarly study of yoga and to situate this book within a broader field of inquiry.

Until recently few yoga texts other than the *Pātañjalayogaśāstra* and its better-known commentaries had been the subject of rigorous philological scholarship. Studies of *haṭhayoga*, which, as we have seen above, is central to yoga's development, have for the most part been reliant on translations of three texts that were published as uncritical editions towards the end of the nineteenth century, namely the *Haṭhapradīpikā*, *Śivasaṃhitā* and *Gheraṇḍasaṃhitā*. In a landmark monograph published in 1994 Christian Bouy, by identifying shared passages in a wide range of *haṭha* texts, was able to demonstrate that these three texts all postdate *haṭhayoga*'s formative period and present convoluted and inconsistent amalgamations of teachings from earlier, more coherent works. These earlier works have only recently begun to be the object of scholarly study. Three have been critically edited, namely the *Khecarīvidyā*, *Amanaska* and *Matsyendrasaṃhitā*. Others are still only available in manuscript form or have been published only in hard-to-obtain Indian editions as simple copies of single manuscripts (e.g. the *Amṛtasiddhi*, *Candrāvalokana*, *Dattātreyayogaśāstra*, *Yogabīja*, *Gorakṣaśataka*, *Vivekamārtaṇḍa*, *Amaraughaprabodha* and *Yogatārāvalī*).[46] The present authors, together with Jason Birch, are working on critical editions of all these texts, and we have included translations of passages from them in *Roots of Yoga*.

Since the early twentieth century the Kaivalyadhama Institute in western India and its offshoot, the Lonavla Yoga Research Institute, have been producing editions of important *haṭhayoga* texts, but these have escaped the attention of most scholars. Their work has concentrated on texts that post-date the fifteenth-century *Haṭhapradīpikā*, such as the *Haṭharatnāvalī*, *Haṭhatattvakaumudī*, *Yuktabhavadeva*, Caraṇ Dās's *Aṣṭāṅgayoga*, the *Ṣaṭkarmasaṃgraha* and Jayatarāma's *Jogpradīpakā*. They have also produced new collations of manuscripts of previously published texts such as the *Haṭhapradīpikā*, *Śivasaṃhitā*, *Gheraṇḍasaṃhitā* and *Siddhasiddhāntapaddhati*. Among their editions of pre-*Haṭhapradīpikā* texts particularly noteworthy are those of the *Vasiṣṭhasaṃhitā* and *Bṛhadyogiyājñavalkyasmṛti*. In addition to these texts (most of which are accompanied by English translations) both institutes have produced very useful manuscript catalogues and encyclopedias, and Kaivalyadhama's *Yogamīmāṃsā* journal continues to include textual studies together with scientific research on yoga's effects.

One-off scholarly studies of yoga texts that we have utilized include the 1920 edition and translation of the Yoga Upaniṣads published by the Theosophical Society's Adyar Library; Kalyani Mallik's verbatim transcriptions of manuscripts of the *Siddhasiddhāntapaddhati*, *Amaraughaprabodha* and *Yogaviṣaya*, published in 1954; and the *Amaraughaśāsana* in the Kashmir Series of Texts and Studies (1918). In 1976 Fausta Nowotny's edition of the *Gorakṣaśataka* was published.[47] It was based on only four relatively late (seventeenth-century) manuscripts; in this book we have based our translations from this text on the readings of a manuscript from 1477 CE not used by Nowotny and which calls the text *Vivekamārtaṇḍa*. Other individual editions of texts from the *haṭha* traditions which we have used in the present volume include those of the *Śivayogapradīpikā*, *Yogayājñavalkya*, *Śrītattvanidhi* and *Śārṅgadharapaddhati*.

The *Pātañjalayogaśāstra* has been the object of scholarly study for nearly two centuries,[48] but advances continue to be made. In particular, recent years have seen very fruitful text-critical studies from Philipp Maas (who, as noted above, was able to make crucial improvements to our dating of the text and the history of its composition) and Kengo Harimoto, who has critically edited parts of the *Pātañjalayogaśāstra* together with its *Vivaraṇa* commentary, demonstrating the importance of the latter for our understanding of the text.

Key to our being able to present new information on the history of yoga has been the remarkable progress made in the study of India's multifarious tantric traditions over the last three decades. The foundations for the study of Śaiva tantra were laid by the publications of the Kashmir Series of Texts and Studies in the first half of the twentieth century and the subsequent work of scholars at the Institut français de Pondichéry, in particular N. R. Bhatt and Hélène Brunner. In recent years great advances have been made by a number of scholars, in particular Alexis Sanderson and his collaborators and students.[49] Many of the critical editions and studies of tantric texts on yoga that we have used in this book have been published in the last two decades; especially noteworthy is the *Niśvāsatattvasaṃhitā*, the earliest known tantric work, a critical edition of which was published in 2015.

Advances in our knowledge of tantra more broadly conceived, including the Buddhist tantric traditions, have been crucial for improving our understanding of the context of tantric yoga.[50] Particularly useful in our analyses has been the ongoing Tāntrikābhidhānakośa Project, which, in a series of volumes, will constitute a comprehensive encyclopedia of Hindu tantric terminology.[51] Tantric studies have benefited from other collaborative projects; special mention should be made of the Nepal-German Manuscript Preservation Project (NGMPP) and the subsequent Nepalese-German Manuscript Cataloguing Project (NGMCP) at the University of Hamburg, which have microfilmed and catalogued a vast range of Nepalese manuscripts, many of which are tantric in orientation.[52] Dependent in part on the NGMPP have been the activities of the Muktabodha Indological Research Institute, which, under the direction of Mark Dyczkowski, has coordinated the transcription of a large number of editions and manuscripts of tantric works; we have used many of their transcriptions in our research.[53]

In tracing the roots and context of the yoga practices taught in the *Pātañjalayogaśāstra* and Śaiva and *haṭha* yoga texts we have utilized passages from the *Atharva Veda*, the early Upaniṣads, the Pali Canon of Buddhist works, the *Mahābhārata* and the *Dharmaśāstras*, and have benefited from the extensive text-critical and analytical scholarship available on these keystones of indology, including that of the Sanskrit commentarial tradition.

There is a great deal more work to be done in establishing the textual roots of the yoga traditions; this book should be seen as a summary of work to date, not a final word. Many tantric and *haṭha* works remain to be critically edited and are only available in manuscripts.[54] A textual corpus whose yoga teachings have so far been very little studied but which promises to be very fruitful is that of the Purāṇas, in particular their earlier sections, which were composed between *c.* 500 and 1000 CE. Usable editions of some Purāṇic passages on yoga are available: we have included translations from the *Skanda*, *Śiva*, *Mārkaṇḍeya* and *Bhāgavata Purāṇas*, together with the *Īśvaragītā* of the *Kūrmapurāṇa*.[55]

Previous general studies of the history of yoga have relied almost exclusively on texts in Sanskrit. As mentioned above, in our translations of passages relevant to the early history of yoga we have included teachings from Buddhist texts in Pali. We have also included a passage from a Chinese translation of the lost Sanskrit original of an early Buddhist tantra, the *Vairocanābhisaṃbodhisūtra*. In addition, when tracing the history of yoga in the second millennium CE, we have included passages from a wide range of works in other languages. These include (in approximate chronological order): the Old Marathi *Jñāneśvarī*, an extensive *c.* thirteenth-century commentary on the *Bhagavadgītā*, which includes beautiful teachings on the ascent of Kuṇḍalinī; the Tamil *Tirumandiram*, a vast compendium of Śaiva lore, which may include older teachings but the similarity of whose yoga sections to certain Sanskrit *haṭha* texts suggests that they were composed in approximately the thirteenth century; the Kashmiri *vatsun* songs of the tantric ascetic Lallā; the Arabic *Ḥawż al-ḥayāt* and Persian *Baḥr al-ḥayāt*; the Tibetan *Rtsa rlung gsang ba'i lde mig*; the Bengali *Gorakṣabijaẏ*; sixteenth- to eighteenth-century texts in Hindi (or, more precisely, its late medieval precursors Avadhi and Braj Bhasha), such as Kutuban's *Miragāvatī*, the *Gorakhbāṇī* attributed to Gorakhnāth, the *Sarvāṅgayogapradīpikā* of Sundardās and Jayatarāma's *Jogpradīpakā*; the anonymous translation into English of the life story of the ascetic Purāṇ Puri;[56] and the *Tashrīh al-Aqvām* (*c*. 1820), a Persian ethnography of northern India, written by Colonel James Skinner.

THE TRANSLATIONS

All of the translations from Pali, Avadhi and Braj Bhasha in this book are ours, as are nearly all of those from Sanskrit. In a few cases, however, we have used translations from Sanskrit by other scholars. We have also used translations by other scholars of passages in languages with which we are not familiar (Arabic, Chinese, Old Bengali, Kashmiri,[57] Old Marathi, Persian, Tamil and Tibetan).[58]

Since this book is intended for a general readership as well as a scholarly one, we have sought to avoid the kind of critical apparatus that is characteristic of indological scholarship. Nevertheless, in the case of many technical terms – and other words for which a knowledge of the Sanskrit clarifies or disambiguates the sense – we have included the original term in brackets after the translation, at least at its first occurrence in the passage in question, e.g., 'The states of the mind are distracted (*kṣipta*), confused (*mūḍha*), agitated (*vikṣipta*), focused (*ekāgra*) and restrained (*niruddha*)' (*Pātañjalayogaśāstra* 1.1). In contrast, words in square brackets are not translations of words in the original text, but are nonetheless suggested by the wider context and therefore must be supplied in order to arrive at a meaningful translation, e.g., '[A yogi], in other words, [is one who must experience] the Śiva-state' (*Mṛgendra Yogapāda* 2a).

A few particularly polyvalent or philosophically complex terms that are resistant to simple translation into English (e.g. *samādhi*) have been left untranslated, with the expectation that the reader will acquire a grasp of their semantic range by reading the introductions and translated passages, and by consulting the glossary and index. Furthermore, certain technical Sanskrit terms that have in recent years been assimilated into the English language – including karma, nirvana, samsara and (again) samadhi – have been kept as Sanskrit terms, complete with italics and diacritical marks (*karma*, *nirvāṇa*, *saṃsāra*, *samādhi*), on the grounds that the semantic slippage and narrowing that occurs when they enter the English dictionary detracts from an appreciation of their actual meanings in their original contexts.

Some of the passages we have translated are obscure to us on account of their esoteric or doctrinally specific nature or because the text has become corrupt in its manuscript transmission. We have enclosed in crux marks (+ . . . +) passages whose original we have been unable to understand as transmitted and for which we have been unable to conjecture a viable emendation. In addition, it is sometimes evident that the redactors of the texts are themselves uncertain of the meaning of their source material and are providing creative interpretations in lieu of complete understanding. We have nevertheless chosen to include some of these difficult passages because this is primarily a source book of important texts on yoga rather than a synoptic textbook, and that while striving for accessibility and clarity of expression we should also allow the selections to reflect some of the diversity, complexity and esotericism inherent in the traditions themselves.

CHAPTER STRUCTURE

The eleven chapters in this book are arranged thematically to reflect important practices of yoga (e.g. posture, breath-control, meditation) and the results of these practices (e.g. yogic powers, liberation). Still other chapters provide additional context for practice and its results (e.g. definitions of yoga, preliminaries, theories of the yogic body). It is important to understand, however, that these themes are not reflective of hard-and-fast categories across the yoga traditions (nor necessarily even within the texts themselves) and that the chapter divisions are to a great degree heuristic, i.e. they illustrate a particular development within yoga traditions. The divisions are also porous to some extent: often a passage that appears in one chapter might equally well be placed in another. For example, a passage on controlling the breath while repeating mantras could arguably be placed in Chapter 4 ('Breath-control') or Chapter 7 ('Mantra'); and a passage on conducting the breath into the central channel might fit in both Chapter 4 and Chapter 5 ('The Yogic Body'). The texts themselves are usually not arranged into such neat categories, and therefore a degree of overlap across the chapters is to be expected. As a result of this arrangement, and the fact that we have extracted all of our passages from much longer texts, the experience of reading this book is inevitably quite different from reading whole texts. Although our approach lends an accessibility to what can be challenging texts to read in their entirety, we hope that these selections will inspire readers to read in full some of the texts from which our translations are taken.

The internal structure of each chapter is as follows: a short introduction providing an overview of the translated material and some historical contextualization, followed by a list of the translated passages and the translations themselves. The translations are arranged in two different ways. In chapters which deal with relatively cohesive and well-defined topics (e.g., Chapter 3 on posture, Chapter 6 on yogic seals, Chapter 7 on mantra and Chapter 10 on yogic powers) the selections progress in chronological order from beginning to end. In other cases, where the topic is broader or more disparate (e.g., Chapter 1 on yoga, Chapter 2 on preliminaries, Chapter 5 on the yogic body), we have further divided the chapter into thematic sections, which are then in turn arranged chronologically. To help the reader contextualize the texts historically, we have included a table that places some of the most important texts in chronological order (see Timeline of Important Texts).

CHAPTER SUMMARIES

The first chapter, simply called 'Yoga', presents a range of definitions of yoga and characterizations of the yogi, as well as various systems of yogic 'auxiliaries' (*aṅga*s) which prepare the practitioner for higher practices or states of yoga, and examples of a common medieval fourfold typology of yoga. Also included here are some criticisms levelled against yoga from prominent figures within the Vedic orthodoxy, as well as censure of particular types and practices of yoga across sectarian yoga-practitioner lines. These criticisms are especially interesting for the snapshots they provide of yoga practices current when they were composed.

The passages in Chapter 2, 'Preliminaries', are all concerned with conditions that must be fulfilled before one begins the practice of yoga proper. These include obstacles to yoga practice, such as mixing with bad company and pride; and aids to yoga practice, ranging from the establishment of a suitable dwelling and a proper diet to listening to philosophical discourses. All texts agree on the necessity of a qualified guru for success in yoga practice and we include several passages on that topic. The haṭhayogic bodily purification practices are also represented here, as are the rules (*yama*s) and observances (*niyama*s) that make up the first two auxiliaries in eightfold (*aṣṭāṅga*) systems.

Chapter 3 concerns the postural practices that have become almost synonymous with yoga in the world today. In early texts the term *āsana* indicates a sitting position, in which other practices (such as breath-control and meditation) are carried out, and the same is true for tantric texts of the first millennium, which do not foreground postural practice. As our selection of texts shows, with the advent of *haṭhayoga* we see the emergence of more complex postures (including non-seated postures), and from the seventeenth century onwards there is a marked increase in the number of postures listed in texts.

If posture (*āsana*) is the most prominent feature of contemporary transnational yoga, breath-control (*prāṇāyāma*) was the defining practice of physical yoga methods in pre-modern India (Chapter 4). Such is *prāṇāyāma*'s importance, indeed, that in some texts other branches of yoga practice – such as fixation and meditation (cf. Chapter 8) and *samādhi* (cf. Chapter 9) – are said to be simply the result of extending the duration of breath-control. The translations begin with some of the earliest descriptions of yogic techniques of breath-control (from the Buddhist Pali canon and the *Mahābhārata*) and include passages on breath-control as purification, as a method of liberation and in combination with mantra (cf. Chapter 7).

Chapter 5, 'The Yogic Body', presents a wide range of texts dealing with the subtle physiology of the yogi, which provides the context and rationale for many of the practices detailed in other chapters of this book. The first three sections treat structures of the yogic body, including channels and winds, the body of the yogi conceived as a microcosm of the universe, and locations in the body (such as *cakra*s, supports and knots). The next two sections concern, respectively, the indwelling force commonly known as Kuṇḍalinī, and the life-giving endogenous liquid known as *bindu*. The chapter concludes with two passages in which the ascetic destruction and desiccation of the body, rather than its preservation, is the goal.

The translations in Chapter 6 deal with the methods of manipulating the breath or vital energies known as 'seals' (*mudrā*s). The first selection, from the earliest known tantra, describes hand gestures, which are the most common type of tantric seal. The second, from a later tantric text, also presents hand gestures, alongside more unusual practices such as howling like a jackal. The remainder of the translations are concerned with haṭhayogic seals, physical techniques fundamental to the earliest systems designated *haṭha*, and whose purpose is to raise the breath or manipulate and preserve the vital energies of the body.

Although it is not mentioned in yoga's earliest descriptions (and is notably absent from some later formulations of *haṭhayoga*), mantra is nevertheless a key feature of almost all Indian religious traditions and, as the passages in Chapter 7 show, it was incorporated into various systems of yoga. Repetition of the upaniṣadic syllable *oṃ* is taught in the *Pātañjalayogaśāstra* and became an important practice in several subsequent yoga teachings. Separately, the repetition of a variety of mantras understood to be vocalized (and sometimes visualized) manifestations of deities became the defining practice of tantric yoga. The magical potential of repeating tantric mantras meant that it flourished in non-ascetic milieus where special powers (see Chapter 10) tend to be foregrounded.

The texts in Chapter 8 treat the three interconnected practices of withdrawal (*pratyāhāra*), fixation (*dhāraṇā*) and meditation (*dhyāna*). The first, withdrawal, is closely related to very early definitions of yoga as the mastery of the mind resulting from its separation from sense objects, a meaning apparent in the texts we have selected. Some texts also present withdrawal as an aspect of advanced breath-control. Fixation may refer to single-pointed concentration on an inner or outer object of choice, or, in tantric texts, a progressive concentration on (and dissolution of) the elements within the body. Finally, we present a range of passages on meditation, beginning with early Buddhism and the *Mahābhārata*. Also included are tantric meditations teaching the active, detailed and empathic visualization of the deity, and texts on meditation without form or focal support.

Chapter 9 is on *samādhi*. Although in Pātañjala yoga *samādhi* is grouped with fixation and meditation in a triadic cluster of practices called *saṃyama*, we give it a chapter to itself here on account of its status as a synonym of yoga in some systems (notably the *Pātañjalayogaśāstra*), and because of the wide variety of different interpretations it is given across texts. Some texts consider *samādhi* as an extension of the meditation stage, sometimes itself conceived as a temporal extension of breath-control. In tantric texts, *samādhi* is usually (though not always) the last of the (six) auxiliaries (*aṅga*s) of yoga, but is still preliminary to the goal, union with or proximity to the deity. In *haṭha* texts *samādhi* may also convey a death-like trance, and some of our selections describe the burial and revival of the yogi in *samādhi* as a kind of ritual display of yogic prowess. The chapter also presents passages on dissolution (*laya*) and the inner sound (*nāda*), both sometimes classified as varieties of *samādhi*.

The passages in Chapter 10 concern the special powers that are said to arise from the practice of yoga. Although often maligned, scoffed at or sidelined, such powers have always been central to textual descriptions of yoga, as the translations in this chapter demonstrate. Yogic powers include the ability to fly, to hear and see across vast distances, to make oneself very small or very large, to have control over other people, and even simply to do whatever one wishes. Belief in the reality of the yogic powers predominates across texts, but the passages presented here also reveal a tension between yogic traditions which embrace the powers as valuable ends in themselves, and those which ultimately judge them as impediments to the higher goal of liberation (even though they may function as markers of spiritual progress).

The final, eleventh chapter of the book is on the topic of liberation (known variously as *mukti*, *mokṣa*, *nirvāṇa*, *kaivalya*, etc.), the final goal and rationale of yoga practice in many (though not all) systems. As our texts show, the precise nature of liberation is subject to significant variation across metaphysical systems. The chapter begins with early descriptions of liberation in a Pali Buddhist sutta and the *Mahābhārata*. It also includes several descriptions of liberation in the Pātañjala yoga tradition, as well as tantric accounts of liberation through accession to the deity. Many texts offer an insight into the vexed sub-category of liberation-while-living (*jīvanmukti*), in which the realized yogi remains indefinitely in corporeal form, enjoying the material fruits of his yogic accomplishments. In contrast, other texts teach the liberation method of yogic suicide (*utkrānti*). Such methods of exiting the physical body can also be used to possess other bodies and thus cheat death, as several texts demonstrate. Finally, we include some passages on the diagnostics of death (*ariṣṭajñāna*), a key skill for the yogi wishing to overcome (or postpone) his mortality.

NOTES

1. We are very grateful to Frederick Smith for reading and commenting on a draft of this Introduction.
2. See United Nations Secretary-General Ban Ki-moon's 'Message on the International Day of Yoga': http://www.unis.unvienna.org/unis/en/pressrels/2015/unissgsm641.html.
3. For the historical contexts of globalized yoga, see De Michelis 2004, 2008; Newcombe 2009; Singleton 2010; Singleton and Byrne 2008.
4. Another factor is a reluctance on the part of scholars to historicize yoga: it is commonly assumed that yoga practice and its social context have remained unchanged over millennia. Such an assumption is apparent in Mircea Eliade's *Yoga: Immortality and Freedom* (1973 [1954]), 'the authoritative standard work' of twentieth-century western scholarship on yoga (Guggenbühl 2008: 5). For example, by mistakenly dating some of the post-haṭhayogic 'Yoga Upaniṣads' as contemporaneous with sections of the *Mahābhārata* (129), Eliade chronologically conflates aspects of the yoga tradition that are in fact separated by more than a millennium. On the a-historical and universalizing tendency of scholarship on Indian

religion, see Green (2008: 284–5): 'Having their intellectual origins in theological notions of the universal, studies of Indian "mysticism" have generally failed to recognize the political dimensions to the physical and psychological acts of conditioning and control that comprise the full variety of Indian meditation systems. Discussions of religion in South Asia have often failed to historicize these practices, in many cases assuming a simple continuity over long periods of time between, for example, Vedic references to Yoga and the famous Yoga practitioners of the colonial period and beyond.'

5. A specific example would be that the practice of abdominal 'churning' called *nauli* can be inferred from the earlier attested *vajrolīmudrā*, which cannot be performed without it (see Chapter 6). More generally, the prior practice of physical postures can be inferred from their appearance and proliferation in later *haṭhayoga* texts. On the other hand, if there is no evidence for a practice in the textual sources prior to contemporary oral accounts or modern texts, then a degree of scepticism is called for.
6. Śivānanda Sarasvatī's sixteenth-century *Yogacintāmaṇi* is an example of a Sanskrit *nibandha* on yoga.
7. On the late composition of the Yoga Upaniṣads, see Bouy 1994.
8. For example, the purported yoga of the Indus Valley civilization (for a summary of this matter, see Samuel 2008: 8). Also excluded here are traditions of mystical and shamanic practice more generally conceived, as well as modern, neo-shamanic re-imaginings of yoga (such as the trope of 'Egyptian Yoga', sometimes claimed to be at the origin of Indian *haṭhayoga*, e.g. Ashby 2005). Similarly, images suggestive of yogic *āsana*s from Mesoamerica, which bear a closer resemblance to the techniques of Indian yoga than the so-called Paśupati seal from the Indus Valley civilization, but which developed in wholly other contexts, are not included.
9. See Mallinson 2011c.
10. As Johannes Bronkhorst puts it, 'The spiritual discipline yoga does not belong to any philosophical system, but may, or may not, get connected with a variety of philosophies, depending on the circumstances' (Bronkhorst 1981: 317).
11. See introduction to Chapter 1 and Vasudeva 2011: 132–7.
12. See Gonda 1963 and Werner 1994 [1977].
13. Heesterman (1962: 2–3) views the *Atharva Veda*'s fifteenth book, on the Vrātyas, as of 'comparatively late date'.
14. The modern yoga guru Shri Aurobindo Ghose (1872–1950) is a case in point. Aurobindo's mystical-intuitive reading method revealed the *Ṛg Veda* to be the ur-document of ancient yogic philosophy and

practice (Aurobindo 1914–20 [1998]), a discovery which was influential on subsequent generations of yoga gurus, notably David Frawley, who has greatly promoted the thesis that the Vedas are the source of yogic knowledge (e.g. Frawley 2001).

15. See White 2009.
16. Thomas McEvilley (1981) has argued that the 'proto-Śiva' represented in some seals is performing a 'shamanic yoga posture'. Feuerstein et al. (1995) follow a similar line of reasoning in their search for 'the cradle of civilization'.
17. See Bronkhorst 2007.
18. Several scholars have argued that yoga developed within the Vedic tradition (e.g. Heesterman 1985). However, although, as we have pointed out above, there is scattered evidence for the use of some yogic methods in Vedic texts, we side with Bronkhorst and others who identify the Śramaṇa traditions as the source of both the metaphysical concepts that frame yogic practice as a whole and its earliest systematic teachings. Countering suggestions that the teachings of the Buddha, for example, are a development from Vedic doctrines, Bronkhorst asserts that Brahmins 'did not occupy a dominant position in the area in which the Buddha preached his message', and that therefore his message cannot be a reaction against (nor either, presumably, an off-shoot of) Brahmanical Hinduism (2011b: 1).
19. See Bronkhorst 1993; 2011a: 319; Silk 1997; 2000. It would therefore follow, as Bronkhorst has surmised, that '*yoga* is the term that the Brāhmaṇical tradition attached to physicospiritual practices that were originally not Brāhmaṇical' (2011a: 319).
20. Bronkhorst (2011a: 321), following Shee (1986), appears to use this distinction to confirm his thesis that 'yoga was used primarily with reference to the religious practitioners of Greater Magadha', rather than to Brahmanical ascetics. He asks 'These Brāhmaṇical ascetics, did they practice yoga?' and appears to conclude, based on Shee, that they did not: '*Yoga*, then, was not the term primarily used for what Brāhmaṇical ascetics practiced in their hermitages [i.e. *tapas*]. As pointed out above, *yoga* was the term primarily used for practices that were associated with the religious currents of Greater Magadha' (ibid.). Bronkhorst's argument at this point has a kind of prescriptive circularity: (1) 'Yoga' refers to a cessative [i.e. leading to the cessation of the cycle of rebirth] technique developed by non-Vedic Buddhists, etc., even though they did not term their practices thus; (2) the yoga-practising *tapasvin*s of the *Mahābhārata* do not share this cessative orientation; and therefore (3) the so-called yoga of the *Mahābhārata*'s ascetics is not really

yoga. The conclusion he draws from Shee's distinction between *tapas* and yoga is also puzzling, insofar as Shee's argument is actually not about 'primary use' at all – if by 'primary' is meant the most common usage of the term as applied to certain practices and goals – but rather about the particular *orientation* of the techniques (this-worldly/power versus liberation). That is, for Shee, *tapas* cannot be yoga even if it is called yoga, because it is power-oriented, and real yoga is liberation-oriented. However, as Shee also points out, the two terms, *tapas* and yoga, are interchangeable in the *Mahābhārata*. Based on this, Bronkhorst might have reached a more balanced conclusion by stating simply that ' "Yoga" was one of the terms commonly used for what Brahmanical ascetics practised in their hermitages, albeit with the qualification that these practices were often distinct from the practices of the Śramaṇas, also commonly known as "yoga".' From this point of view, and bearing in mind the importance of *tapas* within the history of yoga, Bronkhorst's suggestion that 'the Brāhmaṇical contribution to the origins of Yoga is nil!' (2011: 318) would be mistaken.

21. See Mallinson 2015.
22. The commentary (*bhāṣya*) adds that yoga cannot be successful for those who do not practise *tapas*.
23. See also Mallinson 2015.
24. Note that we do not consider all of the teachings on yoga in the *Maitrāyaṇīya/Maitrī Upaniṣad* to be early (see Mallinson 2014: 170).
25. See Larson 1979 and Larson and Bhattacharya 2008.
26. The *Mahābhārata* itself mentions yoga texts (*yogaśāstra*s) in several places. In the *Mokṣadharma* (12.330.30–31, 12.326.65, 12.337.60), after Kapila is said to be the teacher of Sāṃkhya, the *yogaśāstra*s are associated with Hiraṇyagarbha, who elsewhere in the *Mokṣadharma* is identified with Brahmā (12.326.47, 12.335.18). No mention is made here or in any texts from before the composition of the *Pātañjalayogaśāstra* of a teacher of yoga called Patañjali. The (*Bṛhad*) *Yogiyājñavalkyasmṛti* (12.5) also states that Kapila was the first teacher of Sāṃkhya and Hiraṇyagarbha the first of yoga. Vācaspati (in his *Tattvavaiśāradī* commentary on *Pātañjalayogaśāstra* 1.1) says that it is because of the question raised over Patañjali's authorship of the *Yogaśāstra* by this statement in an authoritative *smṛti* treatise that the writer of the first *sūtra* of the *Pātañjalayogaśāstra* called that text a 'further teaching' (*anuśāsana*), i.e. a 'teaching of one who has been taught' (the genitive case of *śiṣṭasya*, 'of one who has been taught', presents the same ambiguity in Sanskrit as in English).

27. See Hopkins 1901; Bedekar 1959, 1962a, 1962b, 1963, 1968; Brockington 2003; Wynne 2003; Malinar 2012; White 2009; Fitzgerald 2011, 2012.
28. See Maas 2008, 2013.
29. See Maas 2013: 61, following Bronkhorst 1985: 194.
30. See Maas 2013: 58.
31. See Chapter 8, n.14 (p. 495) for Franco's summary of de la Vallée Poussin's 1936 list (de la Vallée Poussin 1937a) of the similarities between the *Pātañjalayogaśāstra* and Buddhism; and Larson 1989 for a lexical comparison of the *Pātañjalayogaśāstra* and Vasubandhu's (Buddhist) *Abhidharmakośa*. Similarly, Bronkhurst (1993) argues that the *Pātañjalayogaśāstra* is theoretically dependent on Buddhist sources. See also Coward 1982, Jacobsen 2005: 12, n.15 and Wujastyk forthcoming.
32. See Angot 2012 [2008]: 38–40 for a summary of the *Pātañjalayogaśāstra*'s influence on various later texts which discuss yoga.
33. Yoga is one of ten *darśana*s described in the *c*. twelfth-century *Sarvasiddhāntasaṃgraha*. The later canonical group of six orthodox *darśana*s is commonly divided into three pairs: Nyāya-Vaiśeṣika, Sāṃkhya-Yoga, Mīmāṃsā-Vedānta. See Halbfass 1988: 349–53 for a survey of doxographical literature on the *darśana*s.
34. White (2014) has argued that the *Pātañjalayogaśāstra* was rescued from obscurity by this new extra-Indian interest. While we agree with White's thesis that the *Pātañjalayogaśāstra* has never been important within the practical yoga tradition, evidence in the form of multiple references to the *Pātañjalayogaśāstra* in early modern texts, Sanskrit and otherwise, and catalogue records of several hundred manuscripts of the *Pātañjalayogaśāstra* copied during the early modern period, show that throughout the second millennium CE the *Pātañjalayogaśāstra* remained the most important text on yoga for Indian scholars.
35 Ulrich Timme Kragh's recent extensive edited volume of papers on the *Yogācārabhūmi* (Kragh 2013) shows both the richness of the Yogācāra tradition and the current state of the art of scholarship on it. Kragh notes that the *Yogācārabhūmi* is 'a foundational and systematic overview of Buddhist yoga practice, as announced in the title' (Kragh 2013: 30).
36. By far the most prominent of the tantric traditions – and the source of many of the teachings of the others – was Śaivism, in which Śiva or his consort Śakti are the supreme deities. On the period in which tantra was India's dominant religion, see Sanderson 2009. For a comprehensive overview of the complex structure of the various Śaiva traditions, see Sanderson 1988.

37. See Sanderson 1988: 660.
38. Ritual may take the form of initiation (*dīkṣā*), daily individual and temple worship (*pūjā*), which typically includes ritual sacrifice (*homa*) and mantra-repetition (*japa*), rites of expiation and propitiation (*prāyaścitta*, *śānti*), and so on. See Brunner 1994: 444–5.
39. Brunner (1994) makes this point with reference to '[a]lmost all [Saiddhāntika] Āgamas' (443), noting that 'no hierarchy between the four *pāda*s is recognized, and of course there is no question of the devotee making use of them successively. The *vidyāpāda* has no special status, and in a few texts only is the *yogapāda* presented as a way to liberation in itself. In the vast majority of cases, it is the eminent position of the *kriyāpāda* which is striking: all other teachings converge to make the ritual effective. For ritual action is deemed indispensable [. . .] We have therefore to keep in mind that, even in the texts that possess a *yogapāda*, *yoga* is (with very few exceptions) conceived as subservient to *kriyā*' (44–5).
40. See Sanderson 1988: 687.
41. There is no consensus across texts as to whether this word is spelled *suṣumnā* or *suṣumṇā*. We have opted for the former everywhere in this book.
42. See Vasudeva 2011: 132–7.
43. See Bouy 1994.
44. See Birch 2011.
45. Such transmutations of yoga have been the topic of a number of books over the past decade, including De Michelis (2004), Alter (2004), Strauss (2005) and Singleton (2010).
46. The Gorakhnāth Mandirs in Gorakhpur and Haridwar and the Svāmī Keśavānand Yogasaṃsthān in Delhi have published various such editions, together with Hindi translations.
47. This text was originally called the *Vivekamārtaṇḍa*, which is how we refer to it in this book to avoid confusion with an older text called the *Gorakṣaśataka*. Briggs included a transcription and edition of an abbreviated recension of this text in his 1938 study of the Nāth tradition (Briggs 1989 [1938]). Kuvalayananda and Shukla published an edition of a different abbreviated recension in 1958.
48. For surveys of scholarship on the *Pātañjalayogaśāstra* see Maas 2013 and White 2014.
49. In the field of tantric yoga, the work of the following has been especially important: Gudrun Bühnemann, Dominic Goodall, Shaman Hatley, Harunaga Isaacson, Csaba Kiss, Marion Rastelli and Somdev Vasudeva.

50. For overviews of scholarship on tantra, see Goodall and Isaacson 2011, and Hatley 2013.
51. See *The Tāntrikābhidhānakośa Project: A Hindu Tantric Dictionary*: http://www.ikga.oeaw.ac.at/Tantraproject.
52. On the Nepal-German Manuscript Preservation Project, which came to an end in 2002, see https://www.aai.uni-hamburg.de/en/forschung/ngmcp/history.html. The Nepalese-German Manuscript Cataloguing Project website is at http://catalogue.ngmcp.uni-hamburg.de.
53. See the Muktabodha Indological Research Institute: http://muktabodha.org.
54. The recent identification of the *c.* eleventh-century *Amṛtasiddhi*, the first text to teach many of the principles and practices of *haṭhayoga*, as a tantric Buddhist text (Mallinson forthcoming (b)), and the *Amṛtasiddhi*'s currency in subsequent Tibetan traditions indicate that texts of tantric Buddhism in both Sanskrit and Tibetan may be fruitful sources of further information on the early history of *haṭhayoga*.
55. Further text-critical work on the Purāṇas – some of which is under way, such as the *Skandapurāṇa* Project started by Hans Bakker, and Christèle Barois's work on the *Vāyavīyasaṃhitā* of the *Śivapurāṇa* – together with comparative analysis of their teachings on yoga is likely to shed much more light on these important yoga traditions. Related to both the Purāṇic and Śaiva traditions is a corpus of texts known collectively as the *Śivadharma*. These works on lay Śaivism contain little in the way of direct teachings on yoga, but their prescriptions on how the laity should interact with Śiva-yogins are an important resource on the social reality of first-millennium yoga practitioners. This corpus has yet to be critically edited or accurately dated, but a team of scholars including Peter Bisschop, Nirajan Kafle, Anil Kumar Acharya, Nina Mirnig and Florinda de Simini is currently working on it and their work is certain to be of great importance for the study of first-millennium Indian religion as a whole.
56. See Puri 1810.
57. Our rendition of the Kashmiri songs of Lallā was at first simply a translation of Rājānaka Bhāskara's Sanskrit translation of the text, but then, with help from Sonam Kachru, we revised it so that it followed the Kashmiri more closely.
58. The translations by others that we have used have been altered in minor ways to suit the style of this book. See our Acknowledgements (p. 505) for the scholars whose work we have utilized, and the Primary Sources and Secondary Literature for details of their editions, translations and monographs.

Timeline of Important Texts*

1500–1000 BCE	Vedas (*Ṛg*, *Sāma*, *Yajur* and *Atharva*) (V)
1000–700 BCE	Brāhmaṇas (V)
700–500 BCE	*Bṛhadāraṇyaka* and *Chāndogya Upaniṣads* (V)
3rd century BCE	*Kaṭha Upaniṣad* (V)
1st century BCE	*Cūḷavedalla Sutta* (BC), *Saccavibhaṅga Sutta* (BC), *Satipaṭṭhāna Sutta* (BC), *Muṇḍaka Upaniṣad* (V)
1st century CE	*Mahābhārata Śāntiparvan* (E) completed
2nd century CE	*Rāmāyaṇa* (E) completed, *Pāśupatasūtra* (ŚT)
3rd century CE	*Mahābhārata* (E) completed, *Manusmṛti* (HL)
4th century CE	*Vaiśeṣikasūtra* (HP), *Sthānāṅgasūtra* (J), Patañjali's *Yogaśāstra*, *Pañcārthabhāṣya* (ŚT)
5th century CE	*Visuddhimagga* (B)
6th century CE	*Śvetāśvatara Upaniṣad* (V), *Padārthadharmasaṃgraha* (HP), *Vaikhānasadharmasūtra* (HL)
6th–10th century CE	Early Tantras: *Niśvāsatattvasaṃhitā* (ŚT), *Vīṇāśikha* (ŚT), *Vairocanābhisaṃbodhisūtra* (BT), *Mañjuśriyamūlakalpa* (BT), *Brahmayāmala* (ŚT), *Hevajra* (BT), *Jayadrathayāmala* (ŚT), *Mṛgendra* (ŚT), *Kiraṇa* (ŚT), *Parākhya* (ŚT), *Mataṅgapārameśvara* (ŚT), *Sarvajñānottara* (ŚT), *Siddhayogeśvarīmata* (ŚT), *Mālinīvijayottara* (ŚT), *Svacchanda* (ŚT), *Netra* (ŚT), *Kaulajñānanirṇaya* (ŚT), *Kubjikāmata* (ŚT), *Vimānārcanākalpa* (VT), *Pādmasaṃhitā* (VT)
7th–10th century CE	Early Purāṇas: *Skanda*, *Vāyu*, *Kūrma* (inc. *Īśvaragītā*), *Liṅga*, *Bhāgavata*, *Mārkaṇḍeya*

* It is notoriously difficult to date Indian texts. This timeline should therefore be understood to provide only approximate dates for their composition. Similarly, lists of texts for particular date ranges in the timeline (e.g. 6th–10th century early tantras) are in approximate chronological order only.

8th century CE	*Tantravārttika* (HP), *Brahmasūtrabhāṣya* (HP), *Pātañjalayogaśāstravivaraṇa* (HP)
9th century CE	*Spandakārikā* (ŚT)
10th century CE	*Vijñānabhairava* (ŚT), *Paramokṣanirāsakārikāvṛtti* (ŚT)
11th century CE	Hemacandra's *Yogaśāstra* (J), *Chos drug gi man ngag zhes bya ba* (BT), *Spandasaṃdoha* (ŚT), *Amṛtasiddhi* (H), *Kathāsaritsāgara* (E), *Vimalaprabhā* (ŚT)
12th century CE	*Vajravārāhī Sādhana* (BT), *Viṣṇusaṃhitā* (VT), *Amanaska* (H), *Śāradātilaka* (ŚT)
13th century CE	*Saṃgītaratnākara* (ŚT), *Vasiṣṭhasaṃhitā* (H), *Candrāvalokana* (H), *Matsyendrasaṃhitā* (ŚT), *Vivekamārtaṇḍa* (H), *Gorakṣaśataka* (H), *Dattātreyayogaśāstra* (H), *Jñāneśvarī* (H)
14th century CE	*Tirumantiram* (ŚT), *Aparokṣānubhūti* (HP), *Yogatārāvalī* (H), *Śaṅkaradigvijaya* (VA), *Amaraughaprabodha* (H), *Yogabīja* (H), *Khecarīvidyā* (H), *Śivasaṃhitā* (H), *Gorakṣavijaya* (E), *Śārṅgadharapaddhati* (HC), *Jīvanmuktiviveka* (VA), *Lallāvākyāni* (ŚT), *Reḥla* of Ibn Baṭṭūṭa (T)
15th century CE	*Śivayogapradīpikā* (H), *Rtsa rlung gsang ba'i lde mig* (BT), *Haṭhapradīpikā* (H), *Ḥawż al-ḥayāt* (H), *Mahākālasaṃhitā* (ŚT)
16th century CE	*Baḥr al-ḥayāt* (H), *Miragāvatī* (A)
17th century CE	*Haṭharatnāvalī* (H), *Nādabindūpaniṣad* (H), *Yogaśikhopaniṣad* (H), *Sarvāṅgayogapradīpikā* (H)
18th century CE	*Rājayogāmṛta* (H), *Siddhasiddhāntapaddhati* (H), *Yogamārgaprakāśikā* (H), *Haṃsavilāsa* (HP), *Gheraṇḍasaṃhitā* (H), *Bṛhatkhecarīprakāśa* (H), *Haṭhapradīpikā* (Long Recension) (H), *Haṭhatattvakaumudī* (H), *Jogpradīpakā* (H), *Haṭhābhyāsapaddhati* (H)
19th century CE	*Tashrīh al-Aqvāṃ* (PE)

Abbreviations of categories: A = Avadhi romance; B = Buddhist; BC = Buddhist Canonical; BT = Buddhist Tantra; E = 'Hindu'* Epic/Narrative; H = Haṭhayoga; HC = 'Hindu' Compendium; HL = 'Hindu' Law; HP = 'Hindu' Philosophy; J = Jain; PE = Persian Ethnography; ŚT = Śaiva Tantra; T = Travel Report; V = Vedic; VA = Vedānta; VT = Vaiṣṇava Tantra

* We use quotation marks for the term 'Hindu' because it was not current prior to *c.* 1600 CE, when many of the texts we designate as Hindu were composed.

ROOTS OF YOGA

ONE
Yoga

This chapter introduces definitions and typologies of yoga from a range of traditions and historical periods. Although a complete survey of all interpretations of yoga is beyond our scope, we have sought to present a wide variety of viewpoints, from Brahmanical, Buddhist, tantric and haṭhayogic sources, including criticisms of practices and conducts which are at odds with those recommended by the texts' authors and their lineages, as well as some criticisms of yoga itself. Many of the passages chosen show significant variation in the way yoga is interpreted: however, as well as highlighting some of the challenges inherent in trying to make generalizations about such a broad subject, they also reveal some core features and concepts which remain constant.

Yoga is a particularly polyvalent Sanskrit word, which, in ordinary usage, may signify joining or attaching, a means or method or way, profit or wealth, a trick or deceit, an undertaking or business, mixing, putting together or ordering, suitability, diligence or magic.[1] In this chapter, and in this book as a whole, we focus only on the use of *yoga* in the context of the attainment of liberation or supernatural powers by means of prescribed psychophysical methods,[2] and largely ignore more general religious usages of the word distinct from this restricted sense, such as *yoga* as the accrual of *karma* or as religious conduct broadly conceived, as we find in the early Jain tradition.[3]

Yoga as Practice, Yoga as Goal

In texts that teach yoga in this restricted sense, the word *yoga* may designate either a practice, or body of practices, on the one hand, or the goal of such practices on the other. While today it may be more common to understand 'yoga' as practice (of posture, breath-control, meditation, and so on), in a majority of texts the word *yoga* more commonly indicates the goal achieved through these practices – although the perceived nature of that goal may vary according to the text's doctrinal underpinning.

For example, yoga may be understood as a state of conjunction or union, especially in tantric and non-dual (*advaita*) traditions, although what exactly is being united with what varies according to those traditions' own metaphysical systems. Union may be variously conceived as being with the manifestation of one's own nature (1.1.17); with an element (or 'level of reality', *tattva*) (1.1.16; cf. 1.1.11); with Śiva's power[4] (1.1.10); or as the conjunction of the individual and the supreme self (1.1.15). The *Yogabīja* (1.1.21) states that yoga is the union (*saṃyoga*) of all dualities (*dvandva*).

In opposition to the idea of yoga as union, Patañjali's *Yogaśāstra* and related texts equate yoga with the state of *samādhi* (see 1.1.5), and tend to define yoga in terms of the *separation* or disjunction (*vi-yoga*) of the dualistic Sāṃkhyan categories of *puruṣa* (the spiritual principle) and *prakṛti* (material nature) (e.g. *Pātañjalayogaśāstra* 2.18, 2.23, 2.28, 3.50). Some commentators confirm this view: for example, in the preamble to Bhoja's *Yogasūtrarājamārtaṇḍa* we find a reference to a saying of Patañjali not found in the *Pātañjalayogaśāstra*, but which clearly defines yoga as the disjunction of *puruṣa* and *prakṛti*.[5] Others disagree: another commentator on the *Pātañjalayogaśāstra*, Vijñānabhikṣu, argues in his *Yogasārasaṃgraha* that 'aloneness' (*kaivalya*), the end goal of the *Pātañjalayogaśāstra*'s *sāṃkhyayoga*, is the same as the goal of Vedānta, which he describes as non-separation (*avibhāga*) of the individual self (*jīvātman*) and the supreme self (*paramātman*).[6] The *Īśvaragītā* (1.2.4) presents two forms of yoga: a 'Non-Being Yoga' (*abhāvayoga*), suggestive of the *Pātañjalayogaśāstra*, in which one's own form is meditated upon as being empty; and the superior Great Yoga (*mahāyoga*), in which the yogi focuses on, and unites with, God. In this model, Patañjali's yoga functions as a preliminary to practices leading to union with the deity.

Elsewhere, yoga is identified with equanimity and skill in action (*Bhagavadgītā* (1.1.2)), the condition of *nirvāṇa* (*Liṅgapurāṇa* (1.1.8)), a pleasure- and pain-free state (*Vaiśeṣikasūtra* (1.1.7)), and so on. Also common in early texts is the association of yoga with power (*bala*), such as in the *Mahābhārata* (1.1.3), where Sāṃkhya is said to be unequalled knowledge and yoga to be unequalled power, and in the *Skandapurāṇa* (72.15), where Śiva tells Pārvatī that her son will be endowed with the great power of yoga (*mahāyogabala*).

Doctrinal variation notwithstanding, all of these definitions point to an understanding of yoga as a state, the attainment of which is the goal of the practices associated with it. This meaning of yoga as a goal is by far the more common, although we do find references to 'the practice of yoga' (*yogābhyāsa*) and injunctions to 'practise yoga', in which 'yoga' must indicate the means rather than the end. In the *Gorakṣaśataka*, for example, we read, 'Through practising yoga I have become sick' (69) and the *Dattātreyayogaśāstra* says, 'Not practising yoga gets one nowhere [. . .] one should make every effort to practise nothing but yoga' (106). An exceptional definition of yoga as means is found in the *c.* second-century CE Buddhist *Yogācārabhūmi* (1.1.4).

In some texts the two senses (yoga-as-means and yoga-as-goal) exist side by side. The *Parākhyatantra*, for instance, states that 'Yoga [arises from] the attainment of *samādhi* or it is in the practice of yoga [itself]' (1.1.10), a definition which appears to understand 'yoga' as indicative of both method and goal, with the latter contained within and arising from the former. In *Pātañjalayogaśāstravivaraṇa* 1.1 (1.1.13) yoga is defined as both the goal and the means (*upāya*) for achieving discriminative knowledge (*vivekakhyāti*) and supernatural powers. This dual usage raises similar issues with regard to compound terms such as *haṭhayoga*, which might be translated as either '[the state of] yoga [achieved] *by means of* force (*haṭha*)' or 'the forceful yoga [practice]'. Given the predominance in the texts of yoga-as-goal (rather than method), it makes sense to favour the first translation, in which case we would not be dealing with a *kind* of yoga called *haṭha*, but with methods known collectively as *haṭha* that lead to the goal called 'yoga'. The situation is complicated further when we consider a text such as the *Bhagavadgītā* (see 1.2.1), which teaches a panoply of yogas[7] (or 'means to yoga'?), such as *karmayoga* (yoga of/by actions), *ātmasaṃyamayoga* (yoga of/by self-restraint), *bhaktiyoga* (yoga of/by devotion) and *abhyāsayoga* (yoga of/by repeated practice). That the *Bhagavadgītā*, like the *Parākhyatantra*, sometimes takes 'yoga' to indicate method *and* goal is clear from, for example, its description of *buddhiyoga* (yoga of/by means of the intellect), in which Arjuna is exhorted to 'apply [himself] to yoga' (2.50), by which means he will 'attain yoga' (2.53).

Some texts teach a variety of distinct *types* of yoga method. Our categorization here is by no means exclusive or exhaustive, but rather a presentation of some of yoga's taxonomical variations. Included here is the 'yoga of action' (*kriyāyoga*) of the *Pātañjalayogaśāstra* (an alternative practice for those who have distracted minds) (1.2.2); the 'cosmic yoga' (*prakriyāyoga*) of the *Niśvāsatattvasaṃhitā*, in which one meditates on matter, time, illusion (*māyā*) and other cosmic levels (1.2.3); the twofold yoga of the *Īśvaragītā* where meditation on emptiness ('Non-Being Yoga') leads to a vision of the self as pure and blissful (the 'Great Yoga') (1.2.4); and the yoga of devotion (*bhaktiyoga*) of the *Bhāgavatapurāṇa* (1.2.5). Also of importance here are texts which consider the relationship between yoga and knowledge (*jñāna*), such as the *Bhagavadgītā* (1.2.1), the *Pādmasaṃhitā* (1.2.6), the *Yogabīja* (1.2.7) and the *Jīvanmuktiviveka* (1.2.12).

The Four Yogas

The *Vāyavīyasaṃhitā* of the *Śivapurāṇa* (2.29.5–13) and the *Liṅgapurāṇa* (2.55.7–28) both teach a fivefold yoga consisting of the yoga of mantras (*mantrayoga*), the yoga of touch (*sparśayoga*), the yoga of being (*bhāvayoga*), the yoga of non-being (*abhāvayoga*) and the great yoga (*mahāyoga*).[8] However, from its first appearance in the thirteenth-century *Dattātreyayogaśāstra* onwards, much the most common typology of yoga is a fourfold hierarchy of the yoga of mantras (*mantrayoga* – see Chapter 7), the yoga of dissolution (*layayoga* – see Chapter 9), the yoga of force (*haṭhayoga* – see Introduction, p. xx) and the royal yoga (*rājayoga*). While the hierarchical order of the first three of these four elements varies, there is a general consensus that *rājayoga* is the best of all. The term *rājayoga* begins to occur in texts from the eleventh or twelfth century onwards and is usually identified with either the *practices* of *samādhi* or the *state* of *samādhi* (see Chapter 9).[9]

The *Dattātreyayogaśāstra* also lists four hierarchical stages of practice, called 'inception' (*ārambha*), 'action' (*ghaṭa*), 'accumulation' (*paricaya*) and 'completion' (*niṣpatti*) (1.3.3), a scheme that first occurs in the *Amṛtasiddhi* (19.2) and is found in a number of texts, including the *Sabdī*s of Gorakhnāth (136–9) and the *Śivayogapradīpikā* (5.51). *Rājayoga* seems to be identified here with the completion stage, as it also is in the *Amaraughaprabodha* (52–3) and the *Haṭhapradīpikā* (4.76–7). *Haṭhapradīpikā* 4.3 names *rājayoga* as a synonym of *samādhi* (1.3.8) and points to it as the sole goal of *haṭha* practice (1.3.7; cf. 2.77). The *Śivasaṃhitā* asserts that *haṭha* will not succeed without *rājayoga*, but also claims that *rājayoga* will not succeed without *haṭha* (1.3.6), a claim repeated in the *Haṭhapradīpikā* (2.76). In a handful of texts, *rājayoga* is said to be the union of semen (*retas/bindu*) and uterine fluid (*rajas*)[10] (e.g. *Yogaśikhā Upaniṣad* 1.137ab, *Yogabīja* 1.1.21), the drawing up of seminal fluid during sexual intercourse (e.g. *Sarvāṅgayogapradīpikā* 1.3.5) or ejaculatory sexual intercourse itself (e.g. the *Haṃsavilāsa*). The implication here is that *rājayoga* is the attainment of yoga while still living like a king, i.e. without renouncing the pleasures of worldly existence.

*Yogāṅga*s: Auxiliaries of Yoga

There is also ambiguity around the term *yogāṅga* (a compound of *yoga* and *aṅga*), commonly translated 'limb of yoga', but better rendered 'auxiliary of yoga' when yoga means the goal rather than the method.[11] There, while the *aṅga*s may be indispensable for reaching the goal, they may themselves not be considered as yoga but rather as auxiliary methods for attaining yoga, and may be subsidiary to other methods. This is clearly the case in, for example, the *Mālinīvijayottaratantra*, which teaches a 'six-auxiliary' (*ṣaḍaṅga*) method[12] as a preliminary to the 'conquest of the realities' (*tattvajaya*).

Sixfold methods such as that of the *Mālinīvijayottaratantra* are common in other Śaiva texts, as well as those of non-Śaiva tantric traditions: they are found in scriptures of the Vaiṣṇava Pāñcarātra, such as the *Jayākhyasaṃhitā* (33.6–16b), *Viṣṇusaṃhitā* and *Sanatkumārasaṃhitā*,[13] and many Vajrayāna Buddhist works.[14] It is noteworthy that the *Mālinīvijayottaratantra* unusually places withdrawal (*pratyāhāra*) after *samādhi* as the final and highest auxiliary, suggesting perhaps that withdrawal, rather than *samādhi*, may have been the aim of some early yogas (see Chapters 8 and 9). Other variations in the order, definition and subdivisions of the six auxiliaries are common across Śaiva texts.[15]

Other numerical arrangements of *yogāṅgas* also occur, such as the four-part scheme of the *Śārṅgadharapaddhati*, the five *aṅgas* of the *Vāyupurāṇa*, the seven of the *Mṛgendratantra* and *Gheraṇḍasaṃhitā*, and the fifteen of the *Aparokṣānubhūti* (see pages 9–10 for a presentation of some of these in tabular form). Eightfold soteriological systems have a particularly long history and predate the sixfold systems which first appear in tantric texts. In the context of yoga, by far the most common and influential eightfold scheme is the *aṣṭāṅgayoga* of Patañjali's *Yogaśāstra* and the many texts which replicate its schema. However, notable examples which predate this system may be found in the Pali canon, which teaches the Eightfold Path fundamental to Buddhism (1.4.1), the *Carakasaṃhitā*, the earliest complete, extant text of Āyurveda,[16] and the *Mahābhārata*. The *Mahābhārata* says that an eightfold yoga is taught in the Vedas (12.304.7) and teaches two other eightfold schemata in a single continuous passage (see 1.4.2), the first of which is said to be 'the Eightfold Path of *dharma*' and is akin to the rules (*yamas*) and observances (*niyamas*) of Patañjali's yoga (see Chapter 2), while the second is not given a name other than 'the Path of Eight Auxiliaries', but is more obviously yogic both in its methods, which include restraint of the senses and the stopping of the mind, and its results, which include yogic sovereignty and success in yoga.

Systems of Auxiliaries (*aṅgas*) of Yoga

Fourfold System (*Śārṅgadhara-paddhati*)	Posture	Restraint of the breath	Meditation	*Samādhi*				
Fivefold System (*Vāyupurāṇa*)	Breath-control	Meditation	Withdrawal	Fixation	Recollection			
Sixfold Systems*								
Sixfold 'Tarka class' 1 (*Mṛgendra*, *Raurava*, *Mataṅgapārameśvara*)	Breath-control	Meditation	Withdrawal	Fixation	Discrimination	*Samādhi*		
Sixfold 'Tarka class' 2 (*Mālinīvijayottara*)	Breath-control	Fixation	Discrimination	Meditation	*Samādhi*	Withdrawal		
Sixfold 'Tarka class' 3 (*Viṣṇusaṃhitā*)	Breath-control	Sense withdrawal	Fixation	Discrimination	*Samādhi*	Meditation		
Sixfold 'Posture class' (*Vivekamārtaṇḍa*, *Gorakṣaśataka*, etc.)	Posture	Breath-restraint	Withdrawal	Concentration	Meditation	*Samādhi*		
Sevenfold system (*Mṛgendratantra Yogapāda*)	Breath-control	Withdrawal	Fixation	Meditation	Discrimination	Repetition of mantras	*Samādhi*	[+Yoga itself]

* Our division of sixfold auxiliary systems into 'Tarka' and 'Posture' classes is derived from that of Grönbold (1996).

Eightfold Systems								
The Noble Eightfold Path of Buddhism (*Saccavibhaṅga Sutta*)	Right View	Right Intention	Right Speech	Right Action	Right Livelihood	Right Effort	Right Mindfulness	Right *Samādhi*
Eightfold Path of Dharma (*Mahābhārata*)	Sacrifice	Study	Charity	Austerity	Truthfulness	Patience	Restraint	Lack of greed
	'The Way of the Fathers'				'The Way of the Gods'			
The Path of Eight Auxiliaries (*Mahābhārata*)	Right focus	Right restraint of the senses	Right special observances	Right service of the guru	Right control of diet	Right study	Right renunciation of ritual action	Right stopping of the mind
The eight causes that are said to bring mindfulness (*Carakasaṃhitā, śarīrasthāna*)*	Perception of the cause	Perception of the form	Similarity	Contrast	Attachment to *sattva*	Practice	The yoga of knowledge	What is heard
Eight auxiliaries (*Pātañjalayogaśāstra*)	Rules	Observances	Posture	Breath-control	Withdrawal	Fixation	Meditation	*Samādhi*
	'Outer' Auxiliaries					'Inner' Auxiliaries		
Fifteenfold System (*Aparokṣānubhūti*)	Rules	Observances	Renunciation	Silence	Location	Time	Posture	The root lock
	Equilibrium of the body	Steadiness of gaze	Restraint of breath	Withdrawal	Fixation	Meditation on the self	*Samādhi*	

* See Wujastyk 2011.

That the compound term *aṣṭāṅgayoga* in the *Pātañjalayogaśāstra* and elsewhere should be interpreted to mean 'yoga [attained] by means of the eight auxiliaries', rather than 'the yoga of eight limbs' is clearly implied in Vācaspatimiśra's commentary to *Pātañjalayogaśāstra* 1.1, where he asks how *samādhi* can be identified with yoga itself *and* simultaneously be the last of the eight *aṅgas*. He solves this apparent paradox by proposing that *samādhi* as an auxiliary (*aṅga*) is merely a *part* of the state of yoga, defined in *Pātañjalayogaśāstra* 1.2 as the suppression of the activities of the mind (*cittavṛttinirodha*). Bhojarāja, in his commentary on *Pātañjalayogaśāstra* 2.29, similarly affirms that each of the eight *aṅgas* is subsidiary to the next, ending with *samādhi*. The *Mṛgendratantra* offers a sevenfold *aṅga* scheme, which includes *samādhi* (or perhaps the *practice* of *samādhi*), but adds yoga itself, identified as the state of *samādhi*, as a kind of honorary eighth *aṅga* to which all the others are subservient (1.4.8).

While the exceptions above disprove the statement found in the *Vāyavīyasaṃhitā* (29.14ab) that every yoga is either *ṣaḍaṅga* or *aṣṭāṅga*, sixfold and eightfold yoga systems are the most common. The elements of eightfold systems – rules (*yamas*), observances (*niyamas*), posture (*āsana*), breath-control (*prāṇāyāma*), withdrawal (*pratyāhāra*), fixation (*dhāraṇā*), meditation (*dhyāna*) and *samādhi* – do not vary from text to text,[17] but there is considerable variation in the sixfold schemata. Nevertheless, the latter generally include the former's breath-control, fixation, meditation, withdrawal and *samādhi*. Śaiva sixfold systems are usually distinguished by the inclusion of the *aṅga* of discrimination (*tarka*),[18] the non-inclusion of the rules and observances,[19] theism (the *Pātañjalayogaśāstra* only includes Īśvara ('the Lord') as an option),[20] and quite divergent interpretations of the function and goal of their yogas.[21] In some *haṭha* texts, such as the *Vivekamārtaṇḍa*, we find a sixfold grouping identical to the *Pātañjalayogaśāstra*'s *aṣṭāṅga* sequence, minus the rules and observances (with posture as the first auxiliary), and in which discrimination is absent. This represents a later *ṣaḍaṅga* group distinct from the usual tantric grouping.

Warnings and Criticisms

There is an ancient tradition that yoga is dangerous, even lethally so. The *Mahābhārata* likens the path of yoga to one through a terrifying scorched and pitted wilderness full of snakes and bandits (12.289.50–56); and the *Skandapurāṇa* (180.5) declares yoga's method to be torturous. Yet, despite these warnings, both the *Mahābhārata* and the *Skandapurāṇa* go on to teach yoga. Some texts, however, censure it, or at least its more dangerous practices, which in later works are associated with the *haṭha* method of yoga. In the *c.* tenth-century *Mokṣopāya*, forceful breath-restraint is identified explicitly with *haṭhayoga* (in one of *haṭha*'s first mentions) and *haṭhayoga* is said to cause suffering.[22] Abhinavagupta dismisses all the *aṅga*s of Patañjali's yoga in the fourth chapter of his *Tantrāloka*, noting in particular that *prāṇāyāma* is not to be performed, because it harms the body (4.91a; see Chapter 4). The *Mahākālasaṃhitā* (1.5.5) contrasts *haṭha* with gradual (*krāmika*) yoga and states that many *brahmarṣi*s (sages who have realized the nature of the absolute) have died from the former.[23]

In spite of the close association of *haṭhayoga* and *rājayoga* in *haṭha* texts, there is also a tradition of *rājayoga*, which opposes the forceful techniques of *haṭha* in favour of quietistic methods of *samādhi*. The eleventh- to twelfth-century *Amanaska* (although it doesn't mention *haṭha* by name) declares difficult *haṭha* techniques (*prāṇāyāma*, *mudrā*, *bandha*, etc.) and *ṣaḍaṅga* systems to be superfluous if one practises the easy *rājayoga* techniques of *samādhi*, such as *śāmbhavīmudrā*[24] (1.5.6). Similarly, the *Jīvanmuktiviveka* examines the relative advantages and disadvantages of forceful (*haṭha*) and gentle (*mṛdu*) yoga, arguing that the latter is greatly superior (1.5.7). A much later instance of similar sentiments occurs in the eighteenth-century *Haṃsavilāsa* (1.5.8), which rejects a 'forceful' approach (here *haṭhayoga* is identified with the yoga of Patañjali) in favour of a quietistic *rājayoga* 'conceived of as an esoteric, sensual rapture' whose 'superiority lies in the admission of sexual practices'.[25] *Haṭhayoga* is also identified with the *Pātañjalayogaśāstra*'s *aṣṭāṅgayoga* in the *Yogamārgaprakāśikā* (Chapter 3) and *Aparokṣānubhūti Dīpikā* (143). Given the common modern identification of Patañjali's yoga with a 'mental' or 'spiritual' *rājayoga* that stands in opposition to the merely physical *haṭhayoga* (a notion popularized in the nineteenth and twentieth centuries by Swami Vivekananda and Theosophical Society authors), such references to *haṭhayoga* as the yoga of Patañjali are particularly striking.

So although *haṭhayoga* largely became the de facto method of yoga practice in India in the centuries following the *Haṭhapradīpikā*, it was by no means without its opponents, and there is a strong counter-current – often within Advaita Vedānta traditions – which promotes quietistic practices of *samādhi* over and above the effortful yoga practices.

The criticisms of the *Amanaska* (1.5.6) and the *Siddhasiddhāntapaddhati* (1.5.9) target an impressive array of censured practices. In addition to making clear the preferences of the tradition at hand, these criticisms paint a colourful picture of the kinds of practices that may have been prominent within other yogic systems of the time. Vernacular poets could be equally scathing of what they considered fraudulent yoga practice. Gorakhnāth dismisses the esoteric physiology and *haṭha* breath and body practices of yoga, although he still finds a place for the yogic technique of *khecarīmudrā*,[26] in which the tongue is turned above the palate to drink the nectar of immortality (1.5.10). Noteworthy, too, are criticisms of yoga (viz. Patañjali's *Yogaśāstra*) from within Vedic Hindu tradition, including a refutation of yoga's metaphysical claims in the *Brahmasūtra* (1.5.1), a rejection by Śaṅkara of the use of yoga to suppress the fluctuations of the mind because this is not considered to be a means to liberation (1.5.2), and a statement by Kumārila Bhaṭṭa that yoga is not accepted by those who know the Vedas (1.5.3). As Nicholson points out, the fact that such authoritative authors and texts should reject yoga in this way complicates the claims by certain contemporary Hindu cultural organizations that yoga is Hindu.[27]

Chapter Contents

1.1.4 *Yogācārabhūmi Śrāvakabhūmi* 2.152. Yoga as means.

1.1.5 *Pātañjalayogaśāstra* 1.1–1.2, 3.6. Yoga as the suppression of the activities of the mind.

1.1.6 *Pañcārthabhāṣya* 1.1.43 (on *Pāśupatasūtra* 1.1). Yoga as union.

1.1.7 *Vaiśeṣikasūtra* 5.2.15–16. No pleasure or suffering in yoga.

1.1.8 *Liṅgapurāṇa* 1.8.5a. Yoga as *nirvāṇa*.

1.1.9 *Śivapurāṇa Vāyavīyasaṃhitā* 29.6. Yoga as the state of a mind fixed on Śiva.

1.1.10 *Parākhyatantra* 14.95–7. Yoga as contact.

1.1.11 *Mālinīvijayottara* 4.4–5. Yoga as the union of one thing with another.

1.1.12 *Brahmasūtrabhāṣya* of Śaṅkara 2.1.3. Yoga as the means of perceiving reality.

1.1.13 *Pātañjalayogaśāstravivaraṇa* 1.1. Yoga as means and goal.

1.1.14 *Yogaśataka* 2.4. Yoga as correct knowledge, doctrine and conduct.

1.1.15 *Vimānārcanākalpa* 96. Yoga as the union of individual and supreme self.

1.1.16 Kṣemarāja's *Uddyota* commentary on *Svacchandatantra* 6.45. Yoga as union with an element.

1.1.17 *Mṛgendratantra Yogapāda* 2ab, with the *vṛtti* of Bhaṭṭa Nārāyaṇakaṇṭha. Yoga deriving from √*yuj*, 'to join'.

1.1.18 Hemacandra's *Yogaśāstra* 1.5–7, 15. In praise of yoga.

1.1.19 *Śāradātilaka* 25.1a–3b. Four definitions of yoga.

1.1.20 *Vasiṣṭhasaṃhitā* 1.31. Knowledge consists of yoga.

1.1.21 *Yogabīja* 87a–90b. The union of all dualities.

1.1.22 *Haṃsavilāsa*, p. 47, ll. 15–18. 'He alone is a yogi . . .'

1.2 Types of Yoga Method

1.2.1 *Bhagavadgītā* 3.3, 5.2, 13.25, 14.26, 2.49, 10.10, 8.8, 12.9, 18.52–3, 4.27, 5.4–5. Various yogas.

1.2.2 *Pātañjalayogaśāstra* 2.1–2. The yoga of action.

1.2.3 *Niśvāsatattvasaṃhitā Uttarasūtra* 5.2–3. Cosmic yoga.

1.2.4 *Īśvaragītā* 11.1–10. Non-Being Yoga and the Great Yoga.

1.2.5 *Bhāgavatapurāṇa* 1.2.19. The yoga of devotion.

1.2.6 *Pādmasaṃhitā Yogapāda* 1.1–6. The twofold yoga of action and knowledge.

1.2.7 *Yogabīja* 15–19, 32–5, 60, 71, 73–5. Yoga and knowledge.

1.2.8 *Vimalaprabhā* 4.119. *Haṭhayoga.*

1.2.9 *Haṭhapradīpikā* 1.56. *Haṭha*'s order of practice.

1.2.10 *Haṭharatnāvalī* 1.17–18. *Haṭhayoga.*

1.2.11 *Chos drug gi man ngag zhes bya ba.* The Oral Instruction of the Six Yogas.

1.2.12 *Jīvanmuktiviveka* 3.10.18. The superiority of yoga.

1.3 The Four Yogas

1.3.1 *Amaraughaprabodha* 4–5. The four yogas.

1.3.2 *Yogabīja* 146–52. The four yogas.

1.3.3 *Dattātreyayogaśāstra* 9–11. The four yogas.

1.3.4 *Śivayogapradīpikā* 1.9–12. The typology of *rājayoga.*

1.3.5 *Sarvāṅgayogapradīpikā* 2.13–17, 24. *Rājayoga* as the drawing up of semen.

1.3.6 *Śivasaṃhitā* 5.222. *Haṭha* and *rājayoga* are both needed for success.

1.3.7 *Haṭhapradīpikā* 1.1–3, 2.77, 3.122. *Haṭha* as a stairway to *rājayoga.*

1.3.8 *Haṭhapradīpikā* 4.3–4. Synonyms of *rājayoga.*

1.4 Auxiliaries of Yoga

1.4.1 *Saccavibhaṅga Sutta* 23. The Noble Eightfold Path.

1.4.2 *Mahābhārata* 3.2.71–77. The Eightfold Path of *dharma.*

1.4.3 *Pātañjalayogaśāstra* 2.28–9. The eight auxiliaries.

1.4.4 *Śārṅgadharapaddhati* 4348. The four practices common to all yogas.

1.4.5 *Vāyupurāṇa* 10.76. The five practices of yoga.

1.4.6 *Mataṅgapārameśvarāgama Yogapāda* 1.6. The yoga of six auxiliaries.

1.4.7 *Vivekamārtaṇḍa* 3. The yoga of six auxiliaries.

1.4.8 *Mṛgendratantra Yogapāda* 2c–3d, with the *vṛtti* of Bhaṭṭa Nārāyaṇakaṇṭha. The yoga of seven auxiliaries.

1.4.9 *Aparokṣānubhūti* 102–3. The fifteen auxiliaries.

1.5 Warnings and Criticisms

1.5.1 *Brahmasūtra* 2.1.3, with Śaṅkara's *bhāṣya*. Refutation of the efficacy of yoga.

1.5.2 Śaṅkara's *Bṛhadāraṇyakopaniṣadbhāṣya*. Pātañjala yoga is not a means to liberation.

1.5.3 Kumārila Bhaṭṭa's *Tantravārttika* commentary on *Mīmāṃsā Sūtra* 1.3.4. Yoga is rejected by those who know the Vedas.

1.5.4 Kauṇḍinya's *Pañcārthabhāṣya* on *Pāśupatasūtra* 1.1. Sāṃkhya yogis are beasts.

1.5.5 *Mahākālasaṃhitā Guhyakālīkhaṇḍa* 11.100c–105d. *Haṭha* and gradual yoga.

1.5.6 *Amanaska* 1.3–4, 1.7, 2.29, 2.42. Against effortful, painful yogas.

1.5.7 *Jīvanmuktiviveka* 1.3.27, 3.1.16–18. Forceful versus gentle yoga.

1.5.8 *Haṃsavilāsa*, p. 51, ll. 15–16 and p. 49, ll. 24–7. Patañjali's teaching is not included among true teachings.

1.5.9 *Siddhasiddhāntapaddhati* 6.79–91. Those who do not obtain the supreme state.

1.5.10 Gorakh, *Sabdīs* 31, 133–5. This eightfold yoga is all lies.

1.1

Definitions of Yoga

1.1.1 *Kaṭha Upaniṣad* 6.10–11. Yoga as firm restraint of the senses:

> (10) When the five senses (*jñānāni*), along with the mind, remain still and the intellect is not active, that is known as the highest state. (11) They consider yoga to be firm restraint of the senses. Then one becomes undistracted, for yoga is the arising and the passing away.

1.1.2 *Bhagavadgītā* 2.48, 2.50, 6.23, 6.46. Yoga as equanimity, skill in action and separation:

> (2.48) Perform actions while established in yoga! Abandon attachment, Arjuna, and be equanimous in success and failure. Yoga is said to be equanimity.
>
> (2.50) Yoga is skill in action.
>
> (6.23) Know that which is called yoga to be separation (*viyoga*) from contact (*saṃyoga*) with suffering. It should definitely be practised by one whose mind is not dejected.
>
> (6.46) The yogi is superior to ascetics (*tapasvin*); he is also considered to be superior to those who have knowledge (*jñānin*); and the yogi is superior to ritualists (*karmin*). Therefore, be a yogi, Arjuna!

1.1.3 *Mahābhārata* 12.304.2ab. No power equal to yoga:

> There is no knowledge equal to Sāṃkhya and no power equal to yoga.

1.1.4 *Yogācārabhūmi Śrāvakabhūmi* 2.152. Yoga as means:

> Yoga is fourfold: faith, aspiration, perseverance and means.

1.1.5 *Pātañjalayogaśāstra* 1.1–1.2, 3.6. Yoga as the suppression of the activities of the mind:

(1.1) Now, further instruction on yoga.

[The word] 'now' here is to [express] entitlement, [i.e. because of it] a treatise of further instruction on yoga should be understood to have been authorized.

Yoga is *samādhi*. It is a quality of the mind in all [its] states. The states of the mind are distracted (*kṣipta*), confused (*mūḍha*), agitated (*vikṣipta*), focused (*ekāgra*) and restrained (*niruddha*). Among these [states], when the mind is agitated, *samādhi* is overpowered by agitation. This is not part of yoga.

But that which, when the mind is single-pointed, causes an object to shine forth as it really is and cuts off the afflictions, loosens the bonds of *karma* [and] orients [one] towards suppression [of the activities of the mind] is called 'yoga with cognition (*saṃprajñāta*)'. And this is accompanied by reasoning, reflection, bliss and egoism. We will discuss this later. But when all the activities of the mind are suppressed, that is *samādhi* without cognition (*asaṃprajñāta*).

This [next] *sūtra* seeks to express the defining characteristic of that [i.e. *samādhi* without cognition]:

(1.2) Yoga is the suppression of the activities of the mind.

Because the word 'all' is not included, *samādhi* with cognition is also termed 'yoga'.

(3.6) It is said that 'Yoga is to be known through yoga. Yoga arises from yoga. One who is vigilant by means of yoga delights in yoga for a long time.'

1.1.6 *Pañcārthabhāṣya* 1.1.43 (on *Pāśupatasūtra* 1.1). Yoga as union:

In this system, yoga is the union of the self and the Lord.

1.1.7 *Vaiśeṣikasūtra*[28] 5.2.15–16. No pleasure or suffering in yoga:

(15) Pleasure and suffering [arise] as a result of the drawing together of the sense organs, the mind and objects. (16) When that does not happen because the mind is in the self, there is no pleasure or suffering for one who is embodied. That is yoga.

1.1.8 *Liṅgapurāṇa* 1.8.5a. Yoga as *nirvāṇa*:

By the word 'yoga' is meant *nirvāṇa*, the condition of Śiva.

1.1.9 *Śivapurāṇa Vāyavīyasaṃhitā*[29] 29.6. Yoga as the state of a mind fixed on Śiva:

In sum, yoga is the state of a mind fixed on Śiva, its other states restrained.

1.1.10 *Parākhyatantra*[30] 14.95–7. Yoga as contact:

Pratoda spoke:

(95) Yoga has been defined as contact. That [contact] of the soul is taught to be with what, according to this system? It cannot be union of the soul with a *tattva*, because [the soul is] all-pervading.

Prakāśa spoke: (96) It is connection with [the eight] supernatural accomplishments, such as the ability to become as small as an atom and so forth. Or yoga [comes about] because of the union with [Śiva's] power, or yoga [arises from] the attainment of *samādhi* or it is in the practice of yoga [itself]. (97) Or yoga is immersion into Him arising from the contemplation of His nature. [In fact] union with the Lord is impossible, because He is all-pervading. [When] it is spoken of [in scripture], then [it is spoken of] in a figurative sense.

1.1.11 *Mālinīvijayottara* 4.4–5. Yoga as the union of one thing with another:

(4) They deem yoga to be the union of one thing (*vastu*) with another. A 'thing' is said to be that which must be known in order to ascertain what things are to be rejected and so forth. (5) And it cannot be known in its two forms without [right] knowledge (*jñāna*). The [right] knowledge [thus] mentioned has been taught by Śiva in order to accomplish this.

1.1.12 *Brahmasūtrabhāṣya* of Śaṅkara 2.1.3. Yoga as the means of perceiving reality:

It is said in the treatises on yoga: 'Yoga is the means of perceiving reality.'

1.1.13 *Pātañjalayogaśāstravivaraṇa*[31] 1.1. Yoga as means and goal:

[Objection]: If the removal is the objective, and its means is discriminative knowledge, then [the first *sūtra*] should say 'Now the instruction of discriminative knowledge.' For what purpose does the [first] *sūtra* say '*Now the instruction of yoga*'?

[Answer] Because yoga is the means of obtaining it [i.e. discriminative knowledge]. Precisely the means should be stated. For, if the goal to be obtained is [first] explained, then since the goal presupposes the means [to obtain it], it will furthermore be necessary to speak of the means along with its divisions and in its entirety. On the contrary, when it [i.e. the means, yoga] is denoted, then everything is denoted [. . .] yoga is the result of exercising the divisions of yoga [. . .] yoga is the goal for its own divisions, and it is also the means to obtain discriminative knowledge and [supernatural powers, such as] the ability to become as small as an atom and so forth. Therefore it is more valuable, because it is the cause of two fruits [. . .]

[T]he next *sūtra* [(1.2)], '[*samādhi* without cognition is] yoga [and it is] the termination of the activities of the mind', has the purpose of showing the relationship between discriminative knowledge – whose means is yoga, and which is the means to obtain the removal – and the removal which is the result.

1.1.14 *Yogaśataka*[32] 2.4. Yoga as correct knowledge, doctrine and conduct:

With conviction, the lords of yogis have in our doctrine defined yoga as the concurrence of the three beginning with correct knowledge [i.e. correct knowledge (*sajjñāna*), correct doctrine (*saddarśana*) and correct conduct (*saccaritra*)], since [thereby arises] conjunction with liberation [. . .] In common usage this [term] yoga also [denotes the soul's] contact with the causes of these [three], due to the common usage of the cause for the effect.

1.1.15 *Vimānārcanākalpa* 96. Yoga as the union of individual and supreme self:

> They say that yoga is the union of the individual self and the supreme self.

1.1.16 Kṣemarāja's *Uddyota* commentary on *Svacchandatanta* 6.45. Yoga as union with an element:

> Knowledge is experience of one of the various elements (*tattva*s) which are to be known; yoga is the attainment of union with that [element].

1.1.17 *Mṛgendratantra Yogapāda* 2ab, with the *vṛtti* of Bhaṭṭa Nārāyaṇakaṇṭha. Yoga deriving from √*yuj*, 'to join':[33]

> (2a) To have self-mastery [is] to be a yogi.

The term 'yogi' means 'one who is necessarily conjoined with' (←√*yuj*) the manifestation of his nature. [A yogi], in other words, [is one who must experience] the Śiva-state. It is being a yogi [in this sense] that is the invariable concomitant of self-mastery. It should be understood, therefore, that the term 'yoga' derives its meaning not from √*yuj*, 'to be absorbed [in contemplation]', but from √*yuj*, 'to join'. This is supported by the fact that yoga in the form of *samādhi* is taught [separately] as one of its auxiliaries.

> [And] this (2b) is possible [only] for one whose has conquered his faculties.

One who has failed to bring all his faculties under control is incapable of other [far less difficult] tasks. How can he possibly become a yogi? As [Manu] teaches:

'As a charioteer controls his horses, so a wise man should strive to control his faculties as they roam amid the seductive objects of the senses.'

On the other hand, one who has controlled his faculties will soon realize his own nature. As Sanaka has said:

'When a person has controlled his senses, their objects, the subtle elements, and his mind, he becomes free of all desire and melts into his ultimate identity.'

1.1.18 Hemacandra's *Yogaśāstra* 1.5–7, 15. In praise of yoga:

> (5) Yoga is a sharpened axe for the canopy of creepers that are all calamities, a magical means other than herbs, mantras and tantras for attaining the splendour of *nirvāṇa*. (6) Even the worst deeds are wiped out as a result of yoga, like the thickest and blackest of thick black clouds by a fearsome gale. (7) Yoga destroys sins, even those amassed over a long time, just as fire instantly [destroys] a pile of kindling.
>
> (15) Liberation is the most important of the four aims of man, and yoga is its cause. Yoga is the three jewels that take the form of [right] knowledge, conviction and conduct.

1.1.19 *Śāradātilaka* 25.1a–3b. Four definitions of yoga:

> (1) Now I shall teach yoga, with its auxiliaries, which bestows understanding. The experts in yoga say that yoga is union of the vital principle (*jīva*) and the self (*ātman*). (2) Others say that it is knowledge of Śiva and the self as not being different. Those who know the Śaiva scriptures say that it is knowledge of the nature of Śiva and Śakti. (3) Other wise ones say that it is knowledge of the person (*puruṣa*).

1.1.20 *Vasiṣṭhasaṃhitā* 1.31. Knowledge consists of yoga:

> Vasiṣṭha said:
>
> (31) 'Know knowledge to consist of yoga. Yoga is situated in the self. It has eight auxiliaries and is said to be the duty of all.'

1.1.21 *Yogabīja* 87a–90b. The union of all dualities:

(87) There is no merit greater than yoga, no happiness greater than yoga, [and] nothing more subtle than yoga, for there is nothing higher than the path of yoga.

The goddess said:

(88) Lord, what is the definition of yoga? How is it practised? What happens as a result of yoga? Tell me all of that, O Śaṅkara.

The Lord said:

(89) The union of *apāna* and *prāṇa*, one's own *rajas* and semen, the sun and moon, the individual soul and the supreme soul, (90) and in the same way the union of all dualities, is called yoga.

1.1.22 *Haṃsavilāsa*, p. 47, ll. 15–18. 'He alone is a yogi . . . ':

He alone is a yogi, he [alone] is a teacher, he [alone] is worthy of service whose gaze is steady even without an object, whose breath is steady without effort [and] whose mind is steady without support.

1.2

Types of Yoga Method

1.2.1 *Bhagavadgītā* 3.3, 5.2, 13.25, 14.26, 2.49, 10.10, 8.8, 12.9, 18.52–3, 4.27, 5.4–5. Various yogas:

[The yoga of action]

(3.3) O faultless one [Arjuna], in olden times I proclaimed a twofold perfection in this world: through the yoga of knowledge (*jñānayoga*) of the followers of Sāṃkhya, and through the yoga of action (*karmayoga*) of the yogis.

(5.2) Renunciation and the yoga of action both bring about ultimate bliss, but of the two the yoga of action is superior to the renunciation of action.

(13.25) Some see the self in the self by means of the self through meditation; others through Sāṃkhya yoga; and others through the yoga of action.

[The yoga of devotion]

(14.26) He who serves me steadfastly through the yoga of devotion (*bhaktiyoga*) crosses beyond these *guṇa*s [which I have just told you about] and is ready to become Brahman.

[The yoga of the intellect]

(2.49) O Arjuna, action is very much inferior to the yoga of the intellect (*buddhiyoga*). Seek refuge in the intellect! Wretched are they who are motivated by results.

(10.10) To those who are constantly disciplined, worshipping [me] with love, I give the yoga of the intellect, through which they come to me.

[The yoga of practice]

(8.8) Concentrating with a mind absorbed in the yoga of [repeated] practice (*abhyāsayoga*) and not diverting elsewhere, one reaches the divine supreme spirit, O Arjuna.

(12.9) If you are not capable of keeping your mind absorbed steadily in me, then seek to reach me through the yoga of practice, O Arjuna.

[The yoga of meditation]

(18.52) Living apart, eating little, disciplined in speech, body and mind, always intent on the yoga of meditation (*dhyānayoga*), taking refuge in dispassion, (18.53) giving up egoism, force, arrogance, lust, anger and grasping, unselfish, peaceful: [such a one] is fit for becoming Brahman.

[The yoga of self-control]

(4.27) Others sacrifice all the actions of the senses and the actions of the *prāṇa* in the fire of the yoga of self-control (*ātmasaṃyamayoga*), which is kindled by knowledge.

[Sāṃkhya and yoga]

(5.4) The foolish declare that Sāṃkhya and yoga are separate, not the wise. He who performs even one of them correctly obtains the fruit of both. (5.5) The state attained by followers of Sāṃkhya is that reached by yogis, too. Sāṃkhya and yoga are one: who sees this [truly] sees.

1.2.2 *Pātañjalayogaśāstra* 2.1–2. The yoga of action:

Yoga for him whose mind is absorbed has been described. The following is to explain how one with a distracted mind can become absorbed in yoga.

(2.1) The yoga of action (*kriyāyoga*) is: asceticism, recitation and devotion to Īśvara [the Lord].

Yoga is not successful for one who does not engage in asceticism. Impurity, which is made manifold by beginningless *karma*, afflictions and unconscious impressions and in which the mass of objects of the senses is present, is not broken up without asceticism. This is the use of asceticism. And [because] it does not obstruct clarity of mind, it is considered that [the yogi] should practise it assiduously. Recitation is the repetition of the syllable *oṃ* and other purificatory [formulas] or the study of treatises on liberation. Devotion to Īśvara is offering up all actions to the supreme guru or renouncing their fruits. That, indeed, is the yoga of action.

(2.2) Its purpose is the cultivation of *samādhi* or the attenuation of the afflictions.

For, on being practised assiduously, it brings about *samādhi* and marked attenuation of the afflictions. It will make the markedly attenuated afflictions incapable of propagation like seeds burnt up by the fire of meditation (*prasaṃkhyāna*). Subtle wisdom, however, the discernment of nothing more than the difference between the quality of goodness and the spirit (*puruṣa*), untouched by the afflictions as a result of their attenuation, its duty complete, will bring about a reversal of propagation.

1.2.3 *Niśvāsatattvasaṃhitā Uttarasūtra* 5.2–3. Cosmic yoga:[34]

(2) The goddess spoke: Tell me about *śakti*, great lord, and about the yoga of the cosmos (*prakriyāyoga*), about what should be aimed at and what should not, O lord: on this I have considerable doubt.
(3) The lord spoke: matter, spirit, binding fate, time, illusion, knowledge, the Lord – these should be meditated upon one by one.

1.2.4 *Īśvaragītā* 11.1–10. Non-Being Yoga and the Great Yoga:

The Lord said:
(1) Next I shall teach yoga, which is supremely difficult to obtain [and] by means of which [yogis] see the self as the Lord, shining like the sun. (2) The fire of yoga quickly consumes the entire cage [created by one's] sins. Clear knowledge arises, directly bestowing the attainment of *nirvāṇa*. (3) From yoga knowledge arises; from knowledge yoga is set in motion. The great Lord favours him who applies himself to yoga and knowledge. (4) Those who apply themselves to my yoga, whether once a day, twice a day, three times a day or constantly, are to be known as great lords. (5) Yoga is in fact known to be of two kinds. The first is considered to be Non-Being (*abhāva*) [Yoga]. The second, however, is the Great Yoga (*mahāyoga*), the very best of all yogas. (6) That in which one's own form is meditated upon as empty and without any illusory appearance is said to be Non-Being Yoga, by means of which one sees the self. (7) And that in which one perceives the self as always blissful [and] pure is oneness with me, which is called the Great Yoga of the supreme Lord.[35] (8) Not one of the other yogas of yogis which are heard about in a multitude of books is worth a sixteenth part of the yoga of Brahman [i.e. the

Great Yoga], (9) in which liberated beings directly behold the universal Lord. It is considered to be the best of all yogas. (10) The hundreds and thousands of yogis whose minds are restrained [but] who have been cast out by [me,] the Lord, do not see the one me.

1.2.5 *Bhāgavatapurāṇa* 1.2.19. The yoga of devotion:

'When his mind is purified by the yoga of devotion (*bhaktiyoga)* to the Lord, he who is free from attachment perceives the essence of the Lord.'

1.2.6 *Pādmasaṃhitā Yogapāda* 1.1–6. The twofold yoga of action and knowledge:

Brahmā said: (1) O blessed one, O river of compassion, O supreme spirit, [you] have described the highest good of the man who has knowledge and has applied himself to yoga. (2) Describe that yoga, if there is more to be heard by people like me or if [you] show favour to we who are worshipping [you].

[Yoga's twofold nature.]

The blessed Lord said: (3) O four-faced one, the conjunction (*saṃyoga*) which is the fixing of the undisturbed mind in any sense object is of two kinds.

[The individual characteristics of the two types.]

(4) Constantly fixing the mind only on enjoined actions with the thought that 'action (*karma*) must be performed' is called the yoga of action (*karmayoga*). (5) Continually fixing the mind on the highest goal, on the other hand, is known as the yoga of knowledge, which brings about complete success [and] is auspicious.

[The efficacy in bringing about liberation of the two [yogas] together:]

(6) The mind established in the twofold yoga whose characteristics have been taught quickly goes to the supreme good, which is characterized by liberation.

1.2.7 *Yogabīja* 15–19, 32–5, 60, 71, 73–5. Yoga and knowledge:

(15) Desire, anger, fear, worry, greed, bewilderment, pride, disease, (16) old age, death, poverty, sorrow, sleep, hunger, thirst, hatred, shame, happiness, suffering, despondency, delight, (17) wakefulness, dreaming, deep sleep, doubt and pride: freed from these defects, the individual (*jīva*) is nothing other than Śiva. (18) Therefore, I will describe a means to destroy these defects. Some prescribe knowledge, [but] in this matter it will not succeed on its own. (19) Without yoga, how can knowledge bring liberation, O goddess? And yoga too, without knowledge, is not sufficient to bring liberation. [. . .] (32) My dear, even a god cannot obtain liberation without yoga.

The goddess said: (33) '[Since] for those who have attained knowledge there is nothing more to learn, why doesn't liberation occur for [even] the lowest of those who are detached?'

The Lord said: (34) 'People are considered to be of two kinds: raw and cooked. The raw do not have yoga. People get cooked through yoga. (35) The person who has been cooked in the fire of yoga is alert and free from sorrow. Know the raw [person] to be dull and earthbound, a source of suffering.

(60) 'Those who are detached and have knowledge are always overcome by the body in the end. How can they, those wretched lumps of flesh, be equal to yogis?

(71) 'Yoga is achieved by means of knowledge after many different lives. But through yoga knowledge dawns in a single life. (72) Therefore, there is no better path than yoga at granting liberation.'

The goddess said: (73) 'How is yoga obtained from knowledge after many lives? And how is knowledge attained from yoga in a single life?'

The Lord said: (74) 'A man thinks "After wandering about for a long time, I have become liberated through knowledge." How does he immediately become liberated just by thinking? (75) It is by yoga that a man is liberated after hundreds of rebirths and, because of yoga, birth and death do not occur over and over again.'

1.2.8 *Vimalaprabhā* 4.119. *Haṭhayoga*:

Now *haṭhayoga* is taught. In this system, when the unchanging moment does not arise because the breath is not controlled, [even though] the image has been seen by means of withdrawal and other [techniques], then, having forced the breath to flow in the central channel through the practice of resonance (*nāda*), [the yogi] should accomplish the unchanging moment by being without vibration, as a result of restraining the drops (*bindu*) of semen (*bodhicitta*) in the glans of the penis (*kuliśamaṇi*) in the vagina (*prajñā*).

1.2.9 *Haṭhapradīpikā* 1.56. *Haṭha*'s order of practice:

Posture, breath-retention, then various procedures called seals, and concentration on [internal] sounds: this is *haṭha*'s order of practice.

1.2.10 *Haṭharatnāvalī* 1.17–18. *Haṭhayoga*:

(17) Postures, various breath-retentions, and the divine procedures [i.e. seals] are the auxiliaries of *haṭha* practice, which brings the reward of *rājayoga*.

[Now *haṭhayoga*:]
(18) The ten processes [i.e. seals] beginning with *mahāmudrā*, the eight cleansing techniques, and [the eight] breath-retentions [and] the eighty-four postures: these are considered to [constitute] *haṭha*.

1.2.11 *Chos drug gi man ngag zhes bya ba*. The Oral Instruction of the Six Yogas:[36]

Homage to Glorious Cakrasaṃvara. Take advantage of the karmic process and extract the essence of the human potential.

[Inner Heat Yoga]

The yogic body, a collection of energy channels, coarse and subtle, possessing the energy fields, is to be brought under control. The method begins with the physical exercises. The vital airs [i.e. energies] are drawn in, filled, retained and dissolved. There are two side channels, the central channel *avadhūtī* and the four *cakra*s [i.e. wheels]. Flames rise from the *cāṇḍāli* fire at the navel. A stream of nectar drips down from the syllable *haṃ* at the crown, invoking the four joys. There are four results, like that similar to the cause, and six exercises that expand them. This is the instruction of Caryapa.

[Illusory Body Yoga]

All animate and inanimate things of the three worlds are like the examples of an illusion, a dream and so forth. See this at all times, both in movement and in stillness. Contemplate an illusory deity reflected in a mirror; take a drawn image of Vajrasattva and consider how the reflected image vividly appears. Just as that image is an illusory appearance, so it is with all things. The yogi thus contemplates the twelve similes and sees the reality of how all things are illusory. This is the instruction of Nagarjuna.

[Dream Yoga]

Know dreams as dreams and constantly meditate on their profound significance. Visualize the seed-syllable of the five natures with *bindu*, *nāda* and so forth. One perceives Buddhas and Buddha-fields. The time of sleep is the time for the method that brings realization of great bliss. This is the instruction of Lawapa.

[Clear Light Yoga]

The yogi working with the central channel places the mind in the central channel and fixes concentration on the drop at the heart. Visions arise, like lights, light-rays, rainbows, the sunlight and moonlight at dawn, the sun, the moon, and then the appearances of deities and forms. In this way the myriads of worlds are purified. This most wondrous yogic path is the instruction of Nagarjuna.

[Bardo Yoga]

The yogi at the time of death withdraws the energies of the senses and elements, and directs energies of sun and moon to the heart, giving rise to a myriad of yogic *samādhi*s. Consciousness goes to outer objects, but he regards them as objects of a dream. The appearances of death persist for seven days or perhaps as much as seven times seven, and then one must take rebirth.

At that time meditate on deity yoga or simply remain absorbed in emptiness. After that, when the time comes for rebirth, use the deity yoga of a tantric master and meditate on guru yoga with whatever appears. Doing that will arrest the experience of the intermediate state (*bardo*). This is the instruction of Sukhasiddhi.

[Yogas of Consciousness, Transference and Forceful Projection]

By means of these yogas, at the time of transference and also of forceful projection into another body, the yogi can utilize the mantric seed-syllable of the deity and train in the deity yoga practice in conjunction with the exhalation and inhalation [of the breath], long and short, and project consciousness to wherever is desired. Alternatively, those desiring to transfer to a higher realm can apply themselves to two syllables of *yaṁ*, and also HI-KA and HUM-HU. Consciousness is thrown to the heart of the deity inseparable from the guru, and from there to whatever Buddha-field is desired. This too is the instruction of Sukhasiddhi.

1.2.12 *Jīvanmuktiviveka* 3.10.18. The superiority of yoga:

Because it is a means of attaining the highest realm, yoga is superior to ascetic practices such as fasting according to the phases of the moon, and to rituals like Soma ceremonies. Because it is an internal auxiliary with respect to knowledge and a cause of the cessation of the mind, it is superior even to knowledge. When one knows this, faith in yoga arises. When this faith has been established and one believes [in yoga], vigour arises, a determination to practise yoga as much as possible.

1.3

The Four Yogas

1.3.1 *Amaraughaprabodha* 4–5. The four yogas:

(4) Dissolution (*laya*) of the flow of the mind is said to be 'dissolution'. That which is focused on stopping the breath is *haṭha*. That which is dependent on mantras and divine images is *mantrayoga*. That which is free from fluctuations of the mind is *rājayoga*. (5) *Rājayoga* is sometimes divided into two: medicinal and spiritual. *Haṭha* is also sometimes divided into two: using the breath and using semen.

1.3.2 *Yogabīja* 146–52. The four yogas:

The Lord said:

(146) The breath goes out with a *ha* sound and in with a *sa* sound. This is the mantra *haṃsa haṃsa*. All living beings repeat it. (147) From the teaching of the guru the repetition is reversed in the central channel (*suṣumnā*)[37] and becomes *so 'ham so 'ham*. That is called *mantrayoga*. (148) And conviction arises from the conjunction (*yoga*) of the breath in the rear pathway. The sun is denoted by the syllable *ha* and the moon by *ṭha*. (149) Because of the union of the sun and moon it is called *haṭhayoga*. Indolence arising from [imbalances] of all the bodily humours is consumed by *haṭha*. (150) When the self and the universal self are united, O goddess, the mind dissolves. (151) The breath becomes

fixed when the yoga of dissolution (*layayoga*) occurs. From dissolution happiness [arises], a state beyond the bliss [that can be found] in one's own self. (152) When the powers of becoming as small as an atom and so forth are obtained, one shines forth because of *rājayoga*. Know the four yogas [to arise] when *prāṇa* and *apāna* are joined.

1.3.3 *Dattātreyayogaśāstra* 9–11. The four yogas:

(9) 'Yoga has many forms, O Brahman. I shall explain all that to you: the yoga of mantras (*mantrayoga*), the yoga of dissolution (*layayoga*) and the yoga of force (*haṭhayoga*). (10) The fourth is the royal yoga (*rājayoga*); it is the best of yogas. [The stages] are said to be "inception" (*ārambha*), "action" (*ghaṭa*) and "accumulation" (*paricaya*). (11) And "completion" (*niṣpatti*) is deemed to be the fourth stage. I shall describe these to you in detail, if you want to learn about them.'

1.3.4 *Śivayogapradīpikā* 1.9–12. The typology of *rājayoga*:

(9) Because each of the four yogas is superior to the one that precedes it, one among them is chief: the supremely supreme royal yoga (*rājayoga*). (10) And that is threefold: Sāṃkhya, salvific (*tāraka*) and no-mind (*amanas*). Sāṃkhya [yoga] is knowledge of the twenty-five elements. (11) Yoga which results from experience of the external seal is called salvific. [Yoga] which results from the internal seal is called no-mind. (12) Salvific [yoga] is better than Sāṃkhya and the no-mind yoga [taught] here is better than salvific [yoga]. Because it is the king of all yogas it is known as the royal yoga (*rājayoga*).

1.3.5 *Sarvāṅgayogapradīpikā* 2.13–17, 24. *Rājayoga* as the drawing up of semen:

(13) *Rājayoga* is difficult to fathom. If one does not understand it, nothing is pleasant. *Rājayoga* is better than all [other yogas]. He who masters it is particularly

glorious. (14) Lord Śiva practised *rājayoga*. When he was with Pārvatī, Kāma, the god of love, could not reach him. Ghee not flowing when near fire[38] – this is the great miracle of *rājayoga*. (15) He who pierces the plexus of channels, his semen turns around and rises upwards. This technique is difficult, but very important. [One needs] a woman who will do one's bidding. (16) One may be seen to be attached, but remain free and enjoy the eight kinds of enjoyment. One is not touched by good and bad deeds, like a lotus in water. (17) Always happy, supremely blissful, one is like the moon holding on to its digits every day. Remaining detached in this way: this is the meaning of *rājayoga*. [. . .]

(24) Rare is he who knows the signs of *rājayoga*; he who does not know it must not associate with women.

1.3.6 *Śivasaṃhitā* 5.222. *Haṭha* and *rājayoga* are both needed for success:

Without *haṭha*, *rājayoga* does not succeed, nor does *haṭha* succeed without *rājayoga*. So the yogi should practise both until they are complete. Hence he undertakes *haṭha*, following the path of a good guru.

1.3.7 *Haṭhapradīpikā* 1.1–3, 2.77, 3.122. *Haṭha* as a stairway to *rājayoga*:

(1.1) Salutations to glorious Ādinātha, who taught the science (*vidyā*) of *haṭhayoga*. It is resplendent as a stairway which leads those who wish to ascend to the lofty *rājayoga*. (1.2) Having bowed down to the blessed guru, the Lord, the yogi Svātmārāma teaches the science of *haṭha* solely for the sake of *rājayoga*. (1.3) To those ignorant of *rājayoga* because they are lost in the darkness of multiple doctrines, the compassionate Svātmārāma offers the *Light on Haṭha* (*Haṭhapradīpikā*).

(2.77) At the end of the breath-retention in *kumbhaka*, make the mind free of support. Through practising yoga thus one attains the *rājayoga* state.

(3.122) Posture (*pṛthvī*) without *rājayoga*, breath-retention (*niśā*) without *rājayoga*, the yogic seal (*mudrā*), even though it is wonderful, without *rājayoga* – [these practices] are not good [without *rājayoga*].

1.3.8 *Haṭhapradīpikā* 4.3–4. Synonyms of *rājayoga*:

(3) *Rājayoga*, *samādhi*, the supramental states (*unmanī* and *manonmanī*), deathlessness (*amaratva*), dissolution (*laya*), reality (*tattva*), empty and not empty (*śūnyāśūnya*), the supreme state (*paraṃ padam*), (4) no-mind [state] (*amanaska*), non-dual (*advaita*), without support (*nirālamba*), immaculate (*nirañjana*), liberation in life (*jīvanmukti*), natural (*sahajā*), and the fourth (*turya*): these are synonyms.

1.4

Auxiliaries of Yoga

1.4.1 *Saccavibhaṅga Sutta* 23. The Noble Eightfold Path:

And what, good sirs, is the noble truth of the path that leads to the cessation of suffering? It is this, the Noble Eightfold Path: right view, right intention, right speech, right action, right livelihood, right effort, right mindfulness [and] right *samādhi*.

1.4.2 *Mahābhārata* 3.2.71–77. The Eightfold Path of *dharma*:

(71) Sacrifice, study, charity, austerity, truthfulness, patience, restraint and lack of greed: this is said to be the Eightfold Path of *dharma*. (72) Of these the first group of four is situated on the way of the fathers. One should practise it as a duty, not out of pride, because it has to be done. (73) The second [group of four] is the way of the gods. Good people always observe it.

> Pure of self, he should practise only the Path of Eight Auxiliaries: (74) right focus and right restraint of the senses and right special observances and right service of the guru, (75) and right control of the diet and right study [and] right renunciation of ritual action, [and] right stopping of the mind. By doing these the gods, desiring to overcome transmigration, (76) were freed from passion and hatred [and] attained sovereignty. The Rudras, the Sādhyas, the Ādityas, the Vasus and the Aśvins, equipped with yogic sovereignty, support living beings. (77) In this way, you, too, O son of Kunti, should, attaining great peace, pursue, by means of asceticism, success and success in yoga, O Bhārata.

1.4.3 *Pātañjalayogaśāstra* 2.28–9. The eight auxiliaries:

Discerning cognition, the means of escape, is perfected. And because there is no perfection without method the following [section on method] is begun:

> (2.28) When impurity has lessened as a result of performing the auxiliaries of yoga, the light of knowledge [arises], leading to discerning cognition.

The auxiliaries of yoga are eight [and] will be listed. By performing them, misapprehension, which is of five parts and takes the form of impurity, is lessened [and] disappears. When it is lessened, correct knowledge manifests. The more the methods are performed, the more impurity is attenuated. And the more [impurity] is lessened, the more the light of knowledge increases, in tandem with [impurity's] gradual destruction. It is this increase which experiences transcendence, until discerning cognition arises, i.e. until there is knowledge of the individual natures of the qualities (*guṇa*s) and the self (*puruṣa*).

Performance of the auxiliaries of yoga is the cause of the severance of impurity, as an axe [is the cause of the severance] of the object to be cut. It is what causes one to reach discerning cognition, just as religious observance (*dharma*) alone is the cause of happiness. [. . .]

(2.29) The eight auxiliaries are the rules, the observances, posture, breath-control, withdrawal, fixation, meditation and *samādhi*.

We will explain, in order, their practice and individual natures.

1.4.4 *Śārṅgadharapaddhati* 4348. The four practices common to all yogas:

Posture, restraint of the breath (*prāṇasaṃrodha*), meditation and *samādhi*: know that these four are in all yogas.

1.4.5 *Vāyupurāṇa* 10.76. The five practices of yoga:

Breath-control, then meditation, withdrawal, fixation and recollection (*smaraṇa*) are in this [Pāśupata] yoga declared to be the five practices (*dharma*).

1.4.6 *Mataṅgapārameśvarāgama Yogapāda* 1.6. The yoga of six auxiliaries:

The yoga of six auxiliaries is said be withdrawal, meditation, breath-retention, fixation, reasoning (*tarka*) and *samādhi*.

1.4.7 *Vivekamārtaṇḍa* 3. The yoga of six auxiliaries:

There are six auxiliaries of yoga: posture, breath-restraint (*prāṇasaṃrodha*), withdrawal, fixation, meditation and *samādhi*.

1.4.8 *Mṛgendratantra Yogapāda* 2c–3d, with the *vṛtti* of Bhaṭṭa Nārāyaṇakaṇṭha. The yoga of seven auxiliaries:[39]

How does a person become 'one who has conquered his faculties'? [Śiva] answers:

(2cd) One succeeds in conquering one's faculties gradually by repeatedly practising breath-extension[40] and the other [auxiliaries of yoga].

One achieves conquest of one's faculties gradually, by repeatedly practising the seven auxiliaries of yoga, beginning with breath-extension. Each of these will be defined below. [The word *śanaiḥ* occurs twice. The first, already glossed, means 'gradually'.] The second means 'repeatedly'. Breath-extension and the other [exercises] should be done 'repeatedly', while one 'gradually' increases the number of measures [which is to say, their duration]. These will be explained in due course. This is because if people repeat [these exercises] with too many measures [too soon] various ailments will arise to impede their yoga, such as abdominal swelling produced by the wind element, constipation, expiratory dyspnoea, insanity and loss of consciousness. In order to identify yoga and its auxiliaries, he says:

> (3) Breath-extension (*prāṇāyāma*), withdrawal, fixation, meditation, discrimination (*vīkṣaṇa* [= *tarka*]), repetition of mantras, and *samādhi*. These are the auxiliaries. Yoga itself is the eighth, as that whose purpose they serve.

Breath-extension and the rest are the seven auxiliaries of yoga. Yoga itself should be taken as the eighth, since it is that to which all these are subservient.

1.4.9 *Aparokṣānubhūti* 102–3. The fifteen auxiliaries:

> (102) Rules, observances, renunciation, silence, location, time, posture, the root lock (*mūlabandha*), equilibrium of the body, steadiness of gaze, (103) restraint of the breath (*prāṇasaṃyamana*), withdrawal of the senses, fixation, meditation on the self (*ātmadhyāna*) and *samādhi* are declared to be the auxiliaries, in sequence.

1.5

Warnings and Criticisms

1.5.1 *Brahmasūtra* 2.1.3, with Śaṅkara's *bhāṣya*.[41] Refutation of the efficacy of yoga:

> By this yoga is refuted.

By this the text teaches that one should realize that by the refutation of the Sāṃkhya school, the yoga school is also refuted. In that [school], too, contrary to the revealed texts, matter is said to be an independent cause and the intellect and so forth, which are not known [as such] by people or in the Vedas, are said to be effects.

1.5.2 Śaṅkara's *Bṛhadāraṇyakopaniṣadbhāṣya*. Pātañjala yoga is not a means to liberation:

> And so should suppression of the fluctuations of the mind be practised, because it has a different purpose from the self-realization generated by the sayings of the Vedas, and because it is enjoined in other texts? No, because it is not considered a means to liberation.

1.5.3 Kumārila Bhaṭṭa's *Tantravārttika* commentary on *Mīmāṃsā Sūtra* 1.3.4. Yoga is rejected by those who know the Vedas:

> The treatises on right and wrong accepted in Sāṃkhya, Yoga, Pāñcarātra, Pāśupata and Buddhist texts are not accepted by those who know the three Vedas.

1.5.4 Kauṇḍinya's *Pañcārthabhāṣya* on *Pāśupatasūtra* 1.1. Sāṃkhya yogis are beasts:

> Those who [claim to] have been liberated by Sāṃkhya yoga, the lords of Sāṃkhya and yoga, and everyone from Brahmā to the animals, are considered [unliberated] beasts (*paśus*).

1.5.5 *Mahākālasaṃhitā Guhyakālīkhaṇḍa* 11.100c–105d. *Haṭha* and gradual yoga:

> Yoga is said to be of two kinds: *haṭha* and gradual (*krāmika*). (101) *Haṭha* is called thus because it is performed by using force. Gradual yoga is said to be that which is done by means of application (*yukti*) and the instructions of a guru. (102) Many Brahman sages of old died through *haṭhayoga*, so nowadays one should never practise *haṭhayoga*. (103) Many diseases arise through the retention and inhalation of air, my dear. People die suddenly from them, so one should shun *haṭhayoga*. (104–5) Gradual [yoga] is called [thus] because it is performed in stages. [The use of] medicinal herbs, a measured diet and study, through the instruction of a guru: know these to be the stages (*krama*) of the practices which are useful for yoga. Because it is produced from those [stages, this is] considered to be gradual (*krāmika*) [yoga].

1.5.6 *Amanaska* 1.3–4, 1.7, 2.29, 2.42. Against effortful, painful yogas:

> (1.3) The ultimate reality is not found in the Base and the other *cakra*s, [nor] in the Suṣumnā and the other channels, [nor] in *prāṇa* and the other breaths. (1.4) Some are intent upon *mantrayoga*, some deluded by meditation, [and] some torment themselves with [the practice of] *haṭha*.
>
> (1.7) The magical practices such as sowing enmity, driving away [enemies] and killing, and the use of mantras bring about a proliferation of the multiplicity of phenomena. All the various locks and seals of [*haṭha*] practice produce only the yoga of ignorance. Meditation on the bodily centres, the channels and the six supports (*ādhāra*) is delusion of the mind. Therefore you must abandon all that, which is created by the mind, and embrace the no-mind [state] (*amanaska*).

(2.29) Even though the disappearance of the breath [results from the disappearance of the mind] it cannot be accomplished by practising the yoga of six auxiliaries. The disappearance of the mind is accomplished with ease in the blink of an eye through the grace of the guru.

(2.42) There is no point in spending a long time cultivating the breaths [or] practising hundreds of breath-retentions, which cause disease and are difficult, [or] lots of painful and hard to master seals. When [the no-mind state] has arisen, the mighty breath spontaneously and immediately disappears. In order to reach that [state] whose natural condition is innate, you must constantly serve the one [true] guru.

1.5.7 *Jīvanmuktiviveka* 1.3.27, 3.1.16–18. Forceful versus gentle yoga:

(1.3.27) There are two methods for corralling an ill-behaved beast: [either] showing it green grass [and] stroking it and so forth [or] verbally abusing it and threatening it with sticks and the like. By means of the first of those it can be brought in quickly, [but] by means of the second [the horse], running here and there, can be brought in [only] very slowly. Similarly, thinking with impartiality and happiness of enemies and friends and so forth, [and] individual effort by means of breath-control, withdrawal, etc., are the two methods for pacifying the mind. By means of the first of those, i.e. gentle yoga (*mṛduyoga*), one quickly woos the mind. By means of the second, i.e. forceful yoga (*haṭhayoga*), one does not woo it swiftly, but very slowly.

(3.1.16) But this statement of Arjuna is about forceful yoga (*haṭhayoga*): 'For the mind is unsteady, Kṛṣṇa, destructive, strong and unyielding. I consider restraining it to be as difficult as [restraining] the wind' [*Bhagavadgītā* 6.34]. (17) Because of this, Vasiṣṭha says, 'One who intently sits down over and over again [to meditate] is not able to subdue the mind (*manas*) without irreproachable methods' [*Laghuyogavāsiṣtha* 5.10.126]. (18) 'Just as a vicious elephant in must cannot be subdued without a goad [ibid. 5.10.127ab], the mind [cannot be subdued] without an [appropriate] method [ibid. 5.10.126cd]'.

1.5.8 *Haṃsavilāsa*, p. 51, ll. 15–16 and p. 49, ll. 24–7. Patañjali's teaching is not included among true teachings:

(15–16) 'Dear lady, Patañjali's teaching is nonsense, because there is nothing agreeable in anything achieved by force. A *rājayoga* completed with little effort has been taught by the wise.

(24–7) 'What has been said? That because the teachings of Patañjali cause the vital principle to attain *rājayoga* after forcibly freeing it from [the effects of] accumulated, activated and current *karma*, they are true? The glorious *rājayoga* is attained by the vital principle spontaneously, without forceful methods. There is no point in these extreme exertions. Beautiful lady, *rājayoga* has been revealed, seen and heard by innately sincere, good people. As a result the teachings of Patañjali are not included among true teachings.'

1.5.9 *Siddhasiddhāntapaddhati* 6.79–91. Those who do not obtain the supreme state:

(79) Those who first purify the pathways of the channels by the practice of exhalation, inhalation and breath-retention, forcefully make the mind fully unconscious in the lotus of the heart, and then, with the mind absorbed, observe that which is unchanging [and] indestructible in the flame of the lamp of the syllable *oṃ* in the supreme Kula do not attain the eternal state.[42] (80) All the clever materialists (*cārvāka*) skilled in logic [and] fond of the doctrine that the soul is physical do not cross the unbearable [ocean of suffering], [even] those who are supremely virtuous. All the conquering foreigners (*yavana*), who

revel in sin and are without pity, reap scant reward in this life [and] their truth does not bestow liberation.

(81) Those who concentrate on locations [in the body, such as] Śrīhaṭṭa, the top of the head, the opening in the hollow of the triple hollow, the aperture of Brahman, the forehead, the eye between the brows, the tip of the nose, the sound in the ear canals, the uvula, the throat, the region between the heart and navel, the cavity of the triple lotus, Uḍḍiyāṇa and the root do not, alas, attain the beginningless supreme state. (82) Those who constantly visualize in Gollāṭa, which is a mass of light like the fire at the end of time, or in the adept Jālandhara in Śṛṅgāṭa, a single light flashing like lightning, [and likewise] in the space in the channel of Brahman at the top of the forehead, which looks like lightning, [and] in the peak above that, which is as fiercely hot as ten million suns, do not, alas, attain the beginningless supreme state.

(83) Those who, having pierced the Brahman and other channels as a result of the movement of the mind and the air from the penis into the base of the spine, while leading semen to the secret place of the highest state above the cavity between the temples, struggle to create the internal sound, which is formed of the defining elemental characteristic of space [i.e. sound], in sequence along the spine [and] do not, alas, attain the beginningless supreme state. (84) Those people who insert the tongue, lengthened by means of regular [and] appropriate moving and milking, into [the opening above] the palate, lead it to the Śankhinī [channel] in the middle of the tenth door, [and] drink [the liquid] obtained from the region of the head as a result of the process of [the tongue's] conjunction with the central channel, remain stupefied after being rendered unconscious by drinking the six kinds [of liquor].

(85) Alas, those who practise by blocking both the two pathways behind and in front of the genitals, taking the air to the central [channel] by means of hundreds of

thousands of techniques of meditation and *samādhi*, by the practice of various postures, [and] by the union of *prāṇa* and *apāna* +as a result of correct activity with respect to the *haṃsa* [mantra]+ also drown, unhappy, in the waters of worldly existence.[43] (86) Those who contract the goddess and kindle the fire by pressing the [root] support (*ādhāra*) [and] awaken Kuṇḍalinī, then lead [her] from that place to Pūrṇagiri in the head and then bring her [back] down, delight in defective knowledge [and] for them the innate state is far off.

(87) Those who, through the observance of tranquillity and restraint, bring together the lock, the piercing [and] the seal in which the chin is at the hollow of the throat, fire in the bound pathways, the moon and the sun, equanimity (*sāmarasya*) [and] *nāda*, *bindu* and *kalā*, and who, by means of the experiential mind engage in the yoga of the supramental state (*unmanī*), such people, turned away from their innate happiness, treading the path of unhappiness created by action, bring delusion to the worlds. (88) [Those who practise] the Eightfold Path of yoga, the doctrine of the men of the clan (Kula), the seal of the six openings,[44] the piercing of the *cakra*s, [moving] the breath upwards and downwards in the central channel, [or] who see with the gaze [of yoga a light] like the rays of the sun, pervading every direction, or the sky dark blue like turbulent water: alas, even those who [practise and] visualize thus with controlled minds find misery.

(89) +Those who first practise holding (*dhāraṇa*), then wearing of conch-shell earrings (? *śaṅkhadhāraṇa*),[45] [then] the great holding (*mahādhāraṇa*), [then] complete holding back (*sampūrṇapratidhāraṇa*) +, who from the power of the observance purify the sight, [and] who both practise and cause others to practise +*ardholī*, *bahulī*, *dṛṣṭāsana*, *ghaṇṭī*, *vasan*+ and abdominal churning (*naulikā*): they are for ever deluded and oppressed. (90) Those dullards who practise internal purging, tasting

with the tongue of the fluids at the palate, lips and nose, emesis, *kapāṭa* (?),[46] the drinking of *amarī* (urine), *kharparī* (?),[47] who make use of their own semen after causing it to flow, and eat or massage [themselves with these fluids], they do not obtain the reward of the doctrine [taught in this text]. (91) Those who constantly listen to the sounds of the bell, the *kāhalakāla* (?), the drum, and the kettledrum when they resonate correctly, consisting of the unstruck sound, either when they pervade the body or are in the universe, do not attain the supreme and appropriate condition of the adept.

1.5.10 Gorakh, *Sabdī*s 31, 133–5. This eightfold yoga is all lies:

(31) Don't hurry to eat, nor die from hunger. Day and night contemplate the mystery of the fire of Brahman. Don't practise to extremes (*haṭha*) nor lie about. Thus speaks Lord Gorakh.

(133) Nine channels and umpteen chambers: this eightfold yoga is all lies. Unlock the Suṣumnā with the key by turning back the tongue and holding it at the palate. (134) Don't die fighting the pandits' knowledge. Understand that the supreme level is different, and reach it. Posture and breath cause trouble. Regretting them, day and night, die in the beginning stage [of yoga]. (135) The yogi in the beyond mind state hears the roar of *nāda* and *bindu* at the tenth door. Gorakh bolts the tenth door and searches for another way.

TWO
Preliminaries

The selections in this chapter present some of the conditions and procedures which prepare or entitle the student to practise yoga. As noted in Chapter 1, many of the *practices* that we might today identify as yoga per se are in fact commonly grouped as ancillaries or auxiliaries to yoga, where yoga is defined as the state or goal to be achieved (*samādhi*, *nirvāṇa*, *kaivalya*, etc.). In this sense, all yoga practices (up to and including the *practice* of *samādhi*) could be considered preliminary to yoga itself. In this chapter, however, we will focus predominantly on the procedures that are presented within the texts themselves as being prior to the main body of practice, as well as on the conditions and behaviours that are to be avoided if the practice is to bear fruit. While, as we shall see, the category of 'preliminary' is not a hard and fast one, nor necessarily one that all texts agree on, it is nonetheless useful in illustrating the material, ethical, social and alimentary conditions in which yoga may flourish.

Obstacles and Aids to Yoga Practice

The first section of this chapter (**2.1**) is concerned with the many obstacles standing in the way of progress in yoga. Some of these obstacles are mundane, practical and relatively easy to eliminate (such as eating bitter food, bathing early in the morning or mixing with bad company, e.g. **2.1.3**, **2.1.4**), while others (such as pride and ignorance) are dysfunctions deeply rooted in – indeed, constitutive of – the human condition itself. They are, in other words, the manifest symptoms of the existential problem to which yoga is the solution. It might seem odd, therefore, to present their elimination as *preliminary* to the practice of yoga, insofar as this elimination may itself be coterminous with the accomplishment of yoga. At the beginning of the second *pāda* of the *Pātañjalayogaśāstra* (**2.1.1**), for example, the goal of *kriyāyoga* (see **1.2.2**) is defined as the attenuation of the afflictions of ignorance, egoism, passion, aversion and clinging to life. Once these have been attenuated, subtle wisdom and discernment – the stated goal of yoga practice – can arise. As such, their elimination would appear to be much more than a mere preliminary preparation for yoga. Such 'obstacles' are included within this chapter because they are at the very least *logically* prior to the practices which aim to eliminate them, and to the states of yoga which arise in their absence.

A similar problem presents itself when we consider those conditions which are favourable to success in yoga (section **2.2**). Some conditions are material, mundane and relatively easy to put in place, such as diet, the right season to begin practice, how to sit, and so on. Others, however, may seem more like the results of yoga practice than preliminaries to it. For example, in the *Mālinīvijayottaratantra* it is recommended that one find a quiet, beautiful cave in which to practise yoga (**2.2.4**), a task which requires skills more logistical than yogic. However, prior to engaging in yoga practice one is also expected to have already conquered (among other things) the mind, the vital energy (*prāṇa*), and the senses, accomplishments which in other places are synonymous with the goal of yoga itself. Of course, this apparent paradox can be explained in a similar way to the auxiliaries: here, all the practices of yoga up to and including the practice of *samādhi* are considered preliminary and subsidiary to the state of yoga itself, as well as to the higher practices such as those outlined in the *Mālinīvijayottaratantra*. From this point of view, prior to this moment all yogic activity is merely preparing the ground, much as one would prepare one's practice hut or cave.

Also included in these two sections are advice on how to position the body for yoga practice and initial instructions on what to do with the mind and breath (**2.2.2**, **2.2.3**); statements on what kinds of person are qualified to practise yoga (e.g. **2.2.5**); what to eat and what not to eat (e.g. **2.2.8**); where and how to construct a dwelling (e.g. 2.2.9); when to begin practice (2.2.8); and how to order one's daily practice routine (2.2.10).

Sectarian Observances, Guru, Student and Initiation

In the next section (2.3) are three passages describing the observances, apparel and lifestyle of ascetic yogis. The *c.* second-century CE *Pāśupatasūtra* teaches the rules prescribed for an ascetic yogi of the Pāśupata tradition (2.3.1). The two most influential ascetic yogi traditions of the last millennium are those of the Gorakhnāthīs and Daśanāmī Saṃnyāsīs. Passage 2.3.2 is a verse from the 1503 CE *Miragāvatī*, an Avadhi romance that is an allegory of the Sufi path, in which the hero, on being separated from his beloved, dons the guise of a Gorakhnāthī yogi. Passage 2.3.3 contains a description of the Saṃnyāsīs given by a member of the order in about 1820 CE and recorded by Colonel James Skinner in his *Tashrīh al-Aqvāṃ*, an ethnography of various trades, castes and ascetics in the regions around Delhi.

Following on from this, the selections in section 2.4 consider the role of the guru and initiation in yoga. All texts agree on the necessity of a guru for successful yoga practice. Moreover, according to the *Śivasaṃhitā*, without a guru the practice will be fruitless or even dangerous (2.4.2). References to yoga initiation (*yogadīkṣā*) are rare (a notable exception being the long recension of the *Haṭhapradīpikā*, which mentions it as being essential to success in yoga (2.4.5)). However, if the aspirant wishes to practise yoga in one of the many Indian religious traditions in which it is taught, he or she is necessarily initiated by a guru (or *ācārya*). Especially in the tantric traditions, one needs to be initiated into a lineage before beginning to practise its yoga[1] or to carry out rites which are not in themselves yoga, but in which yoga-type practices may feature (see, for example, the introduction to the yoga section of the *Mṛgendratantra*, 2.4.4).

With the advent of the *haṭha* texts, a non-sectarian ethos emerged in which adherents of all religious traditions were deemed eligible for yoga. Nevertheless, in practice one would still need to be initiated into a particular sect in order to practise yoga with a guru. In other words, in spite of the universalistic spirit and trans-sectarian transferability of the yoga taught in *haṭha* texts, yoga was rarely, if ever, practised in a sectarian vacuum, and initiation from a guru would have been a necessary prerequisite to learning it. The universalism of many popular forms of globalized yoga today – in which initiation, guru and indeed lineage may be altogether absent – thus represents a significant departure from traditional modalities.

In the *Pātañjalayogaśāstra* (1.21–2) aspiring yogis are graded according to the intensity of their method (*upāya*) into three types: gentle/mild (*mṛdu*), medium/middling (*madhya*) and extreme/excellent (*adhimātra*). Each grade is then further divided into three, according to the same schema, giving nine levels of aspirant. An extension of the *Pātañjalayogaśāstra*'s basic threefold schema is found in the *Amṛtasiddhi* (Chapters 15–18), in which there are four grades (very extreme/outstanding (*adhimātratara*) is added to the *Pātañjalayogaśāstra* system).[2] The *Amṛtasiddhi*'s schema is the source of similar schemata found in subsequent *haṭha* texts, including the *Śivasaṃhitā*, in which a particular type of yoga is assigned to each of the four grades of aspiring yogi. The *Śivasaṃhitā*'s teachings are included in this chapter (**2.4.6**).

Purification of the Body

In later *haṭhayoga* texts, beginning with the fifteenth-century *Haṭhapradīpikā*, we find a series of preliminary cleansing techniques which remove gross impurities such as fat and mucus from the body, cure a variety of related diseases and render one fit for the practice of *prāṇāyāma*. Descriptions of some of these practices are included in the fifth section of this chapter (**2.5**). The *Haṭhapradīpikā* terms this set of techniques 'the six [cleansing] processes' (*ṣaṭkarma*) (**2.5.1**) and teaches them as follows: swallowing a long strip of cloth in order to cleanse the stomach (*dhauti*), enema (*basti*), nasal cleansing with thread or water (*neti*), staring until the eyes water (*trāṭaka*), rotating the abdominal muscles to stimulate digestion (*nauli*) and vigorous breathing (*kapālabhāti*). Another technique, described but not listed as one of the six, is vomiting (*gajakaraṇī*). The *Haṭhapradīpikā* thus describes seven rather than six practices, despite calling them the *ṣaṭkarma*s or 'six techniques'. The term *ṣaṭkarma* is older than the *Haṭhapradīpikā* and may refer either to a set of Brahmanical duties or, in tantric traditions, to rituals for curing diseases and controlling other people.[3] This may indicate that Svātmārāma, the *Haṭhapradīpikā*'s compiler, wished to trump these established systems of six processes with a haṭhayogic variety.

Later texts add other methods. For example, Śrīnivāsa, the author of the *Haṭharatnāvalī*, teaches eight techniques (2.5.3), and roundly criticizes Svātmārāma for not including the practice he adds to the *Haṭhapradīpikā*'s seven, the cleansing of the anus (*cakri*). Śrīnivāsa credits each of the cleansing techniques with the ability to purify a particular *cakra*: the *cakri* method, for example, cleanses the Base (*ādhāra*) *cakra*. This is perhaps the earliest instance of physical rather than meditational techniques being said to affect the *cakra*s (on the *cakra*s, see Chapter 5). In this context, he also mentions *vajrolī*, usually classed as a yogic seal (*mudrā*, see Chapter 6) rather than a cleansing technique, as a method for purifying the penis *cakra* (1.62). The *Gheraṇḍasaṃhitā* teaches four versions of *dhauti* (2.5.2), one of which involves prolapsing the lower intestinal tract, rinsing it in water and reinserting it into the body.[4] The addition of such apparently outlandish techniques may indicate a kind of competitive proliferation similar to that which we see in the development of *āsana*s (see the introduction to Chapter 3, below). One particularly striking example is found in the nineteenth-century *Jogpradīpakā* (834–9), which teaches a technique called *mūlaśiśnaśodhana* ('the cleansing of the anus and the penis') in which water is drawn in through the anus and expelled through the penis, a feat which is, of course, anatomically impossible.

Note that although the first textual evidence of the *ṣaṭkarma*s is in the *Haṭhapradīpikā*, this does not mean that the practices themselves are so recent: for example, the *vajrolīmudrā* technique first taught in the *Dattātreyayogaśāstra*, which predates the *Haṭhapradīpikā* by approximately 200 years, can be accomplished only by means of *nauli*.

Ethical Rules and Observances

The final section of this chapter is concerned with ethical rules (*yamas*) and observances (*niyamas*). Their best-known schema occurs in the *Pātañjalayogaśāstra*, which teaches five ethical rules (non-violence (*ahiṃsā*), truthfulness (*satya*), not stealing (*asteya*), sexual continence (*brahmacarya*) and non-acquisitiveness (*aparigraha*)) and five observances[5] (cleanliness (*śauca*), contentment (*saṃtoṣa*), austerity (*tapas*), recitation of sacred texts (*svādhyāya*) and devotion to the Lord (*īśvara-praṇidhāna*)) as the first two components of its eightfold yoga (*aṣṭāṅgayoga*) (2.6.2). These rules and observances are in fact much older than the *Pātañjalayogaśāstra* itself, their forerunners being much in evidence in, for example, the *Mahābhārata* (2.6.1), as well as the earliest surviving Jain text, the *Ācārāṅga Sūtra* (*c.* 350 BCE).[6] However, it is much more common to find a different classification of the *yamas* and *niyamas*, in which there are ten of each. In these lists, which here are exemplified by those found in the *Śāradātilaka*[7] (2.6.4), the rules are non-violence (*ahiṃsā*), truthfulness (*satya*), not stealing (*asteya*), sexual continence (*brahmacarya*), compassion (*kṛpā*), honesty (*ārjava*), patience (*kṣamā*), rectitude (*dhṛti*), moderation in food (*mitāhāra*) and cleanliness (*śauca*). The observances are austerity (*tapas*), contentment (*saṃtoṣa*), belief in the authoritative texts (*āstikya*),[8] charity (*dāna*), worshipping the deity (*devapūjana*), listening to the canonical teachings (*siddhāntaśravaṇa*), modesty (*hrī*), resolve (*mati*), mantra-repetition (*japa*) and the making of sacrificial offerings (*huta*).

In tantric texts the *aṅgas* of yoga are usually said to be six and do not include any *yamas* or *niyamas*. This does not, however, mean that there was no ethical dimension to tantric yoga practice: tantric texts enjoin ethical observances in places other than their yoga teachings, such as in the *caryāpādas* ('sections on behaviour') of certain tantras.[9]

A Note on Householders and Renouncers

In most yoga texts the ideal yogi is an ascetic who has forgone possessions, family and domestic life in order to devote himself to yogic practice. In these renunciant yoga traditions celibacy is held to be an essential prerequisite for yoga practice, as is finding isolated dwelling places away from human society. For ascetic yogis, the goal of liberation can be achieved only by renouncing society. Nevertheless, despite there being few historical accounts of householders practising yoga, some texts indicate that their yoga may also be undertaken by non-renouncers, i.e. married people who live at home with their family. The *Liṅgapurāṇa*, for example, gives instructions on how the householder is to practise sexual continence (**2.6.3**). The *Śivasaṃhitā* repeatedly states that its yoga may be practised by householders; it insists on the necessity of abandoning social interaction during yoga practice, but, once successful, the yogi may reap the rewards of yoga while living as a householder (**2.2.6**).

Displaying more pragmatism than the idealistic depictions of ascetics completely removed from society found in some prescriptive and literary Sanskrit works, other texts teach how the renouncer yogi maintains links with society. For example, the *Gheraṇḍasaṃhitā* recommends that the yogi build his hut inside a walled enclosure in a 'good, devout kingdom' where alms are readily available, but not in a remote area or a forest (**2.2.8**). The yogi therefore lives in only partial isolation from society, remaining close to settlements from which he can obtain food. This verse also suggests that the yogi is reliant on proper societal governance in order to create the conditions for practice. *Haṭhapradīpikā* 1.12 similarly recommends that the yogi inhabit a secluded hut within an enclosure, and shows a comparable concern for proper governance, prosperity and security within the larger society. Here again, the yogi is marginal to society, but nonetheless closely implicated in it.[10]

The yogic techniques taught in the tantric corpus are likely to have developed within ascetic traditions but their practice is also enjoined for householder initiates, both as part of ritual and as an independent body of practice. To what extent householders actually practised these techniques is unclear. Brunner, writing about the Śaivasiddhānta traditions which continue to flourish in South India in particular, suggests that householders only paid lip service to scriptural injunctions to use yogic techniques as part of ritual.[11]

Women Yogis

Texts on yoga are written from the point of view of male practitioners. It can, therefore, be difficult to assess to what extent women have practised yoga in traditional contexts. There are no pre-modern depictions of women practising yogic postures, although there is a small number of depictions of women ascetics and in some they are shown practising the austerity of remaining standing for long periods. Within the Gorakhnāthī yogi order there are, and appear always to have been, very few female ascetics, and there is no record of their practising yoga. Sanskrit and vernacular poems of the Gorakhnāthī and other north Indian ascetic traditions are highly misogynistic, and other Gorakhnāthī legends,[12] as well as current ethnography,[13] suggest that like other male ascetic traditions, the Gorakhnāthīs have always shunned the company of women. Women are never explicitly prohibited from practising yoga, although *haṭha* texts commonly insist that male yogis should avoid the company of women.[14] Note that the *Amṛtasiddhi*, the *Amaraughaprabodha*, the *Haṭhapradīpikā* and the *Gheraṇḍasaṃhitā* specify that this applies only to the beginning stage of yoga practice.[15]

There are some indications within the texts, however, that women did practise yoga. For example, several say that *vajrolīmudrā* – by means of which a man may prevent the loss of semen – may also be carried out by women (for women, generative or menstrual fluid (*rajas*) takes the place of semen).[16] The *Dattātreyayogaśāstra* (156) states that women can obtain *siddhi* through the practice of *vajrolī*, so long as they have no regard for their own and their partner's gender. The *Haṭhapradīpikā* similarly affirms that the practice confers *siddhi* on women, and that a woman who is able through *vajrolī* to preserve her own *rajas* is truly a *yoginī*.[17] These passages also contain indications that women were practising yoga beyond just the context of *vajrolī*. The *Dattātreyayogaśāstra* (155) stipulates that the male practitioner of *vajrolī* should find a woman who is devoted to the practice of yoga, and the *Haṭharatnāvalī* stipulates that a woman should not practise *vajrolī* if she is not familiar with the *Yogaśāstra* (2.109). Both examples suggest that there were women who were seriously engaged in the practice and study of yoga.

The *Arthaśāstra* (e.g. 1.10.7–8, 1.12.10–12) mentions female ascetics (*bhikṣukī*).[18] The *Yogayājñavalkya* states that women and Shudras (the lowest of the four *varṇa*s) can practise breath-control (*prāṇāyāma*) and non-Vedic mantras (6.12, 6.16–19, 6.63–4), which implies that in orthodox Brahmanical society women were allowed to practise at least some aspects of yoga. Moreover, in the *Yogayājñavalkya* it is a woman (Gārgī) who is being taught and initiated into yoga (Yājñavalkya and Gārgī are also interlocutors in the *Bṛhadāraṇyaka Upaniṣad*). Both versions of the *Yogacintāmaṇi* contain a verse which states that women (and men of all four *varṇa*s) may practise yoga, a statement that Birch suggests may derive from the *Viṣṇudharma*.[19] Sanderson notes that in some non-Saiddhāntika tantric Śaiva cults women could be practitioners (*sādhaka*s), and that in the Krama lineage women initiates could be on a par with men.[20] He also points out that there were some female tantric ascetics.[21] Hatley has examined the representation of female practitioners and the divinization of women in the Śākta-Śaiva *Brahmayāmala* or *Picumata*, a text which gives an especially detailed picture of women's participation in tantric ritual and makes reference to women who are 'well-versed in *samādhi*, yoga and the scriptural wisdom'.[22] Noteworthy, too, is the fourteenth-century Kashmiri female poet and wandering ascetic known as Lallā (or Lal Ded), whose songs reveal a deep personal understanding of yoga practice and theory. Finally, Kiehnle notes that Jñāndev's sister Muktābāi was a respected yogi.[23]

While evidence like this leaves no doubt that there were female practitioners of yoga, we know of no further historical sources which might complete our picture of who they were and what practices they were engaged in.

Chapter Contents

2.1

Obstacles and Hindrances to Yoga Practice

2.1.1 *Pātañjalayogaśāstra* 2.3–4. The afflictions (*kleśas*):

What, then, are the afflictions, and how many of them are there?

> (2.3) The afflictions are ignorance, egoism, passion, aversion and clinging to life.

This means that the 'afflictions' are five misapprehensions. By their activity they strengthen the authority of the *guṇas*, render [unwanted] transformation fixed, swell the river of effect and cause and, with the actions and afflictions having become dependent on each other's assistance, bring forth the fruition of actions. [. . .]

> (2.4) Ignorance is the field of the rest, whether they are dormant, diminished, extinct or active.

Of these [afflictions], ignorance is the field, i.e. soil of propagation, of egoism and the rest, whose variations are of four kinds, dormant, diminished, extinct or active.

Of those [kinds] what is dormancy? It is the condition of being a seed found in those [things] in the mind which have only potentiality as their basis. Its awakening [occurs] when it is faced with a support [for the mind or sense organs].

For a person in meditation (*prasaṃkhyāna*) in whom the seeds of affliction have been burnt up, that [awakening] does not happen again, even when faced with a support [for the mind or sense organs]: how can a burnt seed germinate? Thus it is said that the adept man whose afflictions are destroyed is in his final incarnation.

2.1.2 *Amṛtasiddhi* 19.6–7. Fire, women and travelling:

> (6) Whether [the yogi is] a householder or an ascetic, constantly devoted to the practice of yoga and diligently not focusing [on anything else], he should try hard to achieve his aim. (7) When first practising, the yogi should always shun the use of fire, associating with women and constantly travelling.

2.1.3 *Dattātreyayogaśāstra* 51–3, 69c–71b. Various obstacles to yoga:

> (51) In the first period of practice, O sage, various obstacles arise. The first obstacle is laziness, the second is said to be associating with the rogues that were described earlier (52) and the third is magic by means of mantras. The fourth is alchemy, the fifth the science of digging for buried treasures. (53) Various types of delusive obstacles like these arise, O sage, for the yogi whose posture is solid. The wise man should recognize and reject them. [. . .] (69c)[24] Next I shall tell you [some] things that create obstacles to yoga and are to be avoided: (70) salt, mustard, food which is sour, hot, dry or sharp; overeating is to be avoided, as is sexual intercourse with women. (71) The use of fire is to be shunned, and one should avoid associating with rogues.

2.1.4 *Śivasaṃhitā* 5.224–7. Diet, conversation and company:

> (224) Until the practice is complete, the yogi should resort to a restricted diet. Without doing so a wise man will be unable to complete the practice in this life. (225) The clever man should shun conversing with good men in the assembly. He should do so [only] to take care of his person, avoiding excessive chatter. (226) The yogi must avoid all company. He must completely avoid it otherwise he will not get liberation. I have spoken only the truth. (227) The practice is to be performed at home, indoors, shunning company. Outside, people must be met for the sake of everyday business, [but] without attachment.

2.2

Aids and Preconditions for Yoga Practice

2.2.1 *Mahābhārata* 12.232.23–6. When, where and how to practise:

> (23) Adhering to the observances, the sage should make progress in yoga at the three times [dawn, noon and dusk]. He should practise yoga on the top of a mountain, in a shrine or at the foot of a tree. (24) Having restrained all his sense organs, like [a trader] thinking of his wares in the marketplace, he should constantly think with focus and through yoga not disturb his mind. (25) He should assiduously engage in whatever method allows his fickle mind to be restrained and not deviate from it. (26) Focused, he should find empty mountain caves, temples or empty houses to live in.

2.2.2 *Bhagavadgītā* 6.10–18. Preparing the seat and practising moderation:

> (10) The yogi should meditate constantly on the self, in private, alone, with mind and self under control, free from desire and acquisitiveness. (11) In a clean place he should set up a firm seat for himself, neither too high nor too low, with cloth, a deerskin and *kuśa* grass on top. (12) Sitting there on his seat, he should concentrate his mind on a single object and, with the thoughts and senses under control, engage in yoga in order to purify himself. (13–14) Steady, holding body, head and neck straight and unmoving, gazing at the tip of his nose and not looking in (any other) direction, calm, fearless, established in the celibate's vow, he should control his mind and, with his thoughts on me,[25] he should remain engaged in yoga, intent on me. (15) Keeping himself thus constantly engaged in yoga, the yogi whose mind is

restrained attains the peace that is beyond *nirvāṇa* and abides in me.

(16) Yoga is not attained by he who eats too much or nothing at all, nor by he who sleeps too much, nor stays awake, Arjuna. (17) For he who is disciplined in food and enjoyments, disciplined in carrying out activities, and disciplined in sleeping and waking, yoga destroys suffering. (18) When his thoughts are restrained and he abides only in the self, without desire for any pleasures, he is said to be 'yoked' (*yukta*).

2.2.3 *Śvetāśvatara Upaniṣad* 2.8–10. The raft of Brahman:

(8) Having made the body straight with its three parts upright and used the mind to insert the senses into the heart, the wise man may cross all terrifying rivers by means of the raft of Brahman.

(9) With his actions controlled, the wise man should press the breaths in [the body]. When the breath is expended, he should exhale through one nostril. He should restrain the mind vigilantly, as if it were a chariot yoked to badly behaved horses.

(10) In a hidden, wind-free, sheltered [spot], which is flat, clean, free from stones, fire and sand, by quiet, flowing waters and the like, agreeable to the mind, but not oppressive to the eye, he should practise yoga.

2.2.4 *Mālinīvijayottaratantra* 12.5–7. How to practise yoga:

Bhairava said: (5) Listen, oh Goddess: I am explaining how to practise yoga. By becoming steady, the yogi will obtain success (*siddhi*) in this. (6–7) In a hidden cave which is quiet, beautiful [and] free from all disturbances, the yogi who has conquered posture, the mind, the vital energy (*prāṇa*), the senses, sleep, anger, fear and anxiety should practise yoga.

2.2.5 *Dattātreyayogaśāstra* 40–50. Everyone can succeed in yoga if they practise:

(40) [If] diligent, through practice everyone, even the young or the old or the diseased, gradually obtains success in yoga. (41) Whether Brahman, ascetic (*śramaṇa*), Buddhist, Jain, Skull-bearing tantric (*kāpālika*) or materialist (*cārvāka*),[26] the wise man endowed with faith (*śraddhā*), (42) who is constantly devoted to his practice obtains complete success. Success happens for he who performs the practices – how could it happen for one who does not? (43) Success in any form does not arise merely by reading the scriptures. Shaven-headed, bearing a staff or wearing ochre robes; (44) saying 'Nārāyaṇa', having matted hair, smearing oneself with ash, saying 'homage to Śiva' (*namaḥ śivāya*) or worshipping external images; (45) marking oneself in the twelve places or adorning oneself with lots of rosaries: if one does not practise or is hurtful, how is one to get success? (46) The wearing of religious garb does not bring success, nor does talking about it. Practice alone is the cause of success: this is indeed true, Sāṃkṛti. (47) It is a well-known fact that men who wear religious garb but undertake no religious practices deceive people by talking of yoga for purposes of lust and gluttony. (48) Crafty men try various deceits; declaring 'We are yogis', they are fools, intent on nothing but their own satisfaction. (49) Gradually coming to realize that men like that do not practise yoga, but attain their ends through words alone, one should shun those who wear religious garb. (50) These people are always obstacles to your yoga practice. One should take pains to shun them. Such behaviour bestows success.

2.2.6 *Śivasaṃhitā* 5.258–60. The householder yogi:

(258) The householder who is content with whatever he happens to obtain, who has given up inner attachment and who has completed all his duties becomes liberated

by means of the techniques of yoga. (259) Householders intent on the practice of yoga achieve success through worship of the Lord, so a householder should engage himself in the struggle. (260) Living in a house filled with children and a wife and so forth, internally abandoning attachment and then seeing the mark of success on the path of yoga, the householder enjoys himself once he has mastered my teaching.

2.2.7 *Haṭhapradīpikā* 1.16. Qualities needed for success in yoga:

Enthusiasm, boldness, patience, knowledge of the levels of reality, resoluteness and renunciation of contact with people are the six things by which yoga succeeds.

2.2.8 *Gheraṇḍasaṃhitā* 5.2–9, 16–33. Location, season and diet:

(2) The yogi should first get right the location [and] time [for his yoga practice], [his] diet [and] the purification of the channels, and then practise breath-control. (3) He should not undertake his yoga practice in a remote area, a wilderness, a city or near people. When undertaken [in such places], yoga is not successful. (4) In a remote area there is no security, in a wilderness there is no food and among people there is the glare of publicity, so the yogi should avoid these three [places].

(5) In a good, devout kingdom where alms are easily available and which is free from upheaval, the yogi should build a hut and encircle it with a wall. (6) There should be a tank, a well or a pond in the compound, and the hut should be neither too high nor too low and free from insects. (7) The hut should be properly smeared with cow dung and not have any holes. Only in a secluded location of this kind should the yogi practise breath-retention.

(8) He should not undertake yoga practice in winter, in the cool season, in summer or during the rains. Started [at these times], yoga causes illness. (9) It is taught that one should undertake yoga in spring or autumn. Yoga

will be successful then and the yogi is sure to be freed from disease. [. . .]

(16) Should the yogi undertake the practice of yoga without having a measured diet, he will get various diseases and his yoga will in no way be successful. (17) The yogi should eat rice, barley meal, wheat flour and beans such as mung, urad and chickpeas, all clean and without husks, (18) parwal, breadfruit, jackfruit, kakkola berries, śuka grain (?), drāḍhikā (?), cucumber, plantain, ḍumbarī (?), kaṇṭakaṇṭaka (?), (19) raw plantain, young plantain, plantain stalk and root, aubergine, radish and ṛddhi (?). (20) He should eat the five leafy greens: young greens, holy basil, parwal leaf, bathua (fat-hen) and snow-eye (? *himalocikā*).

(21) A measured diet is said to consist of food which is pure, sweet, unctuous, leaves half the stomach empty and is eaten with love for the gods. (22) The yogi should fill half of his stomach with food, a quarter with water and leave the fourth quarter for the movement of air.

(23) Food that is pungent, sour, salty, bitter or parched; curd, buttermilk, an excess of leafy greens, alcohol, palm-nut, jackfruit, (24) horse-gram, masur and white beans, winter melon, the stalks of leafy greens, bottle gourd, jujube, wood-apple, thorny bel, white turmeric, (25) kadamba fruit, lemon, bitter melon, breadfruit, garlic, lotus stalk, *kāmaraṅga* (?), chirauli nut, asafoetida, silk-cotton tree flowers and taro root: (26) these should be avoided by the yogi when undertaking yoga practice, together with travelling, the company of women and the use of fire.

(27) Fresh butter, ghee, milk, jaggery, sugar cane and other sugars, ripe plantain, coconut, pomegranate, *aśiva* (?) juice, grapes, otaheite gooseberry, amla fruit, juice which is not sour, (28) cardamom, nutmeg, clove, *pauruṣa* (?), rose apple, *jambāla* (?), yellow myrobalan, dates: the yogi should eat these.

> (29) The yogi should eat food which is easily digested, agreeable and unctuous, which nourishes the body's constituents, which he wants to eat and which is suitable. (30) The yogi should avoid food which is tough, off, putrid, sharp, stale, too cold or too hot. (31) He should not practise observances that harm the body, such as bathing in the early morning and fasting, nor should he eat only once a day, nor eat at night nor at the end of the night. (32) Following these rules, the yogi should practise breath-control. At first when he starts he should eat milk and ghee every day, and take meals twice a day, at noon and in the evening. (33) Sitting facing east on a thick seat made of either *kuśa* grass, an antelope [or] tiger skin and a blanket, he should cleanse his channels and then practise breath-control.

2.2.9 *Jñāneśvarī* 6.163c–85d and *Bhagavadgītā* 6.11. A place that inspires dispassion and contentment:

> (6.11) In a clean place he should set up a firm seat for himself, neither too high nor too low, with cloth, a deerskin and *kuśa* grass on top.

Therefore, one will have to look for a place (164) where, gladly content, when one has sat down, one does not like to get up, [and,] when one has seen it, dispassion grows twice as great. (165) A place which, [when] one resides there, brings contentment, [and] firmness of mind as armour, (166) where practice is accomplished automatically [and] experience itself teaches the heart, [and where] such greatness of charm [is] constant, (167) coming into the shelter of which, Pārtha, even in a heretic the desire for ascetic exercise arises and devotion takes root, (168) and even a sensual person coming its way expressive of amorous sentiments, affected unexpectedly, forgets to leave. (169) Like that [it] makes one who does not [want to] stay, stay, [and] one who roams about, sit, [and] with a stroke, awakens dispassion. (170) 'This most excellent of kingdoms [should be] abandoned, so that [I may stay] right here, cooling down', this occurs to even a sensual man the moment he sees [it]. (171) Where the abode is openly visible to the eyes it is as [very] beautiful as it is very pure.

(172) One other [thing] should be understood: [it] should be inhabited

by yoga practitioners (*sādhakas*), and it should not be sullied by people coming and going. (173) There should be dense trees at hand, always bearing fruit, their roots sweet like nectar; (174) water at every step, [which remains] clear, however, also at the time of rain; [and] a spring, very easily reached. (175) Yes: it also feels cool [when] a little sun-heat is felt; the wind is very light [and] soft with [its] breeze. (176) [It is] mostly silent, groups of animals do not enter, nor are there [flocks of] parrots [or swarms of] bees. (177) There are geese living on the banks; two or four cranes; there [may be] also a cuckoo, [if he] sits [there only] occasionally. (178) If it is not all the time, so sometimes there may be also peacocks coming and going – we do not say [no to that]. (179) Moreover, it is necessary, Arjuna, [for one] to get such a place. There should be a secluded monastery or a Śiva temple. (180) Of the two that which is acceptable to the mind should be preferred. One should spend most of one's time sitting [there] alone. (181) So one should find a place [like that], [and] watch [whether] the mind is steady [there]. [If] one [intends to] stay, one should install there a seat like this:

(182) On top a pure deerskin, in the middle a folded cloth, on the bottom unbroken *kuśa* shoots, (183) soft, similar [to each other], they [should] remain naturally well-bound; position [them] properly [and] evenly. (184) But, of course, if [the seat is too] high, then the body will sway, if [too] low, [the body] will develop problems from being in contact with the earth. (185) So one should not make [it] like that. It should be steady and level. Much [has been said], let it be; the seat should be like that.

2.2.10 *Jīvanmuktiviveka* 3.8.15. Daily schedule:

> For twenty-four or forty-eight minutes, according to his ability, he should practise yoga. Then for forty-eight minutes he should attend to his guru, either by listening to [his exposition of] the scriptures or by serving him. For forty-eight minutes he should look after his own body. For forty-eight minutes he should reflect upon the scriptures on yoga, and then he should again practise yoga for forty-eight minutes.
>
> Thus making yoga the principal activity and combining with it other activities (carried out quickly) at bedtime one should count the hours of yoga [practised]

that day. Then the next day or over the next fortnight or month, one should increase the time spent on yoga. And thus, when even single instants of yoga are added on to each single period [of practice], within the space of just a year the time spent on yoga becomes greater.

2.3

Sectarian Observances

2.3.1 *Pāśupatasūtra* 1.1–20. The Pāśupata yoga observance:

(1) Next we shall teach the Pāśupata yoga observance of Śiva [Paśupati]. (2) [The aspirant] should bathe with ashes at the three daily junctures [dawn, noon and dusk]. (3) He should rest on ashes. (4) He should bathe again [if he becomes impure for some reason]. (5) He should wear garlands that have been offered [to Śiva]. (6) He should display the attributes [that reveal him to be a Pāśupata in the first stage of practice]. (7) He should live at a temple. (8–9) He should worship an image of Śiva facing the latter's south-oriented face with laughter, song, dancing, bellowing, bowing, chanting and offerings. (10) He should wear one garment (11) or none. (12) He should not look at urine or faeces. (13) He should not talk to a woman or a man of the lowest *varṇa*. (14) If he sees [urine or faeces] or talks to [a woman or a man of the lowest *varṇa*] (15) he should cleanse himself with ashes, (16) perform breath-control (17) and repeat either the Raudrī Gāyatrī or Aghora [mantras].

(18–20) Yoga occurs in one who conducts himself with his mind thus undefiled.

2.3.2 *Miragāvatī* 106. The accoutrements of a yogi of the Gorakhnāthī tradition:

Tightly pulling up his stomach in the *uḍḍiyāna* lock (?), the Gorakhpanthī was wearing wooden sandals on his feet, a girdle and a cloak. He had matted hair, a bladed hoop, earrings, a rosary, a staff, a begging bowl, a tiger skin, a meditation belt, *rudrākṣa* seeds, a meditation crutch [and] ashes [and] was adorned by a trident. He blew the horn whistle and went on the path, reciting that divinely beautiful one's name [Miragāvatī] as his support. He took the ascetic's viol and the puzzle in his hand, and applied his mind (?), playing the strings all alone at night. He was now engaged in yoga, at play on the road to perfection. He called out loud, 'My food is Miragāvatī, give me alms that I may live!'

2.3.3 *Tashrīh al-Aqvāṃ*. Saṃnyāsīs:[29]

This sect of Saṃnyāsīs trace their origins to Dattātreya, whom they call Deva Datta, i.e. a god and an avatar of Nārāyaṇa, whose perfection in breath-control reached such heights that he achieved liberation from death and indeed eternal life. He was also the teacher of Śaṅkara.

This sect worships Sūrya [the sun], Viṣṇu, Devī [the goddess], Gaṇeśa and Mahādeva [Śiva], the five gods, and their main devotion is to Mahādeva. Most of them have a perfect acquaintance with the sciences of the Vedas and the sacred texts, and are pundits and spend their time reading the sacred texts. They have no occupation other than remembering God, being mindful of the unity of all existence and living in seclusion.

They rub ash all over their bodies; the ash is called *babhūt* [Sanskrit *vibhūti*]. Some wear their hair long, [in which case it is] called *jaṭā*, and some shave the hair of their faces and heads. Those with long hair are called *jaṭila* and those who shave their head are called *muṇḍita*. Whatever their devotees give them by way of cloth they dye ochre and wear. They have a white *kaupīna*, i.e. a small loincloth, to cover their private parts. They carry with them a dried gourd for drinking water called a *tumba*. They eat all types of grain and varieties of fruit and sweetmeats, but alcohol and meat are forbidden to them. They do not marry. If by any chance one of their number should get married or fornicate or drink alcohol or eat meat, when he is found out he will be expelled from the sect. Originally they did not accept disciples from any caste except that of the Brahmans; now disciples from the three castes of Brahman, Kshatriya and Vaishya are accepted. Some of them spend their time begging from door to door, some eat only from the households of their devotees and many have land grants and daily allowances for their expenses from the estates of *rājas* [kings].

2.4

The Guru and the Student

2.4.1 *Amanaska* 2.44. Qualifications of the guru:

Only he whose gaze is steady even without a focus, whose breath is steady without effort, [and] whose mind is steady without a support is a yogi, is a guru, is to be served.

2.4.2 *Śivasaṃhitā* 3.10–21. Serving the guru:

(10) Now I shall teach how to succeed quickly in yoga. Yogis who know this do not fail when practising yoga. (11) If it comes from a guru's mouth wisdom is potent. If it does not, it is barren and impotent and brings great suffering. (12) He who zealously makes his guru happy and practises his teachings quickly gains the reward of those teachings. (13) The guru is the father, the guru is the mother, the guru is god. [In this] there is no doubt. For this reason disciples serve him with their actions, thoughts and words. (14) Everything that is good for the self is obtained through the grace of the guru, so the

guru is to be served constantly or else no good will happen.

(15) After walking clockwise around him three times, the yogi should touch his lotus feet with his right hand and prostrate himself before them, touching the eight parts of his body (*aṣṭāṅga*) to the ground. (16) Through faith, success is assured for those who are self-possessed. For others there will be no success, so one should practise zealously. (17–18) Success will never happen for those who are devoted to worldly attachments, who do not have faith, who do not worship their gurus, who are very social, who delight in lying, who speak harshly and who are not content with their gurus. (19) The first mark of success is the conviction that one's practice will bear fruit. The second is having faith, the third is honouring one's guru. (20) The fourth is equanimity, the fifth restraint of the sense organs and the sixth curbing of the diet. There is no seventh.

(21) After finding a guru knowledgeable in yoga and receiving instruction in yoga, the yogi should carefully and resolutely practise in the way taught by the guru.

2.4.3 *Mālinīvijayottara* 4.6. Initiation and yoga:

'There is no right to [practise] yoga without initiation.'

2.4.4 Bhaṭṭa Nārāyaṇakaṇṭha's commentary on the beginning of the *Mṛgendratantra*'s *Yogapāda*:

Now begins the Section on Yoga. The only way to obtain the ultimate isolation [of liberation] is the ritual of initiation. This is established by the following passage of scripture:

'Initiation alone releases from this pervasive bondage which blocks the highest state, and leads [the soul] above [it] to the level of Śiva.'

2.4.5 *Haṭhapradīpikā*, Long Recension, 1.38–9. Initiation:

(38) The fool who wishes to master yoga otherwise, without the process of yoga initiation (*yogadīkṣā*) [and] without a guru, (39) does not obtain success, even after billions of aeons. After [initiation] one should carry out with utmost effort the practices prescribed in the scriptural teachings.

2.4.6 *Śivasaṃhitā* 5.13–28. The four kinds of aspirant:

(13) Know the aspirant to be of four kinds: weak, middling, excellent and outstanding. [The last is] the best and can jump across the ocean of existence.

(14) Lazy, very stupid, sickly, offensive to his guru, greedy, evil-minded, gluttonous, lecherous, (15) fickle, cowardly, diseased, servile, nasty, badly behaved and feeble: know the weak man to be thus. (16) He attains success after twelve years of striving. A guru should be sure to deem him to be entitled to practise [only] *mantrayoga*.

(17) He who is objective, patient, desirous of merit, affable, not too impetuous, confounded by worldly existence, of average valour and strength, (18) level-headed, averagely diligent and of average physique is situated in the middle of the paths of yoga, like those who have reached middle age. (19) Know him to be of middling keenness, middling health and middling valour. For these aspirants yoga becomes established in eight years. (20) He who is of middling merit and middling valour and who is middling in all he does is assuredly a middling aspirant. Recognizing this, gurus should with reason give him dissolution (*laya*) yoga.

(21) Determined, disciplined at dissolution (*laya*) yoga, self-reliant, strong, high-minded, compassionate, forgiving, resolute, (22) brave, in the prime of life, faithful, worshipful of his guru's lotus-feet and devoted to the practice of yoga: know the excellent aspirant to be thus. (23) He can achieve success in six years by means of his

yoga practice. Wise teachers give him *haṭhayoga* in its entirety.

(24) Endowed with great strength, energetic, charming, intrepid, learned, diligent, clear-headed, calm, (25) in the bloom of youth, restrained in his diet, his senses subjugated, fearless, pure, talented, generous, a refuge for all, (26) stable, steadfast, wise, content, patient, good-natured, dutiful, discreet, agreeable, (27) having faith in the sacred texts, worshipful of gods and teachers, averse to company, free from serious illness and experienced in the observances of the excellent aspirant: thus is the practitioner of all yogas. (28) He is sure to achieve success in three years. He is entitled to practise all yogas. In this there is no doubt.

2.5

Preliminary Purification of the Body

2.5.1 *Haṭhapradīpikā* 2.20–38. The six cleansing techniques:

(20) As a result of the purification of the channels, the breath can be held as long as desired, the fire [of digestion] is stoked, the subtle sounds become manifest [and] freedom from disease arises. (21) [The yogi] who has an excess of fat or mucus should first practise the six cleansing techniques, but anyone else, because [their] bodily humours are balanced, should not practise them. (22) *Dhauti*, *basti*, *neti*, *trāṭaka*, *nauli* and *kapālabhāti* are considered to be the six cleansing techniques. (23) These six techniques, which purify the body, should be kept secret. They confer wonderful abilities and are esteemed by the best yogis.

Of them *dhauti* [is taught thus]:

(24) [The yogi] should slowly swallow a damp cloth, about eight centimetres wide and seven metres long,[28] in

the way taught by the guru. Then he should withdraw it. This is taught to be the *dhauti* technique. (25) Cough, asthma, diseases of the spleen, skin ailments and twenty [other] diseases of *kapha* are sure to disappear through the power of the *dhauti* technique.

Now the elephant technique (*gajakaraṇī*):

(26) Having raised the *apāna* breath into the oesophagus, those who have brought all the channels progressively under control vomit up the contents of the stomach. This is called 'the elephant technique' by experts in *haṭha*.

Now *basti*:

(27) Squatting in water up to his navel with a pipe inserted in his anus, the yogi should contract his anus. The [resultant] cleansing is the *basti* technique. (28) Abdominal swelling, diseases of the spleen and all diseases originating in *vāta*, *pitta* and *kapha* are destroyed by the power of the *basti* technique. (29) When it is practised, the water *basti* technique gives clarity to the bodily constituents, senses and mind (*antaḥkaraṇa*). It gives beauty, stokes the [digestive] fire and destroys all imbalances.

Now *neti*:

(30) The yogi should insert a well-oiled thread twenty-four centimetres long into the nostril and draw it out through the mouth. The adepts call this *neti*. (31) It purifies the skull and bestows divine sight. *Neti* quickly destroys all the diseases which originate above the collarbones.

Now *trāṭaka*:

(32) The yogi should focus with unwavering gaze and full concentration on a small object until the tears flow. The teachers have called this *trāṭaka*. (33) It frees [one] from eye diseases and is a door against lassitude (?? *tandrādīṇāṃ kapāṭakam*) and so forth. It should be carefully kept secret, like a casket of gold.

Now *nauli*:

(34) With the shoulders rounded, the yogi should, with a fast and forceful rotation, revolve the belly left and right. The adepts call this *nauli*. (35) It always stokes a sluggish [digestive] fire, fixes the digestion and so on, and brings joy. It removes all imbalances and diseases. This *nauli* is the crown of the *haṭha* techniques.

Now *kapālabhāti*:

(36) Hurried inhalation and exhalation like a blacksmith's bellows is known as *kapālabhāti*.[29] It removes imbalances of *kapha*. (37) [The yogi] whose stoutness and other imbalances and impurities of *kapha* have been removed by means of the six cleansing techniques should then practise breath-control. He easily attains success.

(38) Opining that breath-control alone dries up all impurities, some teachers do not approve of any other [cleansing] technique.

2.5.2 *Gheraṇḍasaṃhitā* 1.9–50, 54–9. Cleansing techniques:

(9) Purification, strength, steadiness, calmness, lightness, realization and abstraction are the seven means of perfecting the body.

(10) The six cleansing techniques bring about purification, and posture (*āsana*) brings about strength; *mudrā* brings about steadiness, and withdrawal (*pratyāhāra*) brings about calmness. (11) From breath-control (*prāṇāyāma*) lightness arises, and from meditation (*dhyāna*) realization of the self. Through *samādhi* are sure to arise abstraction and liberation itself.

(12) *Dhauti*, *basti*, *neti*, *nauli*, *trāṭaka* and *kapālabhāti*; one should practise these six cleansing techniques.

(13) The four types of cleansing (*dhauti*) are called internal *dhauti*, dental *dhauti*, chest *dhauti* and purification of the rectum (*mūlaśodhana*). They purify the body.

(14) Air-flush (*vātasāra*), water-flush (*vārisāra*), fire-flush (*vahnisāra*) and external (*bahiṣkṛta*): there are four types of internal *dhauti* for cleaning the body.

(15) With his mouth like a crow's beak, the yogi should inhale very slowly. He should move his stomach and then slowly expel the air through the rear passage. (16) The great air-flush is to be kept secret. It purifies the body, destroys all diseases and increases the body's [digestive] fire.

(17) The yogi should slowly drink water through his mouth until he is full up to his throat. He should move [the water] through his stomach and expel it downwards from his stomach. (18) The great water-flush is to be kept secret. It purifies the body. The yogi who practises it zealously obtains a divine body.

(19) The yogi should move his navel plexus to his spinal column one hundred times. He gets rid of intestinal diseases and increases his digestive fire. (20) This fire-flush *dhauti* brings about success in yoga for yogis. This great *dhauti* is to be kept secret and never revealed.

(21) Using the crow seal (*kākīmudrā*) the yogi should fill his stomach with air. He should hold it for ninety minutes and move it through the lower passage. (22) Standing in water up to the navel, the yogi should draw out the *śakti* channel(?). He should wash the channel with both hands until the impurity has been removed, then rinse it and put it back in his stomach. (23) This washing is to be kept secret; it is difficult for even the gods to attain. It is certainly only by *dhauti* alone that a divine body may arise. (24) Until a man is able to hold his breath for ninety minutes, he must not practise the great external *dhauti*.

(25) The base of the teeth, the base of the tongue, inside the openings of both ears and the cranial aperture: dental *dhauti* is of these five types. (26) Using resin from the khadira tree or clean earth, the yogi should rub the

base of the teeth until he has removed the impure matter. (27) The [cleaning of the] base of the teeth is an important *dhauti* in the yoga practice of yogis; in order to look after his teeth, the knower of yoga should do it every morning. The cleaning of the base of the teeth is considered to be one of the essential cleansing processes for yogis.

(28) Now I shall teach the technique for cleaning the tongue. A long tongue can get rid of old age, death, disease and so forth. (29) Join together the index, middle and ring fingers, put the three of them into the throat and rub the root of the tongue. By very gentle rubbing the yogi can prevent imbalances of *kapha*. (30) After repeatedly pulling its tip with iron tongs, he should rub it with fresh butter and milk it over and over again. (31) The yogi should do this carefully every day, at sunrise and sunset. When it is regularly done in this way, the tongue becomes long.

(32) Using the tip of the index finger, the yogi should rub the apertures of the ears. By regular practice in this way [the yogi] makes the inner sound manifest.

(33) With his right thumb, the yogi should rub the aperture at the roof of the mouth. By practising thus he can prevent imbalances of *kapha*. (34) The channel [there] becomes clean and divine sight arises. It should be done daily, on waking, after food and at the end of the day.

(35) The yogi should practise three types of chest *dhauti*: with a stick, by vomiting and with a cloth.

(36) He should insert a stick of plantain, turmeric or cane into his gullet, move it about and then slowly withdraw it. (37) He thus expels phlegm, bile and slime through the upper passage. By using the dental *dhauti* technique, [the yogi] is sure to eliminate diseases of the gullet.

(38) When he has finished eating, the wise man should drink water until he is full up to his throat. After

looking upwards for a moment, he should vomit the water. By regularly using this practice he prevents [imbalances of] *kapha* and *pitta*.

(39) The yogi should slowly swallow a piece of fine cloth eight centimetres wide and then withdraw it. This technique is called *dhauti*. (40) Intestinal tumours, fever, diseases of the spleen, skin ailments and [imbalances of] *kapha* and *pitta* are destroyed. The yogi becomes healthier and stronger every day.

(41) Until [the yogi] purifies his rectum he has difficulties with wind. Therefore he should practise purification of the rectum to the best of his efforts. (42) With the help of either a stick of turmeric or his middle finger, the yogi should carefully and repeatedly wash his rectum with water. (43) This keeps intestinal problems at bay and prevents the build-up of undigested matter. It brings about beauty and health, and kindles the [digestive] fire.

(44) *Basti* is said to be of two kinds: wet and dry. The yogi should regularly practise wet *basti* in water and dry *basti* on land.

(45) Squatting in water up to his navel with a pipe inserted in his anus, the yogi should practise wet *basti* by contraction and dilation. (46) He keeps urinary disease, constipation and problems with wind at bay, and he becomes like the god of love, with a body of his own choosing.

(47) Assuming the back stretch pose (*paścimottānāsana*), the yogi should gently move the abdominal area downwards and then contract and dilate the anus using the *aśvinīmudrā*.[30] (48) By practising thus, intestinal ailments do not arise. The yogi increases his digestive fire and eliminates constipation and wind.

(49) The yogi should insert a thin thread twenty-four centimetres long into his nostril and then draw it out of his mouth. This is called the *neti* technique. (50)

Through practising *neti*, [the yogi] can master *khecarī* [*mudrā*]. Imbalances of *kapha* disappear and divine sight arises.

[In verses 51–3 *nauli* and *trāṭaka* are taught as in the *Haṭhapradīpikā*.]

(54) The yogi should practise 'skull-shine' (*bhālabhāti*) in one of three ways: by means of a wind-flush, [drinking] in reverse or a whistle. He [thus] keeps imbalances of *kapha* at bay.

(55) He should inhale through the left nostril and then exhale through the right. Then, after filling himself up with air by inhaling through the right nostril, he should exhale through the left. (56) He should inhale and exhale quickly, and not hold his breath. By practising thus he keeps imbalances of *kapha* at bay.

(57) The yogi should draw in water through the nostrils and then expel it through the mouth. By repeatedly drinking in reverse [like this] he keeps imbalances of *kapha* at bay.

(58) The yogi should drink water through the mouth with a whistling sound and expel it through the nostrils. By using this practice he becomes like the god of love. (59) He does not grow old, he does not get fevers, he has whatever body he wishes for and he keeps imbalances of *kapha* at bay.

2.5.3 *Haṭharatnāvalī* 1.25–31, 52–3, 56–7, 59–64. Additional and alternative cleansing techniques:

(25) In the first stage of practice, *kapha* and other [fluids] flow forth. By neglecting to do the purificatory practices, many diseases will arise. Of these [purificatory practices] we will recount the eight cleansing techniques beginning with *cakri*, according to the tradition of our guru. (26) The eight cleansing techniques are called: *cakri*, *nauli*, *dhauti*, *neti*, *basti*, *gajakaraṇī*, *trāṭaka* and *mastakabhrānti*.[31]

(27) In the *Haṭhapradīpikā* [there is the following verse]: 'They say that there are six cleansing techniques, *basti*, *dhauti*, *neti*, *trāṭaka*, *nauli* and *kapālabhrānti*.' How can such a teaching be taken into consideration when *cakri* is not included? This teaching is wrong, because it goes against the purpose [of giving instruction in the cleansing techniques]. Striving to reject and refute what is taught in the *Haṭhapradīpikā* would be like breaking one's body climbing a high peak. I shall desist: there is no point in cutting fingernails with an axe.
(28) These eight cleansing techniques which function to purify the body should be kept secret. One should not talk about them to anyone, just as [one should not talk about] the sexual life of a respectable woman.

Now the *cakri* technique [is taught]:

(29) Insert a finger halfway into the rectum and move it about fearlessly until the anus dilates. This is called the *cakri* technique. (30) By means of the *cakri* technique disorders of the anus and diseases of the spleen and dropsy are cured, impurities are cleansed and [the digestive fire] is kindled. (31) I proclaim *cakri* to be above all other cleansing techniques, but master Svātmārāma does not recommend *cakri*. [. . .]
(52) As an alternative [to the *gajakaraṇī* taught at *Haṭhapradīpikā* 2.26 (2.5.1)]: Drink water mixed with sesame and jaggery, or coconut water, up to the level of the throat and hold the breath and water in the oesophagus for as long as possible. When the breath has been conquered, completely cleanse the water and breath in the throat using the air variety of *basti*. Experts in *haṭha* call this the elephant technique. (53) Just as the king elephant of a herd is majestic, so is the elephant technique foremost among the techniques of *haṭha*. [. . .]

Now the skull-bellows (*kapālabhastrikā*) [is taught]:

(56) Inhale and exhale rapidly like a blacksmith's bellows. This is called the skull-bellows and dries up all diseases. Alternatively, (57) move the head rapidly left

and right, along with exhalation and inhalation. This is [also] called the skull-bellows. [. . .]

(59) The signs of success in *haṭha* are thinness of the body, radiance of the face, manifestation of the inner sound, clear eyes, good health, conquest of semen, kindling of the [digestive] fire [and] purification of the channels.

(60) When heaviness and impurities such as phlegm and fat have been removed by the eight cleansing practices one should practise breath-control: it is [then] easily mastered.

(61–2) By the power of the eight cleansing techniques the six *cakra*s are completely purified, breath-control is enabled, all diseases are destroyed, one is put on the path to liberation and one gains bodily health. The Base (*ādhāra*) [*cakra*] is purified by *cakri* and the penis [*cakra*] by the *vajroli* technique.[32] (63) The technique called *nauli* [purifies] the Maṇipūra [*cakra*] in the navel. The technique known as *dhauti* [purifies] the heart and throat *cakra*s. (64) Purification is to be performed on the Ājñā [*cakra*] using the techniques of *neti* and *trāṭaka*. *Basti* and the [skull-]bellows purify the whole body.

2.6

Rules and Observances (*yama*s and *niyama*s)

2.6.1 *Mahābhārata* 12.210.17; 12.232.4–7, 10–11; 12.262.37–8. Forerunners of the rules and observances:

(12.210.17) Bodily austerity (*tapas*) is celibacy and non-violence; mental austerity is restraint of speech and mind [and] equanimity.

(12.232.4) One should remove the five problems for yoga which the sages have taught: lust, anger, greed, fear and the fifth, sleep. (5) One conquers anger by means of tranquillity, [and] lust by giving up desire; the resolute [yogi] should get rid of sleep by cultivating the principle of energy (*sattva*). (6) He should guard his penis and stomach [the organs of lust and greed] with willpower, his hands and feet with his eyes, his eyes and hearing with his mind [and] his mind and speech with his actions. (7) He should cast off fear by means of vigilance, and greed by cultivating wisdom.

(10) Meditation, study, charity, truthfulness, modesty, honesty, patience, cleanliness, pure diet and restraint of the senses: (11) by means of these the yogi's vitality increases and he removes sin. He achieves all his aims and develops insight. [. . .]

(12.262.37) Kindness, forebearance, tranquillity, non-violence, truthfulness, honesty, absence of malice, lack of pride, modesty, patience and peace. (38) By means of these the Brahmans on the path reach that highest place which the wise man should use his mind to realize is determined by [one's] actions. [. . .]

2.6.2 *Pātañjalayogaśāstra* 2.30–33, 35–45. Five rules and five observances:

(2.30) The rules are: non-violence, truthfulness, not stealing, sexual continence and non-acquisitiveness.

Of these, non-violence is never causing harm in any way to any creature. The other rules and observances are rooted in it. They are practised in order to practise it, with the aim of perfecting it. They are being expounded only for the sake of bringing about its pure form. And thus it is said: 'Indeed, the more this Brahman here desires to undertake lots of vows, the more he practises that very non-violence in its pure form by desisting from the causes of violence performed out of carelessness.'

Truthfulness is when speech and mind conform with [their] object, [and when] speech and mind are in accord with what is seen [or] inferred. If uttered [in order] to convey one's thoughts to another, speech should not be deceitful, confused or devoid of information. It [should be] undertaken in order to benefit all beings, not to injure beings. And even if [speech] is uttered thus [i.e. truthfully], but with the sole intention of harming beings, there is not truthfulness, only sin. Through this mere appearance of virtue, this counterfeit of virtue, one would end up in terrible darkness. Therefore, after carefully considering the well-being of all, one should speak the truth.

Stealing is unlawfully taking possessions from others for oneself; its rejection, on the other hand, is non-stealing, which takes the form of desirelessness.

Sexual continence is restraint of the hidden organ, the genitals.

Non-acquisitiveness is not taking for oneself the objects of the senses, because one sees the faults of acquiring, protecting, losing, being attached to or harming [them].

These are the rules. But when they are

> (2.31) all-embracing, unlimited by species, place, time or circumstance, they [constitute] the great vow (*mahāvrata*).

Of them, non-violence is limited by species [when, for example,] a fisherman does violence only to fish, and not to any other [creature]. It is limited by place [when one says], 'I will not kill at a sacred bathing spot.' It is limited by time [when one says], 'I will not kill on the fourteenth day of the moon, nor on an auspicious day.' In one who has desisted from [these] three, it is limited by circumstance [when he says], 'I will kill for the sake of gods and Brahmans, and not otherwise.' Similarly, [it is limited by circumstance when] warriors say, 'Violence [is to be carried out] in battle, and nowhere else.'

Non-violence and the other [rules] must be upheld in all respects, without being limited by these [conditions of] species, place, time and circumstance. They are said to be the great vow when they are all-embracing, i.e. when they [are observed] in all situations with regard to all objects in absolutely every way, without exception.

> (2.32) The observances (*niyamas*) are: cleanliness, contentment, austerity, recitation and devotion to Īśvara [the Lord].

Of these, cleanliness is external when brought about by means of earth, water and so on and it is the consumption of pure food, etc.; internal [cleanliness] is the cleansing of the impurities of the mind.

Contentment is not wanting to acquire more than the means at one's disposal.

Austerity is enduring extremes. Extremes are hunger and thirst; cold and heat; standing and sitting [for long periods of time]; not communicating through word or gesture (*kāṣṭhamauna*) and remaining silent (*ākāramauna*);[33] and, as is fitting, [austerity comprises also] the observances of [yogis] such as the *kṛcchra*, *cāndrāyaṇa* and *saṃtāpana* fasts.

Recitation is studying texts on liberation or the repetition of the mantra *oṃ*.

Devotion to Īśvara [the Lord] is dedicating all action to him, the supreme guru.

'He who, whether on a bed or a seat or wandering on the road, is at ease, with all doubts destroyed [and] observes the destruction of the seed of transmigratory existence, remains constantly in *samādhi* [and] enjoys immortality.' From this it is said: [1.29] 'The mind turns inwards and obstacles do not arise' [. . .]

Of these rules and observances [it is said]:

> (2.33) When oppressed by wrong thoughts, [there should be] cultivation of [their] opposite.

When in the Brahman practising thus there arise wrong thoughts of violence and the like, such as 'I shall kill a wrongdoer', 'I shall lie', 'I shall appropriate his wealth', 'I shall have sex with his wife', 'I shall become master of his property', [then,] oppressed by the blazing fever of such wrong thoughts, which lead [him] down a false path, he should cultivate their opposites. He should think thus: 'While being baked in the terrible burning coals of cyclic existence, I have taken refuge in the way of yoga (*yogadharma*) by offering protection to all living beings.' One should cultivate the notion that by taking up wrong thoughts again after renouncing them, one is acting like a dog. By taking up again something [which one has] renounced, one is like a dog which laps up [its own] vomit. [Reasoning] like this should be applied to the other *sūtra*s. [. . .]When his wrong thoughts become incapable of reproduction, because of cultivation of the opposites, the mastery that is created as a result is indicative of the yogi's success. For example:

> (2.35) When non-violence is established [in the yogi], all living creatures [abandon hostility in his presence].

This is [true] of all living creatures.

(2.36) When truthfulness is established [in the yogi] there is correspondence between [his] acts and [their] results.

By telling someone to be virtuous they become virtuous; by telling someone to go to heaven, they go to heaven. His speech becomes efficacious.

(2.37) When non-stealing is established [in the yogi], all jewels come near [to him].

Jewels come to him from all directions.

(2.38) When sexual continence is established [in the yogi], he gains virility,

by gaining which he accumulates unimpeded supernatural powers, and [once] perfected he becomes capable of instilling knowledge in his pupils.

(2.39) When [he is] steady in non-acquisitiveness, complete knowledge of the circumstances of his [previous] births

arises for him. 'Who was I?', 'How did I come about?', 'What might this birth be?', 'How has this [birth come about]?' or 'What shall we become?' or 'How will we be [in the future]?' Thus his desire to know his condition in the past, present and future is automatically fulfilled. These are the supernatural powers [which arise] when one is steady in [one's observance of] the rules (*yamas*). [. . .]

Now we will speak of the observances (*niyamas*):

(2.40) From cleanliness comes disgust for one's own body and non-contact with others.

When there is disgust for one's own body, one practises cleanliness; seeing the shamefulness of the body, one becomes unattached to it, an ascetic. Moreover, there is no contact with others. Seeing the body's true nature, he desires to give up his own body. Failing to see purity in [one's] body even when washing [it] with earth, water and so on, how could one come into contact with the extremely impure bodies of others? What is more:

(2.41) Purity of one's essence, cheerfulness, focus, victory over the senses and fitness for the vision of the self.

[The word] 'arise' completes the phrase. As a result of being firm in cleanliness it is understood that from being clean arises the purification of one's essence, then cheerfulness, then focus, then victory over the senses, then fitness for the vision of the self of the essence of the intellect.

(2.42) From contentment, supreme happiness is attained.

Thus it has been said: 'The pleasure that comes from love in this world and the great pleasure there is in the divine realm are not worth the sixteenth part of the happiness [that comes from] the destruction of desire.'

(2.43) From austerity, there is the perfection of the body and senses as a result of the destruction of impurity.

Just by being carried out, austerity destroys the dirt which constitutes the layer of impurity. As a result of the removal of this layer of dirt, [there arises] perfection of the body by means of the [eight] supernatural powers, beginning with the ability to become as small as an atom and perfection of the senses by means of [powers] such as long-distance hearing and sight.

(2.44) From recitation [arises] union with one's chosen deity.

One practised in recitation sees the gods, sages and adepts, who help him in his task.

(2.45) From devotion to Īśvara [comes] perfection of *samādhi*.

Perfection of *samādhi* [comes to] one whose whole being is dedicated to Īśvara. Through this, he knows everything he desires [to know] as it really is, in other places, other bodies and other times. As a result his wisdom perceives things as they [really] are.

2.6.3 *Liṅgapurāṇa* 1.8.16–19. Sexual continence:

(16) For ascetics practising sexual continence (*brahmacarya*), [sexual continence] is said to be not engaging in sexual intercourse by means of actions of the mind, speech or body. (17) This is in particular reference to hermits who live without wives. I shall also teach you about the sexual continence of householders who live with wives. (18) [For them] sexual continence is said to be performing [sexual intercourse] with their wives according to the regulations and otherwise always restraining from it in thought, deed and word. (19) After

one's ritually pure wife has had sexual intercourse she should take a bath. By behaving thus the disciplined householder is certainly sexually continent.

2.6.4 *Śāradātilaka* 25.7a–9b. Ten rules and ten observances:

(7) The ten rules (*yama*s) are: non-violence, truthfulness, not stealing, sexual continence, compassion, honesty, patience, rectitude, moderation in food and cleanliness.

(8) Austerity, contentment, belief in the authority of the Vedas (*āstikya*), charity, worshipping the deity, listening to the canonical teachings, modesty, resolve, mantra-repetition, and [making] sacrificial offerings: (9) these ten are said by experts in the treatises on yoga to be the observances (*niyama*s).

THREE
Posture

Āsana as a Seated Posture for Breath-control and Meditation

In early yoga texts the word *āsana* denoted either a seat or a way of sitting; later it came to refer to any bodily posture and even repeated dynamic physical movements.[1] In the *Pātañjalayogaśāstra*, the earliest text to give a systematic description of an eightfold yoga practice, *āsana* is a way of sitting and the third of the eight auxiliaries necessary for mastering yoga (1.4.3). The *sūtra*s, i.e. the terse aphorisms that form the core of Patañjali's text, give no details about the nature of *āsana* other than saying that in order to practise breath-control and, by implication, the meditative techniques of yoga, the yogi's *āsana* should be steady and comfortable. The *bhāṣya* or commentary part of the *Pātañjalayogaśāstra* names twelve suitable *āsana*s, adding at the end 'etc.', implying that Patañjali knew more.[2] The twelve *āsana*s that are listed in the *bhāṣya* are not described therein, but later commentaries identify all of them as relatively simple seated postures in which to practise yoga's five remaining auxiliary techniques. Included in this chapter (3.2) is a translation of the passage on *āsana* in the c. eighth-century *Pātañjalayogaśāstravivaraṇa*, a commentary on Patañjali's *sūtra*s and *bhāṣya* attributed to Śaṅkara which is the earliest commentary on the *Pātañjalayogaśāstra* to give descriptions of how these twelve *āsana*s are to be practised.[3] Adopting a posture is a prerequisite for yogic breath-control and meditation, but Patañjali says (2.47) that posture is itself mastered through either the cessation of effort or meditative attainment.

The association of specific postures with yogic meditative practice was not an innovation of the *Pātañjalayogaśāstra*.

Numerous sculptural representations show that seated positions for meditation, in particular the lotus posture, were current in India well before its composition. The texts of the Buddhist Pali canon often instruct the meditator to sit down and cross his legs before beginning his practice[4] and, as will be shown below, meditative postures were taught in early works of the Jain tradition.[5]

The second half of the first millennium saw the composition of a huge corpus of tantric texts, many of which include teachings on yoga, but in them *āsana* is relatively unimportant and not included among yoga's auxiliaries. Many tantric works do, however, instruct the yogi to assume one of various seated *āsana*s when meditating or repeating mantras, or to provide a firm base for the practice of *prāṇāyāma*, which may cause the body to jerk upwards.[6] The *āsana*s taught in first-millennium tantric texts are thus few in number and all relatively simple seated postures.[7] A passage on *āsana* from the earliest known tantra, the *Niśvāsatattvasaṃhitā*, is the third reading in this chapter (3.3).

Postures Other than Sitting Positions

It is not until the composition of Sanskrit texts on *haṭhayoga* in the first half of the second millennium CE that we find systematic descriptions of yogic *āsana*s that are more complex than the seated postures described in earlier texts. The best-known and most influential text on *haṭhayoga*, the fifteenth-century *Haṭhapradīpikā* ('Light on *Haṭha*'), describes fifteen *āsana*s, of which eight are not seated postures (3.8). The *Haṭhapradīpikā* is a compilation and its verses describing complex *āsana*s are taken from earlier texts. The *c*. tenth-century *Vimānārcanākalpa* ('Ritual for Palace Worship'), a text of the Vaikhānasa Vaiṣṇava tradition, includes *mayūrāsana* (the peacock posture) among the nine *āsana*s it teaches and is the earliest text so far identified to include a non-seated posture among the *āsana*s of yoga.[8] Its prose description of *mayūrāsana* is found, in verse form, in subsequent Vaiṣṇava works on yoga, including the *Vasiṣṭhasaṃhitā* ('The Collection of Vasiṣṭha's Teachings'), which adds a further complex *āsana*, *kukkuṭāsana* (the cock). These and other *āsana* descriptions in the *Vasiṣṭhasaṃhitā* were used in the compilation of the *Haṭhapradīpikā*'s section on *āsana*. The *āsana* teachings from the *Vimānārcanākalpa* and *Vasiṣṭhasaṃhitā* can be found in sections 3.4 and 3.6.

Although non-seated postures are not taught in yoga texts until the end of the first millennium CE, Indian ascetics have been using them for at least 2,500 years. In Punjab in the fourth century BCE members of Alexander the Great's entourage came across 'fifteen men standing in different postures, sitting or lying down naked, who continued in these positions until the evening, and then returned to the city. The most difficult thing to endure was the heat of the sun, which was so powerful, that no one else could endure without pain to walk on the ground at mid-day with bare feet.' Two more ascetics called upon the king. 'They came up to Alexander's table and took their meal standing, and they gave an example of their fortitude by retiring to a neighbouring spot, where the elder, falling on the ground supine, endured the sun and the rain, which had now set in, it being the commencement of spring. The other stood on one leg, with a piece of wood three cubits in length raised in both hands; when one leg was fatigued he changed the support to the other, and thus continued the whole day.'[9]

The Buddha lived more than a hundred years before Alexander reached India and, according to the Pali canon, spent time with ascetics who practised a variety of austerities, including physical postures similar to those reported by the Greek historians.[10] Some would never sit down, others would hold difficult squatting positions and a few would undertake the 'bat penance' – hanging upside down from a tree, suspended by their feet.[11] India's greatest epic, the *Mahābhārata*, which was composed during the centuries either side of the beginning of the Common Era, includes several mentions of ascetics who invert themselves, stand on one leg or hold their arms up in the air for long periods.[12] The attitude of the Brahmanical orthodoxy of the time towards such practices was ambivalent, however. In the *Bhagavadgītā*, which is part of the *Mahābhārata*, Kṛṣṇa condemns those who undertake fearsome austerities which are unauthorized by scripture and weaken the body (*Bhagavadgītā* 17.5). Over the course of the first millennium CE, extreme physical asceticism slowly became more acceptable to the Brahmanical tradition, and in the Purāṇas – compendious theistic texts composed during the second half of the first millennium – gods and kings as well as ascetics are said to perform them.[13]

The self-mortifying physical practices of the ascetics with whom the Buddha associated (who were collectively known as Śramaṇas) were means of dealing with the newly theorized problem of *karma*, the accumulated effect of one's actions, which keeps one suffering on the wheel of rebirth. Motionless austerities were understood both to burn away *karma* and to prevent new *karma* from arising, thus bringing about liberation from the wheel of rebirth. These Śramaṇa traditions included the early Jain ascetics and to this day Jains are renowned for the practice of *sallekhanā*, in which they assume a standing or sitting position and fast until death. In a section on ascetic deprivations, a canonical Jain work, the *Sthānāṅgasūtra* (*c.* third–fourth century CE), lists seven postures. A translation of this short passage is included in this chapter (**3.1**). Some of these postures are described in more detail in the eleventh-century CE *Yogaśāstra* ('Yoga Teachings') of Hemacandra, who notes that Mahāvīra, the last great Jain saint, is said to have attained perfect knowledge in *utkaṭikāsana*, a squatting position.[14] In the commentary that he wrote on his own text, Hemacandra describes further *āsana*s (**3.5**), including non-seated postures such as *duryodhanāsana* (named after one of the protagonists of the *Mahābhārata*),[15] a headstand position which is said also to be known as 'the skull technique' (*kapālīkaraṇa*). This name for the headstand does not resurface until the eighteenth century, when it is found in a manuscript of the *Siddhāntamuktāvalī* (a long recension of the *Haṭhapradīpikā*), the *Jogpradīpakā* and the account of Purāṇ Puri (**3.12**).

Hemacandra's *Yogaśāstra* and the texts of the *haṭhayoga* corpus brought to a non-ascetic audience techniques that were developed within ascetic traditions. Among these were non-seated physical postures, for the first time called *āsana*s. Householder practitioners could not be expected to undergo the extreme physical mortifications practised by ascetics and the gods, sages and kings of myth, but they could seek to imitate them with watered-down alternatives. Thus the *kāyotsargāsana* or 'casting-off-the-body posture' taught by Hemacandra is not to be done until death, but simply carried out *kāyānāpekṣam* ('with disregard for the body') (4.133).

The descriptions in Hemacandra's *Yogaśāstra* and the *Vimānārcanākalpa* are the earliest instances of non-seated postures being called *āsanas*. Before long this application of the word became widespread and it is found in texts on subjects other than yoga which were composed at the same time as or shortly after the first *haṭhayoga* manuals. The early twelfth-century *Mānasollāsa* and the *c.* fifteenth-century *Mallapurāṇa* teach a variety of *āsanas* to be practised by wrestlers and elephants trained to fight. The early fourteenth-century Maithili *Varṇaratnākara* uses *āsana* (and another yogic term, *bandha*) to describe positions for lovemaking.

The Proliferation and Triumph of *Āsana*

Hemacandra's inclusion of the standing *kāyotsarga* pose among the *āsanas* of yoga is the earliest example of a process in which various physical practices other than seated postures for meditation were included in yoga texts under the rubric of *āsana*. The *Haṭhapradīpikā* is the first text to teach lying like a corpse (*śavāsana* or the 'corpse pose') among the *āsanas* of yoga; the technique had been taught in the earlier *Dattātreyayogaśāstra* as one of the *saṃketas* or secret methods of *laya*, dissolving the mind into the absolute. The 'bat penance' mentioned by the Buddha resurfaces in the eighteenth-century *Jogpradīpakā* as *tapkāra āsana* (the 'ascetic's posture'). *Mudrās* such as *mahāmudrā* and *viparītakaraṇī*, which involve physical postures and were taught in the *Dattātreyayogaśāstra* and other early *haṭhayoga* texts (see Chapter 6), are taught as *āsanas* in some later works. Thus a *mahāmudrā āsana* is taught at *Jogpradīpakā* 105–7 and the *viparītakaraṇī mudrā*, an inversion which uses gravity to reverse the downward flow of the life force, is found as *narakāsana*, *kapālāsana* or *viparītakaraṇāsana* in texts from the seventeenth to the nineteenth century.[16] And in the twentieth century, postures which became part of modern yoga but which had no Indian precedents were classified as *āsanas*; for example, *trikoṇāsana*, the triangle pose.[17]

Early texts on *haṭhayoga* such as the *c.* thirteenth-century *Dattātreyayogaśāstra* ('Yoga Teachings of Dattātreya') and *Vivekamārtaṇḍa* ('Sun of True Knowledge') declare that there are a huge number of *āsana*s: 8,400,000, according to the *Dattātreyayogaśāstra*, and, according to the *Vivekamārtaṇḍa*, as many as there are varieties of living creatures, from which Śiva has selected eighty-four. Like the *Vivekamārtaṇḍa*, the fifteenth-century *Haṭhapradīpikā* reduces the total number of *āsana*s to eighty-four and this figure has come to be widely accepted, both in texts and within the oral tradition. The first texts to name eighty-four *āsana*s, the *Haṭharatnāvalī* and *Yogacintāmaṇi* (the latter only in an unpublished recension), date from the seventeenth century. The *Haṭharatnāvalī*'s list is included in this chapter, together with a selection from the thirty-six *āsana* descriptions that it gives (3.11).

As the corpus of texts on *haṭhayoga* developed, *āsana* went from being a simple way of sitting for meditation, mantra-repetition and breath-control – taught in passing – to one of its most important, complex, diverse and well-documented practices. The *Dattātreyayogaśāstra* and *Vivekamārtaṇḍa* describe just one and two *āsana*s, respectively; *mudrā* is the most important *haṭha* technique in their teachings. The *Haṭhapradīpikā* teaches fifteen *āsana*s, including eight non-seated postures (it is thus the first text to teach non-seated postures as part of *haṭhayoga*). In texts on yoga from the seventeenth century onwards, in contrast, *āsana* becomes a central concern. The 1660 CE *Yogacintāmaṇi* manuscript mentioned above is the first text to list all eighty-four *āsana*s (in fact, it lists 110 in total); a manuscript of an extended recension of the *Haṭhapradīpikā* dated 1708 CE adds descriptions of approximately eighty *āsana*s to the fifteen found in the earlier recension; the *Rudrayāmalatantra*, a late tantric work, teaches approximately 100 *āsana*s; the 1737 CE *Jogpradīpakā* devotes 314 of its 964 verses to descriptions of all eighty-four *āsana*s; a manuscript in Jaipur dated to 1744 CE and entitled *Āsanayogagrantha* ('The Book of Postural Yoga'), is devoted to descriptions of eighty-four *āsana*s; an eighteenth- or nineteenth-century manuscript from Bikaner of a Jain text catalogued as *Yogāsana* lists 108 *āsana*s;[18] and about two thirds of the *c.* early nineteenth-century *Haṭhābhyāsapaddhati* is taken up with descriptions of 112 *āsana*s, some of which are included in this chapter (3.14).

This proliferation of *āsana* descriptions in Sanskrit and Braj Bhasha sources is mirrored by that seen in texts on yoga written in an Islamic framework. The *c*. fifteenth-century Arabic *Ḥawż al-ḥayāt* teaches five *āsana*s, while its sixteenth-century Persian 'translation', the *Baḥr al-ḥayāt*, adds seventeen more. All the former's *āsana*s and a selection of the latter's are included in this chapter (3.7, 3.10).

The Purposes of *Āsana*

Until the composition of the earliest *haṭhayoga* texts in the first few centuries of the second millennium CE, there were two primary reasons for ascetics and yogis to practise physical postures: as a stable base for breath-control, mantra-repetition and meditation or as a means of stopping *karma* and acquiring *tapas*, ascetic power, which both purifies one's old *karma* and grants supernatural abilities. With the advent of the *haṭha* corpus therapeutic benefits were added. These three reasons for practising *āsana*s will now be looked at in detail.

It is made clear in many texts that *āsana* is a prerequisite for meditation and breath-control. Even as descriptions of *āsana*s proliferated in texts composed in the sixteenth to eighteenth century and their therapeutic benefits come to the fore, they are still often associated with control of the mind. Thus the twenty-two complex modes of sitting taught in the sixteenth-century Persian *Baḥr al-ḥayāt* and illustrated in a manuscript copied in 1602 CE are prerequisites for techniques which have various types of meditation as their main aim. Like the *āsana*s taught in the *Baḥr al-ḥayāt*, most of the eighty-four taught in the eighteenth-century *Jogpradīpakā* are said to have therapeutic benefits, but all are said to require the yogi to gaze in meditation between his eyebrows or at the tip of his nose.

The accumulation of *tapas*, as the heating power generated by asceticism, is not explicitly taught as an aim of yoga in Sanskrit texts,[19] but, from at least the time of the Buddha until the present day, yoga-practising Indian ascetics have sought to acquire *tapas* by holding difficult physical postures for long periods. In a unique and recently discovered first-hand historical account, part of which is included in this chapter (3.12), the ascetic Purāṇ Puri told the collector of Benares, Jonathan Duncan, how, in about 1760 when he was still a boy (but already an initiated ascetic), he went to a festival at Allahabad and learnt from his seniors of the eighteen *Brahmā mudrā*s, various types of ascetic mortification, among which was the practice of the eighty-four *āsana*s, 'different postures in sitting, such as continuing several hours with the feet on the neck or under the arms; after which the members are returned to their natural positions'.[20] That these ascetic practices were not undertaken in order to cow the spirit is exemplified by the story of Purāṇ Puri himself. He chose the *ūrdhvabāhu* austerity and held both his arms in the air for the remaining forty-five years of his life, during which he travelled continuously, reaching as far as Malaysia in the east and Moscow in the west.

Purāṇ Puri's description of the practice of the eighty-four *āsana*s highlights a key difference between traditional and modern *āsana* practice. For traditional yogis it is usually enough to adopt a single position and hold it for a long period (as suggested by the word *āsana* itself, whose root √*ās* means both 'sit' and 'remain [as one is]'), rather than practise several different *āsana*s in succession.[21] Hemacandra, in his *Yogaśāstra*, says that the yogi should use for meditation whichever *āsana* makes the mind steady (4.134). Similar instructions for the yogi to use just one *āsana* are found in a wide variety of texts on yoga, from first-millennium tantric works such as the *Parākhyatantra* (14.7–8) to the *c.* sixteenth-century *Śivayogapradīpikā* (2.14). Travellers to India in the seventeenth century echoed the reports of Alexander's men when they remarked upon Indian ascetics' ability to hold difficult physical positions for hours on end; one such traveller, Peter Mundy, did come across men who moved from the lotus position to a headstand, but these were *bazīgar*s, street performers, not fakirs, holy men.[22]

Sequences of physical postures were included in teachings on yoga in Tibet from at least the fifteenth century onwards. They are part of *'khrul 'khor*, which is sometimes translated as 'magical movement'.[23] There appears, however, to be no direct connection between these posture sequences and the practices of Indian *haṭhayoga*.[24] The absence in Indian texts of clear parallels with these

Tibetan techniques adds weight to the claims found among certain Tibetan traditions that *'khrul 'khor* was either an indigenous Bön practice or originated in China.[25] A systematic teaching of the sequential postures of *'khrul 'khor* found in the fifteenth-century 'Compendium of Enlightened Spontaneity' of Pema Lingpa, Bhutan's patron saint, is included in this chapter (3.9).

Complex sequences of *āsana*s are not taught in any pre-modern Indian texts,[26] but by the eighteenth century Indian yoga texts did start to teach repeated physical movements. The ninth chapter of Sundaradeva's *Haṭhatattvakaumudī* ('Moonlight of the Principles of Yoga') includes various repeated movements among purifications to be performed prior to the practice of *prāṇāyāma* (breath-control). The exercises taught by Sundaradeva are not in the *Haṭhatattvakaumudī*'s section on *āsana* (although they are referred to in one verse as *āsana*s); nevertheless we have chosen to include them in this chapter (3.13). In two closely related texts from the latter part of the eighteenth century or early nineteenth, however, *āsana* does come to include a wide variety of physical exercises, from squat thrusts to rope-climbing. These texts are the *Haṭhābhyāsapaddhati* ('Manual of *Haṭha* Practice') of Kapāla Kuruṇṭaka and the yoga section of the *Śrītattvanidhi* ('Glorious Abode of Truth'), selections from the first of which are included in this chapter (3.14).

In these two texts firmness of the body becomes the sole purpose of *āsana*, as a prerequisite for the practice of the *ṣaṭkarma*s, the six cleansing practices (2.5). The physical benefits of *āsana* practice are occasionally mentioned, in passing, in early works on *haṭhayoga* and several say that *āsana* practice in general gets rid of disease. The *Haṭhapradīpikā* adds that it brings about firmness and nimbleness of the body, and includes specific physical benefits in its descriptions of individual *āsana*s. *Mayūrāsana* (the peacock posture), for example, is said to get rid of all afflictions of the stomach.

These therapeutic effects are an innovation of the *haṭhayoga* texts. Earlier works on yoga mention its physical benefits, but not in the context of *āsana*. And even the earliest works of the *haṭha* corpus put more emphasis on the efficacy of meditational techniques rather than *āsana*s in bringing about improvements in the body. Thus the *Dattātreyayogaśāstra* says that *pratyāhāra* ('withdrawal') brings firmness of the body, and the *Amṛtasiddhi* and *Amaraughaprabodha* say that when the yogi reaches the second of the four stages of yoga his *āsana* automatically becomes firm.

The *Jogpradīpakā*, the *Haṭhābhyāsapaddhati* and the account of Purāṇ Puri all document *āsana* practice during the eighteenth century, the cusp of yoga's engagement with the wider world and the development of modern yoga. They show that the three aims of *āsana* practice were still current, and, in the case of the *Jogpradīpakā* at least, were by no means mutually exclusive. Some authors on yoga did warn against excessive exercise: in his early nineteenth-century commentary on the *Haṭhapradīpikā* Brahmānanda explains that text's admonition against practices that harm the body as referring to 'multiple repetitions of practices such as the sun salutation[27] or the lifting of weights'. Meanwhile, the *Haṭhābhyāsapaddhati*'s *gajāsana* (elephant posture) involves repetitions of what is today known as the *adhomukhaśvanāsana* (downward dog), a constituent of the modern sun salutation. Even in pre-modern India there was no consensus as to which physical practices could be accepted as part of yoga.

Chapter Contents

3.8 *Haṭhapradīpikā* 1.17–18, 24–49, 53–6. The first teaching of non-seated postures as part of *haṭhayoga*.

3.9 *Rtsa rlung gsang ba'i lde mig* ('The Secret Key to the Channels and Winds'). [The first section of] a chapter from Pema Lingpa's *Rdzogs chen kun bzang dgongs 'dus* (*Compendium of Enlightened Spontaneity*). The twenty-three positions of *'khrul 'khor*.

3.10 *Baḥr al-ḥayāt* 4.6.7, 10, 17, 21, 24–5. Knowledge of the Heart and the Character of Discipline.

3.11 *Haṭharatnāvalī* 3.7–20 and selected verses from the rest of the chapter. The eighty-four postures.

3.12 From the life story of the ascetic Purāṇ Puri as dictated to Jonathan Duncan. The eighteen *mudrā*s of Brahmā.

3.13 *Haṭhatattvakaumudī* Chapter 9. Dynamic movements in preparation for breath-control.

3.14 Selections from the *Haṭhābhyāsapaddhati*. Dynamic *āsanas*.

3.1 *Sthānāṅgasūtra* 5.1.396. The five ascetic resolves:

(396) [. . .] There are five further ascetic resolves (*ṭhāṇāi*), as follows: adopting a standing posture (*ṭhāṇātite*), adopting a squatting posture (*ukkuḍuāsaṇite*), adopting the position of an icon (*paḍimaṭṭhātī*), adopting the hero's posture (*vīrāsaṇie*) [and] adopting a seated posture (*ṇesajjite*). There are five further ascetic resolves, as follows: adopting the staff posture (*daṇḍāyatite*), lying in the shape of a club (*lagaṇḍasātī*), generating heat (*ātāvate*), remaining uncovered (*avāuḍate*) [and] not scratching (*akuṃḍuyate*).

3.2 *Pātañjalayogaśāstravivaraṇa* 2.46–8. *Āsana*:

"Together with the supernatural attainments, the rules and regulations have been taught. Now we shall teach posture and the other [auxiliaries of yoga]."* On [posture there is the *sūtra*]

(2.46) A steady and comfortable posture [. . .]

[i.e. the yogi's] posture [should be] steady and comfortable: one should practise a posture in which, for one who is stable in it, steadiness of the mind and limbs arises and there is no discomfort. As examples, names [of postures] made known in other texts, such as the lotus posture, are presented [in the *Pātañjalayogaśāstra* as follows]: the 'lotus' (*padmāsana*), 'hero' (*vīrāsana*), 'good fortune' (*bhadrāsana*), 'lucky mark' (*svastikāsana*),[28] 'stick' (*daṇḍāsana*), 'supported' (*sopāśraya*), 'couch' (*paryaṅka*), 'seated crane' (*krauñcaniṣadanaṃ*), 'seated elephant' (*hastiniṣadana*), 'seated camel' (*uṣṭraniṣadana*), 'symmetrical' (*samasaṃsthāna*), 'steadily serene' (*sthitaprasrabdhi*) and 'whatever is comfortable' (*yathāsukham*), etc.

On that subject (*tatra*): in a pure place such as a temple, a mountain cave or a sandbank in a river, not near fire or water, free from animals [and] clean, one should, in a state of purity, having duly sipped water, bow down before the Supreme Lord, the one ruler of the whole universe, and the venerable lords of yoga and one's own teachers, and then sit on a

* In this passage, we have marked the *bhāṣya* sections of the *Pātañjalayogaśāstra* with double quotation marks.

comfortable mat covered by cloth, an antelope hide and *kuśa* grass, and, facing east or north, adopt one or other posture from among these.

Of them, that called the lotus posture [is as follows]: One should pull the left foot towards oneself and place it on the right [thigh]. In the same way [one should put] the right [foot] on top of the left [thigh]. Keeping the pelvis, chest and neck steady, the gaze focused on the tip of the nose like someone dead or asleep, the mouth sealed like a casket, not touching the [upper] teeth with the [lower] teeth, with the chin and the chest a fist's width apart, the tip of the tongue placed at the front teeth [and] the hands in the tortoise-shell position (*kacchapaka*)[29] on the heels or joined together (*brahmāñjali*).[30] When one sits immediately in this position, without the effort of repeated specific positioning of the body and its parts, that is the lotus posture.

And all this is the same for the other postures, too, [but] they have some distinguishing characteristics.

Thus when one puts the right foot on top of the left [thigh] and the right hand on top of the left [hand] and sits like that, it is the 'good fortune' posture. The rest is the same [as the lotus posture].

Thus the 'hero' posture is when one of the legs is bent and the knee of the other leg is placed on the ground.

In each case only the distinguishing characteristics are being explained.

When one sits with the right toe made invisible by holding it between the left thigh and lower leg, and the left toe made invisible by holding it between the right thigh and lower leg, in such a way that the heels do not press the testicles, that is the 'lucky mark' posture.

When one sits like a staff, with the legs extended and the ankles, big toes and knees together, that is the 'stick' posture.

A 'supported' [posture] has a support such as a yoga belt or crutch.

The 'couch' posture is lying with the arms extended as far as the knees.

The 'seated crane', 'seated elephant' [and] 'seated camel' postures are to be understood from their similarity to the seated positions of the crane, etc.

The 'symmetrical [pose]' is when the thighs and lower legs are placed on the ground.

'Steadily serene'. 'Steadily serene' is [sitting] in any other way, having thought of it oneself. A posture in which one is free from exertion is also called 'steadily serene'.

And 'whatever is comfortable': that form in which the sitter is comfortable is 'whatever is comfortable'.

From the word 'etc.' must be understood any other posture taught by a teacher.

Now the method of mastering those postures is given:

> (2.47) [. . .] from the cessation of effort or the [meditative] attainment of infinity.

"[The word] 'arises' completes the sentence."

The addition [of the word 'arises'] gives the meaning 'a firmly established posture arises'. "[A posture] is perfected as a result of the cessation of effort" for the period after the posture has been adopted or from not making any effort [at all]. "By means of which the body does not tremble." 'By means of which' means by means of cessation of effort. Because effort makes the body tremble. The meaning is that one's posture becomes unmoving. "Alternatively, [a posture is perfected] when [the mind] has attained infinity." The universe is infinite; infinity is the state of being infinite. Having attained that, i.e. being all-pervasive, the mind, established in the state of being the universe, perfects, i.e. makes firm, the posture.

> (2.48) As a result of that there is no trouble from the pairs of opposites.

'As a result of that' means as a result of posture becoming steady. The following is understood as being an automatic consequence: "as a result of mastering posture, one is not troubled by pairs of opposites such as cold and heat".

3.3 *Niśvāsatattvasaṃhitā Nayasūtra* 4.11–17, 104–6. The earliest tantric teaching on *āsana*:[31]

The goddess said:

> (11) And how can there be meditation on Śiva, who is supportless? And how can one become Śiva when one already has the same essence as Him?

The Lord said:

> (12a–14b) The things which might be seen by the eye, spoken about, thought by the mind, discerned by the intellect, considered one's own by the ego or endowed

with form: wherever they are not to be found, there one should seek Śiva, in one's own body, whatever country or stage of life one is in.

(14c–15d) The lucky mark, lotus (*padmaka*), good fortune, half-moon (*ardhacandra*), extended (*prasārita*), supported (*sāpāśraya*), joined-hands (*añjalika*) and yoga belt (*yogapaṭṭa*) ([or one that is] comfortable): these eight principal postures have been proclaimed in brief.

(16–17) Focused and self-controlled, the user of mantras should assume one of these postures, worship Śiva with actions and thoughts, pay homage to the previous teachers of his tradition and continuously cultivate the absence [of external objects]. He should fix his thoughts in his head and turn his eyes upwards. [. . .]

(104–6) He should worship repeatedly the god of gods and the lord of obstacles, pay homage to the previous teachers of his tradition, engage in yoga and concentrate on meditation. He should assume the lotus pose or the lucky mark, good fortune, moon (*candra*), supported (*sāpāśraya*) or yoga-belt (*yogapaṭṭa*) pose, or sit in a comfortable posture. With his tongue at his palate, his teeth not touching, his body upright and his gaze on the [tip of] his nose, he who speaks the truth, does no harm and constantly practises yoga will achieve success.

3.4 *Vimānārcanākalpa* Chapter 96. The earliest teaching of a non-seated *āsana*:

There are nine varieties of yoga posture: the sacred (*brāhma*), lucky mark, lotus, cow's mouth (*gomukha*), lion (*siṃha*), the liberated (*mukta*), hero's, good fortune and peacock (*mayūra*) postures.

With the right foot on top and the left foot underneath, conceal the big toes behind the knees. Put the left hand in the lap and the right hand, palm upwards, on top of it. Keep the body straight and the gaze between the eyebrows. That is the sacred posture.

Place the ankles on either side of the perineal seam and position the rest of the body as before. That is the lucky-mark posture.

Place the soles of the feet on top of the thighs and the palms as before. That is the lotus posture.

Put the right knee on top of the left knee. That is the cow's-mouth [posture].[32]

As before, put the ankles on either side of the perineal seam, below the scrotum, extend the hands and put them on the knees [and] look at the tip of the nose with the mouth closed. This is the lion posture.[33]

Put the left ankle over the penis and the right over that. This is the posture of the liberated.

Put the right foot on the left thigh and the right thigh on the left foot. This is the hero's posture.

Put the heels to either side of the perineal seam, below the scrotum, and hold the feet with the hands. [This is] the blessed-good-fortune posture.[34]

Fix the palms of the hands on the floor, place the elbows on either side of the navel, raise the head and feet and remain in the air like a staff. This is the peacock posture.

It is recognized that of these postures the best are the sacred, the auspicious lucky mark and the lotus. The cow's mouth, the lion and the posture of the liberated are middling. The hero's pose, the good fortune and the peacock are the lowest.

3.5 Hemacandra's *Yogaśāstra* 4.124–34, with selected passages from the *Svopajñavṛtti* auto-commentary. Various seated and non-seated *āsanas*:

(124) The postures are the couch, hero's, thunderbolt (*vajrāsana*), lotus (*abjāsana*), good fortune, stick, squatting (*utkaṭikāsana*), milkman (*godohikāsana*) and casting-off-the-body (*kāyotsargāsana*).

To each of the words 'couch' and so forth the word 'posture' (*āsana*) is [to be] joined.

He explains the postures in sequence:

> (125) The couch pose is when the lower parts of the lower legs are placed on the feet and the hands are at the navel, palms upwards, with the right hand on top.

This is the *āsana* of the eternal ascetics and the blessed Mahāvīra at the time of liberation. In the same way that a couch is on feet, so is this couch [pose]. The followers of Patañjali say 'the couch [pose] is resting with the arms extended to the knees' (*Tattvavaiśāradī* 2.46).

> (126) The posture in which the left foot is placed on the right thigh and the right foot on the left thigh is known as the hero's pose. It is suitable for a hero.

This hero's pose is suitable for ford-makers (*tīrthakaras*) and other heroes, not for the timid. The placement of the upper hand is as in the couch pose. Some call this the lotus position. When just one foot is put on top of a thigh it is the half-lotus (*ardhapadmāsana*).

> (127) The thunderbolt pose is assumed when one sits in the hero's pose and, with both arms behind the back in the cross shape of a thunderbolt, holds the big toes of both feet.

Others call this the ghoul pose (*vetālāsana*).

> (128) Others say that the hero's pose is when one sits as if on a chair [*siṃhāsana*], [but] with the chair having been taken away.

When one sits on a chair with the feet[35] on the ground and the chair is taken away and one remains as one was, that is the hero's pose. The 'others' who say this are orthodox teachers (*saiddhāntikas*) who have taught it in the context of austerities which bring suffering to the body. The followers of Patañjali, on the other hand, say, 'The hero's pose is when one is supported on one foot placed on the ground, with the other above, its leg bent back at the knee' (*Tattvavaiśāradī* 2.46).

> (129) Yoga experts say it is the lotus position when the middle part of one lower leg touches the other.

> (130) The good fortune pose is when one makes the soles of the feet into a bowl shape in front of the testicles, and puts the hands on top of them in the shape of a tortoise shell.
>
> (131) When one sits down and extends both feet with the toes and ankles touching and the thighs touching the ground, it is called the stick pose.
>
> (132) They call it the squatting pose when the buttocks touch the heels. The milkman pose is when the heels are off the ground.

The glorious Lord [Mahā]vīra obtained perfect knowledge (*kevalajñāna*) in the squatting pose. It has been taught because it is used by those who undertake the intensive course of asceticism (*pratimākalpikas*) and others.

> (133) Remaining indifferent to the body while holding a standing or sitting position with both arms hanging down is called the casting-off-the-body [pose].

The casting-off-the-body [pose] of those who stand up is that of those who have taken vows such as that of a Jina (*jinakalpikādīnām*) and those who have nearly become ford-makers (*chadmasthatīrthakarāṇām*); they stay standing up straight. On the other hand, [the casting-off-the-body pose] of those who have taken the [lesser] vow of the elders (*sthavirakalpikānām*) is, by implication, undertaken either standing, sitting or lying down, according to one's capability. Casting off the body (*kāyotsarga*) [usually] means the casting off or abandonment of the body while it is engaged in an activity other than remaining still, meditating or observing silence.

Here, merely as examples, brief descriptions of other *āsana*s will be given.

The 'curved-like-a-mango' pose (*āmrakubjāsana*) is a posture that has the shape of a mango [and is] how Lord Mahāvīra, when he was observing the single-night vow, endured the twenty torments devised by the lowliest of deities, Saṅgamaka.

And there is the 'lying on one side [pose]' (*ekapārśvaśāyitva*), in which one may look upwards, downwards or sideways.

And the 'lying stretched out like a stick [pose]' (*daṇḍāyataśāyitva*) occurs when one holds the body straight with the legs extended and does not move.

And the 'lying like a club (*lagaṇḍa*)[36] [pose]' (*lagaṇḍaśāyitva*) occurs when one's head and heels are touching the ground, but [the rest of] one's body is not.

And the 'symmetrical [pose]' is when the two [feet] are contracted and the heels and toes are pressed together.

And the Duryodhana pose (*duryodhanāsana*) is when the head is on the ground and the legs are pointing upwards. It is also known as the skull technique (*kapālīkaraṇa*).

In that same [pose], when the thighs are as in the lotus position, it is [called] the stick-lotus position (*daṇḍapadmāsana*).

And in the lucky-mark pose the left [leg] is bent and the [left] foot put between the right lower leg and thigh, and the right [leg] is bent and [the foot] put between the left leg and thigh.

And the supported [pose] occurs when a yoga belt (*yogapaṭṭaka*) is used.

Postures such as the ways of sitting (*niṣadana*) of the crane (*krauñca*), goose (*haṃsa*), dog (*śva*), elephant (*hasti*) and eagle (*garuḍa*) are to be learnt by observing how such creatures sit. Thus how they are performed is not set out [here].

> (134) Whichever of these postures produces mental steadiness when adopted should be used to practise meditation.

3.6 *Vasiṣṭhasaṃhitā* 1.67–81. *Āsana*, including early teachings of non-seated postures:

> (67) I shall teach the postures. Listen carefully, son. [They are] the lucky mark, cow's mouth, lotus, hero's, lion, peacock, cock (*kukkuṭa*), turtle (*kūrma*), good fortune and the posture of the liberated. I will explain their characteristics one by one.
>
> (68) Place the soles of both feet directly between the calves and the thighs, and sit up straight. This is called the lucky-mark pose.
>
> (69) Put the ankles of both feet on either side of the perineal seam. This is a variant of the lucky-mark posture, and it destroys all sins.
>
> (70) Place the right ankle beside the left buttock, and the

left ankle beside the right buttock. This is called the cow's-mouth posture.

(71) Place the soles of the feet on the thighs, O chief of Brahmans, cross the hands and from behind take a firm hold of the big toes. This is the lotus posture. It is praised by everyone.

(72) Place one foot on one thigh, and the other foot under the other thigh. This is known as the hero's pose.

(73–5) Place the ankles under the scrotum on either side of the perineal seam, with the left ankle on the right, and the right ankle on the left. Place both hands on the knees and splay the fingers. Open up the mouth and gaze with deep concentration at the tip of the nose. This is the lion pose. It is for ever praised by yogis.

(76–7) Press the palms of both hands firmly on the ground and put the elbows on either side of the navel. Lift up the head and the feet, and remain in the air like a stick. This is indeed the peacock pose. It destroys all sins.

(78) In the lotus posture slide both hands between the calves and thighs, put them on the ground and lift the body into the air. This is the cock pose.

(79) Place the ankles under the scrotum on either side of the perineal seam. With both hands take a firm and very steady grip on the sides of the feet. This is the good-fortune pose. It destroys all diseases.

(80) Press the anus with both crossed ankles and meditate. Yoga experts know that this is the turtle pose.

(81) The left ankle is placed above the penis and the other heel is laid on top of it. This is known as the posture of the liberated.[37]

3.7 *Ḥawż al-ḥayāt* 4.2–9. The five pre-eminent postures:[38]

(2) Know that the body is like a waterskin filled with water and dirt. If you want to inflate it to make it float

on water, it will not have room enough for air, since it is full of both [water and dirt], so it prevents you from attaining the goal. The body is similar when it is full of water and food; it is unable to control any of these things. There is no doubt concerning [the need to] empty and cleanse the 'skin', which means squeezing it out delicately and gently, inasmuch as it is not to be torn apart. That [is to be accomplished by] the positions established by 'the folk' [i.e. the yogis], and there are eighty-four positions reliably transmitted by eighty-four men, who relate of each position its special characteristic and purpose. We shall mention in this book five of them, the use and knowledge of which are indispensable to the wayfarer.

(3) One needs at the beginning to fast, inclining even to excess, and at that time one performs one's practices in secluded places seen by no one. In the beginning of the striving (*mujahada*), one's powers are exhausted and the body is weakened, but do not worry about that, because the first period of striving is like summer and winter, and the end of it is like spring and fall.[39] One therefore sets obligatory times for oneself every day and night.

(4) The first position is for the strengthening of the nerves, the kidneys, the back, the digestion of food, and the extraction of cold humours concealed in the nerves and joints. One sits cross-legged, then places one's left foot with the lower leg on the right thigh, and similarly with the right [foot] on the left [thigh]; one strives gently and moderately until one is able to do it, and it becomes habitual, painless and effortless. This is difficult in the beginning, but once one is able to do it, one can gradually do all the positions. Then [one sits with] back erect and places the hands on the knees, supporting the upper arm and leaning forward, and one gazes at the navel while seated without moving. One is not diverted from this until he imagines that he is a tree firmly rooted in

the earth, and he says the word *alakh* (which means God, who is great and mighty) continually in the heart, not with the tongue. This is repeated in all of the positions. When one reaches this station, one attains the quality of 'little food, little speech and little sleep'.

(5) The second position is that one sits as described in the first [position] and puts the right hand on the nape of the neck, up to the left shoulder blade, and the left likewise on the right shoulder blade. And he sits upright and turns his head, along with his body, in the four directions, not merely turning his face, continually repeating in his heart the previously mentioned repetition [i.e. *alakh*]. When he wants to remain still, he places his hands on his knees and sits with upper arms supported. If he never forgets the chant in the heart, he may attain awareness. When he is [fully] present in his chanting, he witnesses something from the hidden world that brings him joy and delight and incites him to increase his effort. When he attains this station, he will be free from elephantiasis, leprosy, haemorrhoids and fever, which in the opinion of physicians are incurable diseases. He will [likewise] be free of [any] remaining cases of illness from his prior state. Whoever has any of these illnesses, and who practises this and persists in this, will be rid of it. This is well known and often experienced among them.

(6) The third position is that one sits as we have explained in the first [position] and inserts the hands between the lower leg and the thigh up to the elbows. He then extends the hands [to the ground] and holds himself up by the strength of the hands. He does not forget his previously mentioned chant. When he attains this station, the watery matter in him is reduced, and the fiery, airy and earthy matter are increased. This is the station intermediate between human and angel.

(7) The fourth position is that he sits as we have described in the first [position] and inserts the hands between the lower leg and the thigh, then leans forward and places

the hands on the nape of the neck, locking the fingers together, without interrupting the previously mentioned chant. When he attains this station, he will have no fear or dread of either jinn or humanity. If, for example, the sky were to fall upon the earth, he would not fear. This is indeed a mighty rank.

(8) The fifth position is that he first places his hands firmly on the earth, and he places the section between the big toe and the other toes of the right foot on the right elbow, and his left foot similarly on the left elbow. He holds himself up by the power of the hands and is especially [careful] not to interrupt his previously mentioned chant. As a special property in this state, when he attains this station, and he is so steady and experienced that he passes the entire night in this condition, he attains levitation and he becomes a member of the company of spirits.

(9) These five positions make the remaining ones superfluous.

3.8 *Haṭhapradīpikā* 1.17–18, 24–49, 53–6. The first teaching of non-seated postures as part of *haṭhayoga*:

(17) Posture, being the first auxiliary (*aṅga*) of *haṭha*, is taught first. It gives steadiness, good health and lightness of limb.

(18) I will describe some postures accepted by *muni*s such as Vasiṣṭha and yogis like Matsyendra.

(24) While in the cock pose, take the neck tightly in both hands and lie back like an upturned turtle. This is the upturned-turtle pose (*uttānakūrmaka*).

(25) Grasp the big toes with the hands and bring them all the way to the ears, as if one were drawing a bow. This is called the bow pose (*dhanurāsana*).

(26) Place the right foot at the root of the left thigh and the left foot by the outer side of the [right] knee. Taking hold of the [left] foot, twist the body. This is the pose taught by the glorious Matsyendra.

(27) Matsyendra's posture stokes the digestive fire and is a weapon that will destroy a whole array of terrible diseases. Through its practice Kuṇḍalinī is awakened and a man's moon [i.e. semen] becomes steady.

(28) Stretch the legs out on the ground like sticks, and grasp the toes with both hands. Place the forehead on the knees and remain in that position. This is called the back-stretch pose.

(29) This is the back-stretch pose, chief among postures, which sends the air along the rear channel. It stokes up the digestive fire, slims the belly and gives [people] good health.

(30) With both hands on the ground taking the weight of the body, and the elbows placed either side of the navel, lift the body up into the air like a stick. They call this the peacock pose.

(31) The splendid peacock posture rapidly takes away all diseases of the spleen and stomach, and overcomes imbalances of the humours. If one has eaten a lot of bad food, it burns it all away and it stokes up the digestive fire so that poison can be digested.

(32) The corpse pose (*śavāsana*) is when one lies supine on the ground like a corpse. The corpse pose takes away fatigue and relaxes the mind.

(33) Śiva taught eighty-four postures. I will describe four which are essential.

(34) The best four among them are the adept's pose (*siddhāsana*), the lotus position, the lion pose and the good-fortune pose. One should regularly sit in a comfortable adept's pose.

(35) Press one heel against the perineum, fix the other foot above the penis and firmly place the chin on the chest. Motionless and with the senses restrained, gaze unwaveringly between the eyebrows. Known as the adept's pose, this bursts open the door to liberation.

(36) The adept's pose can [also] be when the left ankle is placed above the penis and the other ankle is laid on top of it.

(37) This [version of] the adept's pose is known by some as the thunderbolt pose; others say it is the posture of the liberated, and still others call it the secret pose (*guptāsana*).

(38) The adepts know the adept's pose alone to be chief among all the *āsana*s, just as moderation in food is chief among the rules (*yama*s) and non-violence among the regulations (*niyama*s).

(39) Out of all the eighty-four postures, it is the adept's pose that one should regularly practise. It cleans out impurities from the 72,000 channels.

(40) The yogi who contemplates the self and eats sparingly for twelve years obtains perfection (*niṣpatti*) from regular practice of the adept's pose.

(41) With the adept's pose mastered, there is no need for lots of other postures. When the breath is carefully held in unaccompanied retention (*kevala kumbhaka*), the supramental state (*unmanī*) arises automatically, without any effort.

(42) When just this adept's pose is steady and perfect, the three locks (*bandha*s) happen automatically, without any effort.

(43) There is no pose like the adept's, no breath-retention (*kumbhaka)* like the unaccompanied (*kevala*), no *mudrā* like *khecarī*, and no method of dissolution (*laya*) like listening to the internal sounds (*nāda*).

(44) Place the right foot on the left thigh, and the left foot on the right thigh. Passing both hands around the back, firmly grasp the big toes. Place the chin on the chest and gaze at the tip of the nose. This is called the lotus position: it destroys diseases in those who restrain themselves.

(45–6) Carefully place the upturned feet on the thighs and the hands palm up in the lap. Fix the gaze on the tip of the nose and the tongue at the uvula. Rest the chin against the chest and gently draw the breath upwards.

(47) This is known as the lotus position. It destroys all diseases. It is hard for anyone to learn, but the wise can learn it here on earth.

(48) Cup the hands, assume a very rigid lotus position and firmly place the chin on the chest. By focusing the mind on the ultimate reality, repeatedly raising the lower breath (*apāna*) and sending the inhaled air downwards, a man gets unparalleled knowledge thanks to the power of the goddess (*śakti*).

(49) The yogi who sits in the lotus position and retains the air inhaled through the channels is liberated. In this there is no doubt.

(53) Place the ankles under the scrotum on either side of the perineal seam, with the left ankle on the left and the right ankle on the right.

(54–5) Take hold of the sides of the feet firmly and steadily with both hands. This is the good-fortune pose. It destroys all diseases. Some accomplished yogis call this Gorakṣa's pose (*gorakṣāsana*).

(56) When the master of yoga is comfortable in postures (*āsanas*) and locks (*bandhas*), he should practise purificatory techniques such as seals (*mudrās*) in order to cleanse the channels.

3.9 *Rtsa rlung gsang ba'i lde mig* ('The Secret Key to the Channels and Winds'). [The first section of] a chapter from Pema Lingpa's *Rdzogs chen kun bzang dgongs 'dus* (*Compendium of Enlightened Spontaneity*). The twenty-three positions of *'khrul 'khor*:[40]

Homage to Innate Enlightenment, Samantabhadra!

I, the Powerful Skull-Garlanded Lotus, have composed this 'Secret Key' to elucidate the [nature of the] Inner Winds in order to help practitioners to open their subtle energy channels, balance the three humours of wind, bile and phlegm, and ensure vibrant health.

In an isolated place free from disturbances, abide in the non-conceptual space of 'leaping over the skull' and generate boundless love and compassion for all beings.

Magical Movements [for Clearing Hindrances]:

First, expel the stale winds three times [from the two side channels]. Then rub the palms of the hands together and massage the left and right sides of your body.

Second, turn the feet outward and alternate turning them to the left and right.

Third, apply [sesame] oil [to the body] and shake.

Fourth, churn the abdomen three times to the left and three times to the right.

Fifth, as if pushing a thunderbolt (*vajra*), hold the breath [in the lower abdomen] and firmly press out both arms.

Sixth, like throwing a rock, fling the left and right arms outwards three times.

Seventh, rotate the wrists inwards and outwards three times each.

Eighth, while holding the breath [in the lower abdomen], rotate the entire body and the heart centre three times to the left and right and exclaim *Ha Ha*.

Ninth, with hands [crossed in front and] holding the upper arms, rotate to the left and right and then strike the heart centre.

Tenth, while holding the breath [in the lower abdomen], rotate the left and right shoulders in and out three times each [with the arms straight and the fists pressing against the thighs].

Eleventh, strongly strike the fists nine times against the navel.

Twelfth, join the palms at the heart centre and alternate striking the elbows against the sides of the ribs and then bang both [elbows against the body] simultaneously.

Thirteenth, interlacing your fingers, push against the back of the neck and rotate [the head] three times to the left and three times to the right.

Fourteenth, like drawing a bow, pull three times to the left and three times to the right and, while crossing the arms, strike the point of the shoulder.

Fifteenth, rotate the head and eyes three times to the right and three times to the left. Then stretch the head nine times to the back and front, and nine times from side to side. Then, shaking [the head] nine times, expel all stagnant air.

Sixteenth, the 'lion's frolic': seal the eyes with the two index fingers, block the ears with the two thumbs, block the nostrils with the middle fingers and, with the small and ring fingers, seal the lips. Rotate the head three times to the left and three times to the right. Then shake [the upper body] three times.

Seventeenth, while standing up, shake the legs to the back and front and from left to right. Turn the arms to the left and right and shake them to the front.

Eighteenth, bend forward and touch the hands to the ground. Standing up, repeat nine times.

Nineteenth, while standing up strike the heels [on the ground] then, rising up, jump. Then alternate shaking the arms and legs.

Twentieth, sit in [full lotus] *vajra* posture and lift up the body [with the hands pressing against the ground], then drop the body against the floor. Do this three times, shaking the body into wakefulness.

Twenty-first, while lying back, hold the breath [in the lower abdomen] and raise the body three times.

Twenty-second, bend forward and touch the forehead to the ground. Then, rolling back, touch the toes to the ground. Shake the body and utter a strong *Ha* three times.

Twenty-third, sit comfortably in the seven-point posture of Vairocana.

I, Pema [Padmasambhava], wrote down these twenty-three secret yogic movements. I pray to my heart son [Pema Lingpa] that they will be of benefit for all beings.

This completes the first section, the stage of *'khrul 'khor* [the yogic movements].

Samaya. Sealed! Sealed! Sealed!

3.10 *Baḥr al-ḥayāt* 4.6.7, 10, 17, 21, 24–5. Knowledge of the Heart and the Character of Discipline:[41]

(6) The word of recollection of *kahkī*. When the meditator wants to do this practice, he should sit in the *karbat* posture. *Karbat* is the expression for the sitting position of the turtle. The turtle has two manners of sitting. In the first, gathering the hand and foot and head to oneself, one sits in forgetfulness of oneself. Here the posture is not the goal; the goal is a uniform posture. With the left foot on one knee, and the sole of the left foot placed beneath the buttocks, one holds the right knee straight and attaches the toes of the left foot to the right heel, and places the right hand on the right knee and the left hand on the left knee. Then one goes from the right knee, saying *hī hī* to the left knee, but one doesn't bow the head. One tilts the shoulder blade a little and then straightens it. One does this firmly so the veins of the neck stand out, with the lips separated by a finger's breadth and the teeth tightly clenched. One inhales firmly from the breast and exhales firmly, until one departs from oneself and reaches the Real.

(7) The word of recollection of *nirañjan*. When the seeker wishes to perform this activity, he should learn the womb pose (*garbha āsana*). They call it the womb pose because when the child is in the womb of the mother it accomplishes it. One places the left foot on the right foot, holding the buttocks on both feet, holding the head evenly between the two knees, placing both elbows under the ribs, putting the hands over the ears, bringing the navel towards the spine. The breath of life that appears from the navel they call *nirañjan*, which is an expression for the undifferentiated. One holds the breath; one brings it in the midst of the belly. One takes it above from below,

and below from above, in this exercise to such a degree that the inner eye, winged imagination, wandering reflection and incomparable thought – all four – emerge from their restrictions. They enter witnessing of the spiritual state and become one.

(10) The word of recollection of *gorakhī*. If the wayfarer wants to purify his interior, with the recollections (*adhkār*) of the Jogis he performs the *gorakhī* practice with the posture of the lotus position, in this form. He brings the soles of both feet together, placing the tips of the feet beneath the genitals. He twists the hands behind the back and then meditates. He tilts the head slightly and agitates the body a little. Evenly, he holds the breadth of the tongue tightly to the teeth. From time to time he shuts his eyes. As soon as he forcefully exhales by the nostrils with complete effort, he inhales two such [breaths]. With difficulty he completes this and does it in succession. After dawn and after midday, the benefit of this activity will be revealed.

(17) The word of recollection of *tarāwat*. When one wishes to perform the *tarāwat* recollection, one sits cross-legged, entwining the fingers of both hands together and holding them over the shins. One inhales the breath upward; when the breath arrives near the palate, one exerts pressure upon it, in inhaling towards the base of the brain by way of the nostrils. One grasps the nose quickly with the thumb and forefinger, to make the air flow in the base of the brain. The hand was held out even as one holds it. One maintains this thought until the air is in the entire base of the brain. Whatever is in control of the head goes to the extremes. Unveiling both sublime and base is attained, and from this one obtains witnessing.

(21) The recollection of the *sahasa āsana*, for the strengthening of the foot, the veins, the shoulders, the back, the digestion of food and the drying out of hidden moistures that are in the chain of the body. One holds this position,

placing the right foot and shin on the left thigh and holding the left foot and shin on the right thigh, slowly and gently, until it becomes a habit, though it is difficult in the beginning. One holds the back straight and both hands under the knees, holding the arms straight, with the hair sticking to the body. Whoever arrives at this station has three qualities appear in him: little sleep, little food and little speech.

(24) The recollection of the thunderbolt pose. One sits cross-legged, just as has been recalled. One introduces both hands in between the shin and the thigh and bows down, placing both hands on the neck, so that the fingers of both hands are intertwined on the neck. One does not forget the recollection. When one reaches this station, one leaves fear of demons, jinn, fairies, humans and animals. If heaven fell on earth, it would not be a problem. This is a mighty rank.

(25) The recollection of the emptiness pose (*sun āsana*). First, one clenches both fists and places them on the earth, placing the toes of the right foot on the right elbow and the toes of the left foot on the left elbow. One performs the recollection. Whoever reaches this station becomes capable of flight and becomes one of the spiritual entities – and God knows best.

3.11 *Haṭharatnāvalī* 3.7–20 and selected verses from the rest of the chapter. The eighty-four postures:

(7–8) Śiva has taught eighty-four postures, having chosen them one by one from among the 8,400,000 types of living beings. I will describe the features of some of those eighty-four postures. Postures were taught by Śiva the primal lord (Ādinātha) and bring physical health and well-being.

(9–20) 1. Adept's, 2. good fortune, 3. thunderbolt, 4. lion, 5. craft (*śilpāsana*), four kinds of lotus position: 6. bound lotus (*bandha-padmāsana*), 7. hand lotus (*kara-padmāsana*), 8. cupped lotus (*samputita-padmāsana*),

9. pure lotus (*śuddha-padmāsana*), six kinds of peacock pose: 10. stick peacock (*daṇḍa-mayūrāsana*), 11. side peacock (*pārśva-mayūrāsana*), 12. natural peacock (*sahaja-mayūrāsana*), 13. bound peacock (*bandha-mayūrāsana*), 14. compact peacock (*piṇḍa-mayūrāsana*), 15. one-foot peacock (*eka-pāda-mayūrāsana*), 16. Bhairava (*bhairavāsana*), 17. burner of the god of love (*kāma-dahanāsana*), 18. hand-bowl (*pāṇi-pātrāsana*), 19. bow (*kārmukāsana*), 20. lucky mark, 21. cow's face (*go-mukhāsana*), 22. hero's, 23. frog (*maṇḍūka*), 24. monkey (*markaṭāsana*), 25. Matsyendra (*matsyendra*), 26. side Matsyendra (*pārśva-matsyendra*), 27. bound Matsyenda (*baddha-matsyendra*), 28. supportless (*nirālambana*), 29. moon (*candra*), 30. neck (?*kāṇṭhavaṃ*),[42] 31. one-foot (*eka-pādaka*), 32. lord of snakes (*phaṇīndra*), 33. back stretch, 34. lying-back stretch (*śayita-paścima-tāna*), 35. wonder-worker (*citra-karaṇī*), 36. yoga-sleep (*yoganidrā*), 37. shaking (*vidhūnana*), 38. foot-pressing (*pādapīḍana*), 39. swan (*haṃsa*), 40. stomach (*nābhi-tala*), 41. sky (*ākāśa*), 42. raised sole (*utpāda-tala*), 43. foot-at-the-navel (? *nābhi-lasita-pādaka*), 44. scorpion (*vṛścika*), 45. wheel (*cakra*), 46. jump (*utphāla*), 47. upturned turtle (*uttāna-kūrma*), 48. turtle, 49. bound turtle (*baddha-kūrma*), 50. crooked (*nārjavam*), 51. belly (*kabandha*), 52. Gorakṣa's pose, 53. thumb (*aṇguṣṭha*), 54. fist (*muṣṭika*), 55. graced by Brahmā (*brahma-prāsādita*), five kinds of cock: 56. five-crested cock (*pañca-cūli-kukkuṭa*), 57. one-footed cock (*eka-pādaka-kukkuṭa*), 58. summoned cock (? *ākārita-kukkuṭa*), 59. tied-crest cock (*bandha-cūlī-kukkuṭa*), 60. sideways cock (*pārśva-kukkuṭa*), 61. half-woman Śiva (*ardha-nārīśvara*), 62. heron (*baka*), 63. earth-bearer (*dharā-vaha*), 64. moonstone (*candra-kānta*), 65. shower of nectar (*sudhāsāra*), 66. tiger (*vyāghra*), 67. king (*rāja*), 68. Indrāṇī's pose (*indrāṇī*), 69. *śarabha*,[43] 70. jewel (*ratna*), 71. wonderful (*citra*), 72. bound bird (*baddha-pakṣī*), 73. Śiva's pose (*īśvara*), 74. multi-coloured lotus (*vicitra-nalina*), 75. beloved (*kānta*), 76. pure bird (*śuddha-pakṣī*), 77. mellifluous (*sumandraka*),

78. Caurańgi's pose (*caurańgī*), 79. crane (*krauñca*), 80. firm (*dṛḍha*), 81. bird (*khaga*), 82. Brahmā's pose (*brahma*), 83. snake-person (*nāga*), 84. corpse.

These together make the eighty-four postures. [. . .]

(44) The stick-peacock pose is when the peacock pose is practised like a stick. The side-peacock pose is when the peacock pose is practised on both sides.

(45) When the peacock pose is done in the lotus pose, it is called the bound-peacock pose.

(46) Stretch one foot out in front and make the other like a peacock. This is known as the compact peacock. It destroys all diseases.

(47) Extend one leg to the neck and stretch out the other. This makes the one-foot-peacock pose.

(49) Sitting comfortably in the good-fortune pose, invert both feet. When practised like this, it becomes the burner of the god of love (*kāma-dahana*).

(50) Carefully place both ankles on the navel and put the hands on them in the shape of a bowl. This is known as the hand-bowl pose.

(55) The frog pose is when both ankles press the buttocks, the knees are like a girdle and the hands are placed on the soles of the feet. It removes disorders of the legs.

(61) The wise [yogi] should make the hands into a lotus shape and lift up the face, supporting [it] on the elbows. This is the supportless pose.

(64) Place one leg on the neck and lift up the other like a stick. Cup the hands. This is called the one-foot pose.

(65) Wrap both legs around the neck, put the head in the hands and look upwards. The lord-of-snakes pose destroys all ills and constantly brings happiness.

(68) Lie down and stretch. This is the lying-back-stretch pose.

(69) In the lying-back-stretch pose, extend the arms and make the legs like sticks. This is the wonder-worker.

(70) Wrap the legs around the neck and lock the hands around the bottom. Lie down. This yoga-sleep pose brings happiness.

(71) Sitting on one heel, stretch out the other leg and take hold of its toes with that hand. Hold the other heel with the other hand. This is the shaking pose. Practise it on both sides.

(72) Stand on the sole of one foot, put the other on the bottom and take a firm hold of it, having wrapped both hands around the body. This is the foot-pressing pose. [. . .]

(75) Supporting the body with both hands on the ground, place the feet on the forehead and look up at the heels above the head. This is known as the scorpion pose.

3.12 From the life story of the ascetic Purāṇ Puri as dictated to Jonathan Duncan.[44] The eighteen *mudrā*s of Brahmā:

The beginning of Purāṇ Puri's account of his life as an ascetic in the second half of the eighteenth century:[45]

I then went to Prayāg [Allahabad] on the occasion of a *melā* or assembly held at that place; a great concourse of fakirs were assembled on that occasion; among whom I heard various discussions; as, that such-and-such *tapasyā* or devotional discipline had such-and-such peculiar advantages; and they described the eighteen penances, which are in the manner following:

1. *Ṭhāḍeśvarī* ('Lord of Standing'): standing upright during life and never sitting down.

2. *Ākāś Muni* ('Sky Sage'): fixing one's regards towards heaven and never looking down towards the earth.

3. *Med'ha-Muni* (? 'Sacrificial Sage'): keeping both hands fixed on the breast.

4. *Phersa-bahan* (?): keeping both hands extended horizontally.

5. *Dhūmrapāna* ('Smoking'): tying the feet with a cord to the branch of a tree or other high place and swinging with the head downwards with a fire underneath, the smoke of which is taken in at the mouth.

6. *Pātāl Muni* ('Underworld Sage'): looking always towards the earth, the reverse of *Ākāś Muni*.

7. *Muni* ('The Sage'): observing constant silence.

8. *Caurāsi Āsan* ('Eighty-four Postures'): different postures in sitting, such as continuing several hours with the feet on the neck or under the arms; after which the members are returned to their natural positions.

9. *Kapālī* ('The Skull'): placing a betel nut on the ground and standing with the head on the nut and the feet in the air.

10. *Pātālī* ('Of the Underworld'): burying oneself underground up to the breast with the head downwards, having from the middle of the body to the heels in the air, and in that situation to be engaged in the ceremony termed *jap* or silent repetition of the names of God.

11. *Ūrdhvabāhu* ('Arm-in-the-air'): having both arms forcibly raised up above the head and extended for ever in that position.

12. *Baiṭheśvarī* ('Lord of Sitting'): to preserve constantly a sitting posture, without ever rising or lying down.

13. *Nyāsa-dhyān* ('The Meditator'): to keep in the breath: this is necessary for those who become eminent in science. Such persons when they practise meditation as a devotional exercise, so confine their breath that there appears to be no respiration in the corporeal frame, whence they are elevated to beatific visions of the deity.

14. *Caurangī Āsan* ('Caurangi's Pose'): to sit down many hours on the knees, bringing the right foot over the left shoulder, and the left over the right, with the arms in like manner over the back, so as to hold the toes of the feet on both sides in the hands.

15. *Paramahaṃsa* ('Ultimate Ascetic'): to go naked and not to hold conversation or connection with any person whatsoever. If any person brings you food, you are to receive and eat it, or otherwise to remain immersed in contemplation on the divinity, and not stand in awe of any one.

16. *Pañca Agni* ('Five Fires'): to be immersed in smoke from fire on all sides, and having, fifthly, the sun above; thus to live naked and to remain fixed in meditation on the deity.

17. *Tribhaṅgī* ('With Three Bends'): standing always on one foot.

18. *Sūrya Bhāratī* ('Sun Saint'): he who eats only after seeing the sun.

Of these eighteen kinds of devotional discipline, I chose that of the *Ūrdhvabāhu*, on entering into which it is necessary to be very abstemious in eating and sleeping for one year, and to keep the mind fixed, that is, to be patient and resigned to the will of the deity. For one year great pain is endured, but during the second less, and habit reconciles the party; the pain diminishes in the third year; after which no kind of uneasiness is felt. These are the eighteen *mudrā*s or ways of Brahmā, whose sons have performed them, and various other penances. As to the fruits or consequences, God alone is thoroughly acquainted therewith; what can I, an ignorant mortal, know, so as to describe what benefits each penance has already produced or what rewards will be obtained by those who may hereafter undertake them?

3.13 *Haṭhatattvakaumudī* Chapter 9. Dynamic movements in preparation for breath-control:

(1–6) Sit in the adept's or lucky-mark poses, put the hands on the thighs, keep the spine upright and straight, and bend the neck downwards and to the side, so that it brushes the shoulders. Bend the neck and make it gently touch the throat, as in *jālandharabandha*, then repeatedly move it forcefully and firmly to the right side. Move it fifty times on the right side and then the same on the left. Move the neck in such a way that the region from the navel, chest, back, waist and stomach moves. This is called the movement of Mount Meru (*meru-cāla*[*na*]). It removes air in the waist and back, destroys phlegm in the throat, cures problems of wind in the stomach and chest, and completely gets rid of diseases of phlegm (*kapha*). It straightens the central channel (*suṣumnā*), stimulates Kuṇḍalinī and loosens all the channels. One should practise it until one is tired.

That is the stimulation of Mount Meru, [to be performed] when beginning breath-control (*prāṇāyāma*). Now the wheel lock (*cakrī-bandha*):

(7–9) First stretch out both legs straight and flat along the ground, +then gently place the hands halfway down the thigh of each leg+ and, lying back, raise both feet and quickly take them backwards above the head, over and over again. Raise the bottom high with the hands and rapidly move it [?] in a circle. Practise this repeatedly every day until tired. It is the lock (*bandha*) called the wheel (*cakrī*) and it gets rid of all diseases. The wheel lock (*cakrī-bandha*) stimulates Kuṇḍalinī, stretches the midriff, fans the digestive fire, loosens all the channels (*nāḍīs*) and gets rid of problems such as constipation, indigestion and intestinal pain.

That is the wheel lock (*cakrī-bandha*). Now the practice of stretching (*tāna*).

(10) Seated in the easy posture (*sukhāsana*) with the hands joined together on the lower part of the stomach, gaze at the navel and repeatedly stretch the region five fingers above the navel and below the heart.

(11) By doing this while carefully and constantly holding the back, neck and head straight, the breath soon enters the rear pathway, and the bulb (*kanda*) and the goddess [Kuṇḍalinī] move.

(12) Alternatively the wise yogi should every day repeatedly practise stretching solely in the region of the navel. This stimulates the bulb (*kanda*) of the sage.

That is the practice of stretching (*tāna*). Now the *cāraṇā*[46] exercise. The following is said in the *Siddhāntaśekhara*:

(13) A *cāraṇā* is a rotation of a limb in both directions. There are ten principal *cāraṇā*s. Others are considered lesser by the wise.

(14) The ten [main] *cāraṇā*s are considered to be those of the head, stomach, arms, legs, thighs and knees.

(15) Of the lesser *cāraṇā*s the most important are those of the wrists, feet, fingers and other joints in the body.

(16) The wise man should meditate on dancing Śiva +and touch the chest+ when he practises *cāraṇā*.

(17) The lesser *cāraṇā*s should be performed in this way fifty or twenty-five times [a day] for three months.

(18) The yogi should practise *āsana*s thus. His channels are purified, he becomes strong, diseases are cured and his breath and fire are awakened.

(19) He loses weight, his lifespan increases and he overcomes untimely death. These and other benefits arise from regular practice of *cāraṇā*.

That is *cāraṇā*.

3.14 Selections from the *Haṭhābhyāsapaddhati*. Dynamic *āsana*s:

(1) Lie down on the back, bind the neck with the fingers, put the elbows together and, keeping the bottom in contact with the ground, stretch out each of the feet in turn, while rotating the other clockwise and anticlockwise. This is the bull kick (*vṛṣapādakṣepa*).

(6) Lie like a corpse, put the knees together and bring them to the navel. Hold the neck with the hands and rotate the knees. This is the lying-on-the-back-like-a-dog pose (*śvottānāsana*).

(21) Lie down on the back, place the knees on the chest, wrap the arms around the joined lower and upper legs and rock to the left and right. This is the millstone pose (*dṛṣadāsana*).

(22) Lie down on the back. Pass the feet over the head and put them on the ground. Lie face down. Roll on to the side and then repeat the process over and over again. This is the rolling pose (*luṭhanāsana*).

(23) Lie face down. Keeping the navel on the ground, rest the arms on the ground like pillars, purse the lips and hold the position, whistling like a flute. This is the lizard pose (*saraṭāsana*).

(24) Lie face down. Move the elbows up to the sides, rest the palms on the ground and lift the body over and over again. This is the fish pose (*matsyāsana*).

(25) Lie face down. Put the toes pointing downwards on the ground, plant the palms of the hands at the crown of the head, raise the bottom and look at the navel. Bring the nose to the ground and take it up to the hands. Do this over and over again. This is the elephant pose (*gajāsana*).

(26) Assume the elephant pose. Repeatedly put the head on the right and then the left side of the abdomen. This is the hyena pose (*tarakṣvāsana*).

(27) Assume the elephant pose after bending each leg in turn. This is the bear pose (*ṛkṣāsana*).

(28) In the elephant pose bend both knees over and over again. This is the rabbit pose (*śaśāsana*).

(29) In the elephant pose rotate each leg in turn in front of the body. This is the chariot pose (*rathāsana*).

(30) In the elephant pose strike each arm in turn on the ground. This is the ram pose (*meṣāsana*).

(31) In the elephant pose put both feet in the air and touch the ground with the head. This is the goat pose (*ajāsana*). [. . .]

(37) Put the palms of the hands on the ground and kick the soles of the feet upwards, then fall on to the ground. Do the same action over and over again. This is flying-upwards-like-a-cock (*kukkuṭṭoḍḍāna*). [. . .]

(43) Plant the palms on the ground and, pointing the feet upwards, dance on the palms. This is the inverted dance (*viparītanṛtya*). [. . .]

(64) Intertwine the fingers of the hands, pass the entire body between the arms and remain in the resulting position. This is body-wringing (*aṅgamoṭana*).

(67) Put the soles of the feet in the palms of the hands and stand and walk about. This is the sandals pose (*pādukāsana*). [. . .]

(81) Place a foot on the neck and stand up. This is the three-steps[-of-Viṣṇu]-pose (*trivikramāsana*).

(82) Stand up and sit down repeatedly. This is repeated standing (*utthānotthāna*).

(83) Standing three handwidths[47] away from a wall, touch it with the chest, push the chest out and then touch it again. This is the embrace pose (*āliṅgāsana*).

(84) Stand while hugging one knee to the chest. This is the child embrace (*bālāliṅgana*).

(85) Hold the scrotum and penis tightly between the thighs and stand on tiptoes. This is the loincloth pose (*kaupīnāsana*).

(86) Join the hands, put both feet inside them and then take them out and in by jumping. This is jumping-across-the-threshold (*dehalyullaṅghanaṃ*).

(87) Jump up and kick the bottom with the heels. This is the deer posture (*hariṇāsana*).

(88) Stand up straight, raise the arms and jump repeatedly. This is the pestle pose (*musalāsana*).

(89) Stretch out one leg like a stick and hold its foot with one hand. Keep the sole of the other foot on the ground

and spin around quickly. This is the Pole Star pose (*dhruvāsana*).

(90) Extend the arms and spin around. This is the potter's-wheel pose (*kulālacakrāsana*). [. . .]

The rope poses.

(94) Hold a rope with both hands, pass both feet together between them and over the head, and put them on the ground. Repeat. This is the cockroach pose (*paroṣṇyāsana*).

(95) Support the abdominal region with a rope and hold the body rigid like a stick. This is the stick pose.[48]

(96) Place the buttocks on a rope and be rigid like a stick. This is the weight pose (*bhārāsana*).

(97) Hold a rope with both hands and climb upwards. This is the Nārada pose (*nāradāsana*).

(98) Assume the lotus pose, take a rope in both hands and climb it. This is the heaven pose (*svargāsana*).

(99) Assume the cock pose, take a rope in both hands and climb it. This is the spider pose (*ūrṇanābhyāsana*).

(100) Hold a rope in both fists and place the soles of both feet on top of them. This is the parrot pose (*śukāsana*).

(101) Holding the upper part of a rope with the two big toes and the lower part with the hands, climb it. This is the centipede pose (*tṛṇajalūkāsana*).[49]

(102) Hold a rope in one fist and climb it. This is the caterpillar pose (*vṛntāsana*).

(103) Pass each fist between a thigh and knee, and hold a rope in either hand. Carry a weight with the teeth and climb up. This is the crane pose (*krauñcāsana*).

FOUR
Breath-control

Breath-control (Sanskrit *prāṇāyāma*) has been central to the practice of yoga since the earliest descriptions of yogic techniques. The Buddha practised extended breath-retention (4.3); *prāṇāyāma* is mentioned by name as one of two types of *dhyāna* ('meditation') in the *Mokṣadharma* of the *Mahābhārata* (8.3.5);[1] it is one of the eight auxiliaries of yoga of the *Pātañjalayogaśāstra* (1.4.3); it is included in all tantric six-auxiliary yoga systems (see 1.4.6–7); and when in the fifth century CE India's finest poet Kālidāsa described Śiva in meditation, he devoted a verse to his mastery of breath-control (4.8).

Today, the physical practice of yoga is popularly identified with bodily postures, but in pre-modern India it was breath-control that was the defining practice of physical yoga. Thus, the *Amaraughaprabodha* defines *haṭha*, the yoga method in which difficult physical techniques predominate, as 'addiction to stopping the breath',[2] and the *Haṭhapradīpikā* (2.75) says that it is through breath-retention that *haṭha* is mastered. Furthermore, a wide range of texts teach that breath-control's efficacy is such that it can accomplish all the auxiliaries of yoga. The *Mṛgendratantra*, for example, says that fixation is achieved by twelve rounds of holding the breath, meditation by twelve fixations, and *samādhi* by twelve meditations (4.11; see also Chapter 8).[3] Elsewhere, breath-control is said to bestow liberation directly upon the yogi (e.g. *Gorakṣaśataka* 4.16; *Jogpradīpakā* 4.23).

But breath-control is not seen as an easy way to master yoga. Indeed, it is often equated with *tapas*, ascetic practice. In critiques of yoga, breath-control is singled out because of its difficulty and danger. The tenth- to eleventh-century Śaiva scholar Abhinavagupta taught that breath-control should not be practised insofar as it harms the body,[4] and his disciple Kṣemarāja advocated an easy method to realization, which is easy by virtue of not including breath-control (or seals or locks).[5] In his *Yogaśāstra* (6.2) Hemacandra dismisses mastery of the breath by means of painful methods,[6] because it alone cannot bring about liberation.[7] The wording of these criticisms suggests that the target for these scholars was the still unformalized *haṭhayoga*; the *haṭha* texts that were subsequently composed themselves teach that breath-control is dangerous and must be practised carefully or will harm the yogi (*Vivekamārtaṇḍa* 99–102). Similarly, in his commentary on the *Mṛgendratantra* – one of the many Śaiva works that does teach breath-control – Nārāyaṇakaṇṭha warns that excessive practice of it may lead to abdominal swelling, prolapse, laboured breathing, insanity and epilepsy (1.4.8).[8]

Early References to Breath-control

The word *prāṇāyāma* is a compound of *prāṇa* ('life-breath') and *āyāma* ('control').[9] In the many typologies of the breaths found in Sanskrit texts *prāṇa* is both the first breath and a generic name for all the breaths (on which, see Chapter 5). Other breaths have specific bodily functions, but *prāṇa* sustains life and is sometimes equated with *jīva*, the vital principle.

Prāṇa as life-breath is mentioned from the beginning of India's literary record. Within the Vedic sacrificial tradition it is often one among other elements of the sacrifice.[10] The three older Vedas and the older Upaniṣads make no mention of controlling *prāṇa*, but the *Atharva Veda* (4.1) appears to prescribe the joining together of two breaths in order to attain immortality and the *Jaiminīya Upaniṣad Brāhmaṇa* (3.3.1) includes an instruction not to breathe during the recitation of the Gāyatrī chant (with no indication of its purpose). These two brief and obscure early references to breath-control may be forerunners of the two traditions of *prāṇāyāma* practice which subsequently developed. In one, that of the *Atharva Veda*, the union and sublimation of breaths leads to mystical ends; in the other, that of the *Jaiminīya Upaniṣad Brāhmaṇa*, holding the breath is an ascetic practice, often associated with the internal repetition of sacred formulas.[11]

In a list of the breaths of the Vrātya, a nebulous figure on the fringes of Vedic society, the *Atharva Veda* gives a typology of seven *prāṇa*s ('upward breaths'), together with seven *apāna*s ('downward breaths') and seven *vyāna*s ('pervasive breaths') (4.1). The breaths are identified with aspects of the cosmos and its temporal cycles, and the entry of the seasons (which are the fifth pervasive breath) into the sun (the fourth upward breath), for the full moon (the first downward breath) and new moon (the third downward breath) is said to lead to immortality. An echo of this is found in much later tantric and haṭhayogic descriptions of yoga as the union of the sun and moon, in which the upward-moving breath (*prāṇa*) is the moon and the downward-moving breath (*apāna*) is the sun.[12]

Breath-control as Expiation and Purification

Directly positive benefits of breath-control are not taught in subsequent texts until those of the tantric corpus; in textual descriptions in the intervening centuries *prāṇāyāma* is an expiatory or purificatory technique. Thus the *Dharmasūtra*s and later texts on *dharma* prescribe *prāṇāyāma* as a method of expiation (*prāyaścitta*) for a variety of wrongdoings;[13] a similar prescription is found in the *Pāśupatasūtra* (4.7; Kauṇḍinya's commentary adds that it brings about meditation). This expiatory capacity of breath-control is connected with its identification as a means of cultivating *tapas*, the inner heat generated by ascetic practice. When the Buddha tried breath-control (before ultimately dismissing it as futile) he said that it was as painful as if his head were being squeezed, his stomach stabbed and his body roasted over hot coals (4.3). In a passage echoed in several subsequent texts, the *Baudhāyanadharmasūtra* says that *prāṇāyāma* is the best *tapas* (4.4), as does an unidentified quotation in Patañjali's *Yogaśāstra* (4.6). In addition to expiation, *tapas* may bring about purification, and both these passages which identify *prāṇāyāma* as *tapas* also say that it purifies the yogi.[14] In the *Dharmasūtra*s breath-control is taught as one of various purificatory rituals in a Brahman's daily worship[15] (where specified, it is said that the breath is to be held for as long as possible or until exhaustion).[16]

The *Mānavadharmaśāstra* expands upon these notions, saying that *prāṇāyāma* burns up faults in the sense organs, and adds, in a verse that is found in several other texts,[17] that other auxiliaries of yoga, namely fixation, withdrawal and meditation, burn up sins, attachment to the senses, and base qualities respectively (**4.5**).

It is this understanding of *prāṇāyāma* as purificatory that is most prominent in texts dedicated to expounding yoga. Breath-control may be able to bring about yoga's highest aims, but in its basic form it is a preliminary, purificatory technique. Thus in tantric texts three rounds of *prāṇāyāma* are often prescribed before ritual in order to purify the body.[18] More specifically, *prāṇāyāma* is said to bring about *nāḍīśuddhi* ('purification of the channels'). This is first stated in the *Niśvāsatattvasaṃhitā Nayasūtra* (**4.9**) and is taught in several subsequent tantric works.[19] In *haṭhayoga* texts purification of the channels is the primary aim of the simple method of *prāṇāyāma* (in contrast with the more *siddhi*- and liberation-oriented *kumbhaka*s or 'breath-retentions', on which see below, p. 132). In Hemacandra's *Yogaśāstra*, *prāṇāyāma* is said to be for acquiring good health, because it purifies the channels, and for knowing the time of death (**4.14**).[20]

Simple *Prāṇāyāma*

In the *Dattātreyayogaśāstra* the procedure for the practice of *prāṇāyāma* is as follows (see **4.15**). The yogi assumes a steady posture and inhales[21] through the left nostril. He holds his breath for as long as possible, then exhales through the right nostril, before inhaling again through the right nostril, holding the breath and exhaling through the left nostril. He should perform twenty repetitions of this procedure four times a day. After three months the channels will be purified and physical indications of progress will appear: perspiration, trembling and, in the higher stages, levitation. In the *Vasiṣṭhasaṃhitā* a similar method is taught, but the breath is not to be held after inhalation and six repetitions of the cycle are to be performed three times a day (see **5.1.9**).

Equivalent procedures are taught in earlier tantric works and other haṭhayogic texts. Some texts also teach breath-retention after exhalation,[22] and there is considerable variety in prescriptions of the duration of inhalation, retention and exhalation, the ratios between them and the number of repetitions.[23] Many texts teach a threefold hierarchy of breath-control based on the duration of its elements (e.g. the *Pātañjalayogaśāstra* (4.6), *Dattātreyayogaśāstra* (4.15) and *Jogpradīpakā* (4.23)).[24]

'Accompanied' and 'Unaccompanied' Breath-retention

Once the channels are purified, the yogi is qualified to practise more advanced breath-control techniques. In the *Dattātreyayogaśāstra* the only advanced technique is spontaneously retaining the breath for as long as one wishes, with no regard for inhalation or exhalation. This practice, which is called *kevala kumbhaka* ('unaccompanied breath-retention'), echoes the 'stopped' (*stambhavṛtti*) *prāṇāyāma* of the *Pātañjalayogaśāstra* (4.6). *Kevala kumbhaka* produces a variety of supernatural capabilities; indeed, the *Dattātreyayogaśāstra* says that it can enable the yogi to do whatever he wants. In the *Vasiṣṭhasaṃhitā*, purification of the channels qualifies the yogi to practise breath-control, accompanied by meditation on the syllable *oṃ* (7.6) and a pure breath-retention similar to that taught in the *Dattātreyayogaśāstra*. While this is the extent of the teachings specifically on *prāṇāyāma* in these two texts, all the subsequent practices in their yogas involve holding the breath, often in particular locations in the body.

In later *haṭha* texts, pure breath-retention remains the ultimate breath practice, but its preliminary practice, which is called *sahita kumbhaka* ('accompanied breath-retention') because it is accompanied by inhalation and exhalation, is developed considerably. In the *Gorakṣaśataka* there are four *sahita kumbhaka*s (4.16) and the *Haṭhapradīpikā* adds four more (4.20). These techniques, although classified as *kumbhaka*s ('breath-retentions'), are in fact distinguished by their methods of inhalation and/or exhalation. Thus in *bhrāmarī kumbhaka*, for example, the yogi is to make the sound of a bee while breathing in and out. The benefits of these techniques are predominantly physical. The *sūryā kumbhaka*, for example, in which the yogi inhales through the right nostril and exhales through the left, alleviates imbalances in the wind humour (*vāta*). Others, however, act upon the structures and processes of the yogic body (see Chapter 5). Thus *bhastrī kumbhaka*, which involves forceful exhalation, is said to awaken Kuṇḍalinī and pierce the three knots along the central channel, and the *Haṭhapradīpikā* says that practising the various *kumbhaka*s will make the breath enter the central channel (**4.20**). The yogi is often instructed to apply certain locks (*bandha*s) while holding the breath; these, as well as some of the haṭhayogic seals (*mudrā*s), assist the yogi in steadying the breath and making it enter and rise up the central channel (see Chapter 6).[25]

Prāṇāyāma for Liberation

The *Pātañjalayogaśāstra*, Kauṇḍinya's *Pañcārthabhāṣya* on the *Pāśupatasūtra*, and several tantric texts,[26] together with the *Viveka-mārtāṇḍa* (but no other *haṭhayoga* works), teach that holding the breath results in *udghāta* or 'eruption' (see **4.6**, **4.7**, **4.9**, **4.11**).[27] The precise meaning of this term varies from text to text. Bhojarāja, in his eleventh-century commentary on the *Pātañjalayogaśāstra*, defines *udghāta* as 'the wind's striking the head when it has been propelled upwards from its source in the navel'.[28] Analysing *udghāta* in Śaiva texts, Vasudeva writes: 'To summarize, *udghāta* appears to be the yogic term for the sensation of a spontaneous upward surge of vital energy brought on in the early stages of self-induced asphyx-iation.'[29] An *udghāta* (or a series of *udghāta*s) can pierce the *granthi*s ('knots') along the central channel, and in the *Svacchandatantra* (5.54ff.) this enables the yogi to become Śiva.[30]

These notions of *udghāta* and its results, as well as the rather more elliptic teaching from the *Atharva Veda*, provide evidence for the positive benefits of breath-control beyond the purificatory and preparatory. Likewise, *prāṇāyāma* can also steady the mind. This is predicated on the notion that the mind and breath are inextric-ably linked. This connection, which is first taught in the *Chāndogya Upaniṣad* (**4.2**), appears to underpin teachings in the *Pātañjala-yogaśāstra* and tantric texts (e.g. the *Mataṅgapārameśvara Yogapāda* 2.10c–11d (**4.12**), Hemacandra's *Yogaśāstra* 5.2–3 (**4.14**) and *Gorakṣaśataka* 9 (**4.16**)).[31] Controlling the mind by controlling the breath is said to lead directly to liberation (Hemacandra's

Yogaśāstra 5.3 (4.14); *Gorakṣaśataka* 10 (4.16); *Yogabīja* 87 (4.18); *Jogpradīpakā* 412 (4.23)).

In its section on yogic powers, the *Pātañjalayogaśāstra* says that *jaya* ('conquest') of the *udāna* breath allows the yogi to perform *utkrānti* ('yogic suicide'), which leads to final liberation (3.39). In tantric texts *prāṇāyāma* is said to lead to – or be equated with – *prāṇajaya* ('conquest of the breath'), which is sometimes used as a synonym for *nāḍīśuddhi* ('purification of the channels').[32] Once the breath is conquered, the yogi can move it to wherever he wants in his body.[33] In a broad range of texts from different traditions, this ability is said to enable the yogi to accomplish multifarious aims, including several of the other auxiliaries of yoga. Thus, by moving the breath through the eighteen vital points (*marmans*), the yogi masters withdrawal (*Vimānārcanākalpa*, 5.1.6). Or by fixing it at certain points and simultaneously practising a particular meditation, he masters fixation (*Niśvāsatattvasaṃhitā Nayasūtra* 4.99–118 (4.9); on fixation, see Chapter 8).[34] The master of breath-control may also unite the different breaths found in the body. In particular, many texts of the tantric and haṭhayogic traditions teach that the yogi should join *prāṇa* ('the upper breath') and *apāna* ('the lower breath'), and then make them move up the central channel to the head, where the yogi attains his goal (e.g. *Niśvāsatattvasaṃhitā Uttarasūtra* (5.1.3), *Vivekamārtaṇḍa* (5.1.11); cf. *Lallāvākyāni* (4.17)). *Utkrānti* or 'yogic suicide' is accomplished by moving the breath to the head and then making it exit the body through the top of the skull.[35] *Utkrānti* is often taught together with *parakāyapraveśa* ('entering another's body'), in order to perform which the yogi projects his breath outside of his body and into a corpse.[36]

Prāṇāyāma with Mantra-repetition

In many systems breath-control is to be accompanied by internal mantra-repetition. Such breath-control is commonly denoted as *sagarbha* ('full')[37] in contrast with breath-control without mantra-repetition, which is *agarbha* ('empty'). The notion of *sagarbha prāṇāyāma* can be traced back to some of the earliest teachings on *prāṇāyāma*, such as that from the *Jaiminīya Upaniṣad Brāhmaṇa*, described above, in which the recitation of Vedic mantras is to be accompanied by breath-control. This continuity is clear in, for example, the *Īśvaragītā*, which, in its definition of *sagarbha prāṇāyāma*, quotes, without attribution, the *Baudhāyanadharmasūtra*'s definition of *prāṇāyāma* as the recitation of Vedic mantras while the breath is controlled (4.4). The same verse is quoted, with attribution, in the *Haṭharatnāvalī* (3.96). In some texts, such as the *Mṛgendratantra* (4.11) and the *Vāyavīyasaṃhitā* of the *Śivapurāṇa* (37.33–4), *sagarbha prāṇāyāma* also includes visualization. The *sagarbha prāṇāyāma* is superior to its *agarbha* form; the *Kiraṇatantra*, for example, says it is one hundred times better (15.34). In the yoga systems of tantric works, such as the *Mṛgendratantra* and *Kiraṇatantra*, tantric rather than Vedic mantras are to be used. With some exceptions, haṭhayogic texts do not teach the use of complex Vedic or tantric mantras in *prāṇāyāma*; most commonly it is the syllable *oṃ* that is to be internally repeated (e.g. *Vasiṣṭhasaṃhitā* (7.6)). The haṭhayogic texts are somewhat ambivalent towards mantra and, developing an earlier tantric practice, many of them teach the Ajapā Gāyatrī, a yogic appropriation of Vedic mantra-repetition in which the mere act of breathing is said to be an involuntary chanting of the *haṃsa* form of the famous Vedic Gāyatrī mantra (on mantra, see Chapter 7).

Prāṇāyāma has remained a key element of yoga practice since the earliest descriptions of yoga practices. In 1318 CE, when the poet Amir Khusraw praised the supernatural attainments of Indian ascetics in his Persian *Nuh sipihr*, he emphasized the yogis' mastery of breath-control.[38] Muslim interest in yoga grew rapidly and texts on its practices (often reworked to fit an Islamic context) were composed in Arabic and Persian. These texts give extensive treatments of *prāṇāyāma*. Here we reproduce the chapter on *prāṇāyāma* found in the fifteenth-century Arabic *Ḥawż al-ḥayāt*. Despite *prāṇāyāma*'s continuing importance in yoga practice, textual descriptions of its techniques did not proliferate over the sixteenth to nineteenth century in the same way as those of *āsana* and *mudrā*: the number of *kumbhaka*s taught in *haṭha* texts remained fixed at eight.[39] In the nineteenth century the arrival of printing techniques made *prāṇāyāma* practices available to the general public in an unprecedented way; a situation which, as Nile

Green (2008) has argued, transformed the role of breathing practice by reinscribing it within the political-colonial context of modern India.

Chapter Contents

4.1 *Atharva Veda* 15.16–18. The breaths of the Vrātya.

4.2 *Chāndogya Upaniṣad* 6.8.2. The connection between the breath and the mind.

4.3 *Mahāsaccakasutta* (*Majjhimanikāya* I, Book 9, abridged). Non-breathing meditation.

4.4 *Baudhāyanadharmasūtra* 4.1.22–4, 28–30. Purificatory breath-control.

4.5 *Mānavadharmaśāstra* 6.69–72. Purificatory breath-control.

4.6 *Pātañjalayogaśāstra* 2.49–53. Breath-control.

4.7 *Pañcārthabhāṣya* on *Pāśupatasūtra* 1.16. Purificatory breath-control.

4.8 *Kumārasambhava* 3.44–50. Śiva in meditation.

4.9 *Niśvāsatattvasaṃhitā Nayasūtra* 4.109c–118d. The four types of breath-control.

4.10 *Parākhyatantra* 14.13c–15b. Breath-control and fixation.

4.11 *Mṛgendratantra Yogapāda* 4, 12a–24b, 27c–30b, 33c–36b, 44c–51b, with selections from the *vṛtti* of Bhaṭṭa Nārāyaṇakaṇṭha. Breath-extension.

4.12 *Mataṅgapārameśvara Yogapāda* 2.10c–11d. Breath-control.

4.13 *Īśvaragītā* 11.30–37. Breath-control with and without mantra-repetition.

4.14 Hemacandra's *Yogaśāstra* 5.1–35, with selections from the *Svopajñavṛtti* auto-commentary. Breath-control.

4.15 *Dattātreyayogaśāstra* 54ab, 58c–69d, 72c–83d. Accompanied and unaccompanied breath-control.

4.16 *Gorakṣaśataka* 8–10, 28c–49b. The four breath-retentions.

4.17 *Lallāvākyāni* 4, 56–7. Knowledge through breath-control.

4.18 *Yogabīja* 76–77, 80–86. *Prāṇa* and *apāna*.

4.19 *Ḥawż al-ḥayāt* Chapter 5. The breath and its control.

4.20 *Haṭhapradīpikā* 2.37–43, 54–6, 68–70. Breath-control and the four additional breath-retentions.

4.21 *Gheraṇḍasaṃhitā* 5.47–57. Seeded and unseeded breath-control.

4.22 *Gheraṇḍasaṃhitā* 5.79–91. The Ajapā Gāyatrī.

4.23 *Jogpradīpakā* 393–432. Breath-control.

4.1 *Atharva Veda* 15.16–18. The breaths of the Vrātya:

(16.1–2) The Vrātya has seven upward breaths (*prāṇa*), seven downward breaths (*apāna*) [and] seven pervasive breaths (*vyāna*).

(3) His first upward breath is called 'upper'. It is fire. (4) His second upward breath is called 'fully grown'. It is the sun. (5) His third upward breath is called 'brought near'. It is the moon. (6) His fourth upward breath is called 'all-pervading'. It is air. (7) His fifth upward breath is called 'source' (*yoni*). It is these waters. (8) His sixth upward breath is called 'dear'. It is these domestic animals. (9) His seventh upward breath is called 'unlimited'. It is these creatures.

(17.1) His first downward breath is the time of the full moon. (2) His second downward breath is the eighth day after the full moon. (3) His third downward breath is the time of the new moon. (4) His fourth downward breath is faith. (5) His fifth downward breath is initiation. (6) His sixth downward breath is sacrifice. (7) His seventh downward breath is these payments to the priests.

(18.1) His first pervasive breath is this earth. (2) His second pervasive breath is the atmosphere. (3) His third pervasive breath is heaven. (4) His fourth pervasive breath is the constellations. (5) His fifth pervasive breath is the seasons. (6) His sixth pervasive breath is the groupings of the seasons. (7) His seventh pervasive breath is the year.

(8) The gods go through the year and the seasons go through the Vrātya in succession for the same reason. (9) When they enter into the sun for the new moon and the full moon, (10) then they attain one and the same immortality. It is the sacrificial offering.

4.2 *Chāndogya Upaniṣad* 6.8.2. The connection between the breath and the mind:

> Just as a bird tied by a string flies off in all directions and, on not reaching any other place to stay, returns to where it is tied, in the very same way, dear boy, the mind flies off in all directions and, on not reaching any other place to stay, returns to the breath. For the mind, dear boy, is tied to the breath.

4.3 *Mahāsaccakasutta* (*Majjhimanikāya* I, Book 9, abridged). Non-breathing meditation:

> The Buddha said, 'Then, Aggivessana, this occurred to me: "Suppose I meditate the non-breathing meditation." So I stopped the passage of the breath in and out of my mouth and nose. When that was stopped there was a loud noise of winds coming out of my ears, just like the loud noise when a blacksmith's bellows are pumped. But although, Aggivessana, unsluggish energy arose in me and unmuddled mindfulness came about, my body was impetuous, not calmed, while I was being troubled by that painful exertion. And this painful feeling that arose in me, Aggivessana, remained, [but] without taking over my mind.
>
> 'Then it occurred to me to try the non-breathing meditation again. Extreme winds slashed my head as if a strong man were attacking my head with a sharp sword. [It had the same result as before, but I tried it again.] I got extreme headaches, as if a strong man were squeezing my head with a tight leather headband. [It had the same result as before, but I tried it again.] Extreme winds stabbed my stomach, like a slaughterman – or his pupil – stabbing a cow's stomach with a sharp butcher's knife. [It had the same result as before, but I tried it again.] An extreme heat arose in my body; it was as if two strong men were to take a weaker man by the arms and roast him over hot coals. [It had the same result as before.]
>
> 'Then some gods saw me and said, "The ascetic

Gotama is dead." Others saw me and said, "The ascetic Gotama is not dead, but he is dying." Other deities said, "The ascetic Gotama is not dead, nor dying. He is a saint and this is how saints behave."'

[The Buddha then fasts until the skin of his belly touches his backbone, he falls over from fainting, his hair falls out and, finally, he loses his fair complexion. At this point, he declares:]

'Then, Aggivessana, this occurred to me: "The ascetics or Brahmans of the past who experienced painful, sharp [and] severe sensations due to [self-inflicted] torture [experienced] this much at most, not more than this. And those ascetics or Brahmans who in the future will experience painful, sharp [and] severe sensations due to [self-inflicted] torture [will experience] this much at most, not more than this. And those ascetics or Brahmans who in the present experience painful, sharp [and] severe sensations due to [self-inflicted] torture [experience] this much at most, not more than this. But I, indeed, by means of this severe and difficult practice, do not attain to greater excellence in noble knowledge and insight which transcends the human condition. Could there be another path to enlightenment?'

4.4 *Baudhāyanadharmasūtra* 4.1.22–4, 28–30. Purificatory breath-control:

(22) Sitting with purificatory *kuśa* grass in his hand, he should practise breath-controls [and recite] the purificatory texts, the utterances, *oṃ*, and the obligatory sections of the Veda.

(23) Constantly engaged in yoga, he should practise breath-controls repeatedly, generating extreme heat as far as the ends of his hair and the tips of his nails. (24) As a result of holding [the breath] wind arises; from wind fire arises; by means of heat the waters arise. Through these three he is then purified internally. [. . .]

(28) Breath-control is said to be when one recites three

times the [Vedic] Gāyatrī [mantra], together with the utterances *oṃ* and the Śiras chant with the breath extended.

(29) Sixteen daily breath-controls, together with the utterances and *oṃ*, purify even an abortionist within a month.

(30) The best austerity (*tapas*) has this as its beginning; this signifies *dharma*. For destroying all faults it is this which is pre-eminent, it is this which is pre-eminent.

4.5 *Mānavadharmaśāstra* 6.69–72. Purificatory breath-control:

(69) In order to cleanse [himself of the deaths] of those creatures whom he injures unknowingly by day or by night the ascetic should perform six breath-controls. (70) One should know that for the Brahman, three breath-controls performed correctly together with the great utterances [*bhūr*, *bhuvaḥ* and *svaḥ*] and *oṃ* are the ultimate austerity (*tapas*). (71) For just as metals' impurities are burnt up when they are smelted, so faults in the sense organs are burnt up by restraint of the breath. (72) By means of breath-controls one burns up faults, by means of fixations, sins, by means of withdrawal, attachment to the senses, [and] by means of meditation, qualities which are not those of the Lord.

4.6 *Pātañjalayogaśāstra* 2.49–53. Breath-control:

(2.49) Breath-control is stopping the flow of inhalation and exhalation when in [an unwaveringly comfortable posture].

Inhalation is the drinking in of external air when one has mastered posture. Exhalation is the expulsion of abdominal air. The stopping of their flow, i.e. the absence of both of them, is breath-control.

(2.50) [Breath-control] is external, internal or stopped; regulated according to location, time and number; [and] long and subtle.

[Breath-control] in which the absence of flow is preceded by exhalation is external. [That] in which the absence of flow is preceded by inhalation is internal. In the third [breath-control], namely 'stopped', absence of both [inhalation and exhalation] arises as a result of sudden effort. Like when water completely contracts when placed on a heated stone, so [in 'stopped' breath-control] there is immediately an absence of the flow of both [inhalation and exhalation].

These three are regulated according to location; location is the sphere of operation of [the breath]. Their being regulated according to time means that they are limited by a restriction on how many moments [they last]. [The three types of breath-control are also] regulated according to number: the first eruption (*udghāta*) results from a certain number of inhalations and exhalations, the second eruption of the restrained [breath] likewise results from that many, [and] the third is the same. Because breath-control is thus said respectively to be mild, middling and intense, it is 'regulated by number'. When it is practised thus, it is long and subtle.

(2.51) The fourth [breath-control] casts aside the external and internal spheres of action.

[The breath-control] regulated in the external sphere of action according to location, time and number is cast aside. [The breath-control] regulated in the internal sphere of action in the same way is cast aside. In both [breath-control] is long and subtle. The fourth breath-control is the absence of the flow of both [inhalation and exhalation] preceded by those [breath-controls] and resulting from gradual conquest of the levels. The third [breath-control], on the other hand, is an absence of flow undertaken all of a sudden without regard for the sphere of activity. Regulated according to location, time and number, it is long and subtle. But the fourth is an absence of flow [of inhalation and exhalation], preceded by the casting aside of both [the external and internal domains] and resulting from limitation of the sphere of activity of inhalation and exhalation, and from gradual conquest of the levels. This is what distinguishes the fourth breath-control.

(2.52) As a result, the covering of the light is lessened.

For the yogi who practises [these] breath-controls, activity which veils discriminatory knowledge is lessened. That [activity] is explained as covering the naturally luminous essence of goodness (*sattva*) with a magical net made of the great delusion and then engaging that same essence of goodness in what is not to be done. So through the practice of breath-control action which covers the light of this [yogi] and binds [him] to the wheel of rebirth becomes weak and is continuously diminished. Thus it is said: 'There is no austerity superior to breath-control. It results in the cleansing of impurities and the illumination of knowledge.'

Moreover,

> (2.53) [As a result of breath-control] the mind becomes capable of the fixations.

[This is] as a result of the practice of breath-control, from the teaching [at *Pātañjalayogaśāstra* 1.34] that '[mental steadiness] may also result from the exhalation and retention of breath'.

4.7 *Pañcārthabhāṣya* on *Pāśupatasūtra* 1.16. Purificatory breath-control:

> Question: If, having bathed, the impurity [that arises from seeing urine, faeces, a woman or a low-caste man (*śūdra*)] were not removed, then what must be done to get rid of it?
>
> Answer: Because an absolutive verb form [such as *upaspṛśya* ('having bathed')] requires [another verb], breath-control must be performed.
>
> Because of this, the text says 'by performing breath-control (*prāṇāyāma*)'.
>
> Here 'breath' means the breath which is the air that flows out from the mouth and nostrils.
>
> Its control, i.e. its restraint or suppression, is breath-control. And that is to be seen to be intentional. Why? Because breath-control is preceded by knowledge, desire and effort.
>
> It consists of one eruption (*udghāta*) or two eruptions.
>
> And it lasts twenty measures (*mātrās*), twenty-four measures or thirty measures. A measure is the time taken to blink.
>
> Breath-control is to be performed according to one's ability and strength.
>
> Therefore, after bathing one should sit facing east or north in one or other of the postures such as the lotus, lucky mark, hands joined at the loins, half-moon,

small seat, stretched out like a stick and complete good fortune, and, having performed these ancillary actions, one should lift up the neck and, beginning with either an inhalation or an exhalation, perform [breath-control] until the breaths are restrained and one is in meditation.

Of those [results], being in meditation is when the body is full inside, like an elephant, while the sign of [the breaths] being restrained is when exhalations and inhalations occur in the body, like a turtle, and one's sense organs are purified: then the breaths should be considered to be restrained. After that they are to be released very gently through the nose, so that even a lotus petal [held] at the nostrils does not flutter.

4.8 *Kumārasambhava* 3.44–50. Śiva in meditation:

(44) Kāma, the god of love, his body about to fall,
saw Three-Eyed Śiva in meditation,
seated on a cedarwood dais covered by a tiger skin;

(45) his upper body held steady by his yogic posture,
straight and erect, his shoulders rounded,
seeming, from the placing of his upturned hands,
to have an open lotus in his lap;

(46) his crown of dreadlocks bound up by a snake,
a double-stringed *rudrākṣa* rosary hanging from his hand,
he was wearing a knotted deerskin made a bluer black
by the glow cast from his neck;

(47) with his eyes gazing downwards,
their fierce pupils dimmed and stilled,
holding the brows steady, lashes unflickering,
he was focusing on his nose;

(48) as a result of restraining his inner winds
he was like a cloud without the rage of rain,
like a pot of water without a ripple,
like an unflickering lamp in a place without wind;

(49) with the beams of light from his head,
which had found a way out of the eyes
of the skull on his crest,
he was dulling the splendour,
more delicate than a lotus thread,
of the young moon;

(50) controlling his mind in *samādhi*,
checking its motion through the nine doors
and fixing it in his heart,
he was gazing on the self in the self,
which the sages know to be the imperishable.

4.9 *Niśvāsatattvasaṃhitā Nayasūtra* 4.109c–118d.[40] The four types of breath-control:

He should meditate through controlling the breath. (110) He should inhale through the left [channel] and exhale through the right. This is the purification of the channels of one whose path is the path to liberation. (111) Exhalation, inhalation [and] retention make up the threefold breath-control. (112) He should exhale internally, inhale internally and perform a motionless breath-retention [internally]: these are the three internal [practices]. (113) There is a fourth breath-control, known as the Very Tranquil (*supraśānta*), [achieved] by moving [the vital energy] from the heart into the navel and [by moving] the mind away from the sense objects. (114) Once he has completed this cessation of breathing, having brought the breath to the navel he should raise it and gently exhale it through the left nostril. (115) He should perform the wind fixation in his [left] big toe, the fire fixation in the navel, the earth fixation in the region of the throat, the water visualization in the uvula (116) [and] in the head the ether fixation, which is said to bring about all supernatural powers. He masters [these fixations] through one, two, three, four and five eruptions. (117) Yogis should always understand that it is called 'eruption' (*udghāta*) when the breath, having been restrained, goes to the head and back. (118) By maintaining these breath-controls, attachment and hatred cease. Through the fixations [one is freed] from all sins. Through withdrawal the senses are controlled.

4.10 *Parākhyatantra* 14.13c–15b. Breath-control and fixation:[41]

(13c–14b) The repeated stretching of the entity inside the body that moves to and from the [heart] lotus called the breath, once it is controlled, is called breath-control (*prāṇāyāma*). (14cd) By [these] stretchings the inner spaces are purified; by this purification one conquers the fixations. (15) The fixations have their own *maṇḍala*s, seed-syllables, and locuses, and they are associated with (?) the [characteristic] functions of the [five] elements.

4.11 *Mṛgendratantra Yogapāda* 4, 12a–24b, 27c–30b, 33c–36b, 44c–51b, with selections from the *vṛtti* of Bhaṭa Nārāyaṇakaṇṭha. Breath-extension:[42]

(4) Breath (*prāṇa*) is the vital wind (*vāyu*) already defined. Its extension (*āyāma*)[43] is the strenuous exercise of that wind by expelling it, drawing it in and holding it. Its effect is to remove any defects in the faculties.

The vital wind is single; but because of its different functions (propulsion and so forth) it has five aspects. These five, beginning with the outgoing (*prāṇa*) and the down-going (*apāna*), as well as their [various] functions, have been explained in the Section of Doctrine. Breath-extension is vigorous exercise of the out-breath and other aspects of this vital energy. It consists of exhalation, inhalation and the pause [thereafter]: the vital wind is exercised by being expelled for longer than if it were occurring freely; it is then drawn in again in the same way, and held.

The word *kratu* ('faculties') refers here either to the [ten] faculties [of sense perception and action] or to the [faculty of] volition/attention [i.e. the mind, which is the eleventh]. [Breath-extension] repels, eliminates, any defects in these caused by not doing what is prescribed or by doing what is forbidden. This is confirmed in the following (*Manusmṛti* 6.71):

'The repeated practice of breath-extension destroys any defects in the faculties, just as impurities are burnt away when ores are smelted in a furnace.' [. . .]

At this point the sage [Bharadvāja] puts a request [to Indra]:

> (12–13) Working the breath (*prāṇa-khedana* [= *prāṇāyāma*]) causes the mind to cease contact [and this] cessation is the source of [all the other auxiliaries], beginning with fixation. It is therefore the basis of the whole. Describe it at length, O best of the gods, and whatever else [even further] removed is a means of success in yoga.
>
> [Indra's] reply to this:
>
> (14) It cannot be taught at length for fear of the effect that would have on [the scale of] this treatise. Nonetheless, since a request must not go unanswered, I shall teach an outline.
>
> (15–16) When he has evacuated his urine and the rest according to the ordinances, he should clean his penis, anus, left hand and both hands with one, five, ten and seven pieces of soil, twice [if he is an] ascetic. Then, having thrice drunk water and twice wiped his face, he should touch the openings, his arms, his navel, his heart and his head; and he should wipe his lips twice or thrice.
>
> (17–20b) If he observes a diet of wholesome food [eaten] when he has digested, and is [therefore] sound in body, he should sit facing north on a good seat in a house enclosed by three walls or in some untroubled place, such as a forest. He should do obeisance to Maheśvara, Umā, Skanda and the Leader of the Gaṇas. Then with his neck, head and chest straight, with his eyes on the tip of his nose, protecting his testicles with his heels, not allowing his two rows of teeth to touch, well balanced, with his body upright, he should place his tongue at the top of his teeth and exhale the air through one nostril as far as he can.

[. . .] he should sit upon a fine seat (*āsana*) such as a raised wooden platform or board covered with a cloth or an antelope skin. Alternatively, the text means that he should sit in one of the various yoga postures (*āsana*s) which are defined in certain other scriptures, such as the lotus, the lucky mark and the half-moon. Such a posture will be 'good' if, as a result of repeated practice, it enables him to remain still and comfortable. Then, facing north and having bowed to Parameśvara, Devī, Skanda and Gaṇeśa, keeping his head, throat and chest perfectly straight, his gaze fixed on the tip of his nose, keeping apart his upper and lower rows of teeth, using his heels to protect his testicles from painful pressure that may occur if he jerks upwards as a result of the ascent of the vital breath (*udghāta*), not allowing his body to slump, well balanced and placing his tongue at the top of his teeth, he should exhale in order to purify the energy channels, expelling the air within his body through the right nostril for as long as he can.

> (20c–21b) This is the exercise of exhalation (*recaka*). By its repeated practice one gradually becomes successful in rites of piercing or dispersing, even when the targets of these [actions] are remote.
>
> (21c–22b) Inhalation (*pūraka*) is to fill one's body with the air outside, to the limit of one's power. By repeatedly practising this [exercise] one will be able to draw towards one even the heaviest [of objects].
>
> (22c–23b) Breath-retention (*kumbhaka*) is defined as immobilizing [the breath] by neither releasing nor drawing [it] in. By repeatedly practising this, one realizes a power to immobilize which nothing can resist.
>
> (23c–24b) If the yogi understands the [breath] as it moves, and recognizes the affinities of the qualities which it manifests in the paths of the moon, the sun and the Lord, he can accomplish whatever he wishes.

By practising [these exercises] the yogi gains control over his breath and becomes aware of how it circulates. He thereby comes to understand the correspondences between the effects he wishes to bring about and the breath's movement in the central, left and right channels. He becomes aware that when the right breath is active it is best for this supernatural effect, the central for that, and the left for another; and so is able to achieve whatever he desires. [. . .]

(27c–28b) [Breath-extension] is [of three grades. It is] inferior, intermediate or superior, according to whether it lasts twelve or more *tāla*s. One *tāla* equals twelve circuits round the knee cap. The span of time termed a *tāla* is what it takes to move [the palm of] one's hand round the circumference of one's knee cap twelve times.

The shortest [kind of] breath-extension lasts for twelve such *tāla*s, the intermediate for twenty-four and the superior for forty-eight.

(28c–29b) If it is accompanied by a visualization and the repetition of [a] mantra it is termed 'full' (*sagarbha*), and the opposite if it isn't. The latter is less conducive to stability of awareness than the full is.

(29cd) In the morning [it destroys any] sin committed during the night, and in the evening [any] done during the day.

(30ab) As for the empty [form], that too [has no small virtue; for it] destroys the fickleness of the racing senses. [. . .]

(33c–34b) In order to master the fixations and the rest, and the functions of the vital energy, the wise [yogi] should adopt the full [form of] breath-retention (*kumbhaka*), [doing it] with untiring concentration.

(34c–35b) If its time span is multiplied by the [number of the] suns [i.e. twelve] it will stop the mind. It then receives the name fixation, because it bestows the Perfections of Fixation.

(35c–36b) The word fixation means stasis; [but] it also refers by extension to the focus [of this stasis]. For the beginner, the only appropriate focus is one of these [levels] beginning with the Earth.

[There follows a detailed description of the meditative process of fixation, which is given in Chapter 8 of this book.]

The sage [Bharadvāja] now questions [Indra] in order to learn about these matters, namely the location and holding of the functions of the outgoing and other breaths, and the results [thereof]:

> (44c–45b) Tell me, O you who are greatest among the gods, where in this wretched body are the functions of the outgoing and other breaths to be located, and what is the effect of mastering them?

The answer:

> (45c–46b) By holding it in the heart, navel, chest, throat and back the yogi conquers projection and the other functions.

The vital energy described above exists as the outgoing and other breaths. By holding it in these five places from the heart to the back the yogi masters projection and the other functions of those breaths. As for that yogi,

> (46c–49b) When he has mastered projection he maintains his body at will. When he has mastered expulsion he eats but does not excrete. When he has mastered elevation he achieves such virtues as the mastery of language. By mastering the function of the 'breath' of equal distribution he conquers ageing and is master [of his body]. If he has mastered deflection, he is able to roam through his body. He is untouched by mud, water or thorns and has an extraordinary, inexhaustible vigour.

A yogi who has conquered the function of the outgoing breath termed 'projection' maintains his body at will, only as long, that is, as he wishes to, because it has been stated above that the nature of projection is that it keeps one alive: 'The function of projection is defined as life.'

If a yogi masters expulsion, the function of the down-going breath, he can eat, yet have a body which is free of waste matter. For as a result of mastering the down-going breath his food and drink are not transformed into waste matter (urine, faeces and the like), but only into the nutrient fluid. Consequently, he becomes entirely free of faeces and other food waste. For [normally] a creature's food and drink are transformed into both waste matter and the nutrient fluid.

One who masters elevation, the function of the ascending breath (*udāna*), achieves such virtues as mastery of language in the form of a supernatural poetic power and eloquence. One who masters the function of the *samāna* breath [which serves to distribute nourishment equally throughout the body] becomes permanently free of the process of ageing, with a body that can endure anything and is entirely at his command. One who masters deflection, the function of the circulatory breath (*vyāna*), roams at will in his body. The text means that he is able, for example, to expel or withdraw the breath through his Brahmā-aperture, through the passages of his ears and so forth. Furthermore, he is untouched by mud, water, thorns and the like. He need not come into direct contact with these, even when he sits down upon them. He also develops inexhaustible physical strength.

Thus he has answered this incidental question. He now returns to the main subject:

> (49c–50b) Twelve fixations [equal one] meditation, and this causes a divine radiance to occur. Twelve of these [equal one] *samādhi*, and that brings about the ability to become as small as an atom and other such [supernatural powers].
>
> (50c–51b) Once a yogi has thus mastered himself, he achieves the said virtues immediately when he practises. This is so even if he doesn't do the [exercise of] breath-extension, [provided he can establish himself] in the [appropriate state of] mind [without it].

4.12 *Mataṅgapārameśvara Yogapāda* 2.10c–11d. Breath-control:

> *Prāṇa* is that which is known as the breath (*vāyu*) and it is on the path of transmigration. (11) It is seen to be indivisibly united with consciousness. Breath-control is said to be the complete restraint of its motion.

4.13 *Īśvaragītā* 11.30–37. Breath-control with and without mantra-repetition:

> (30) The rules and regulations have been taught. [Now] learn about breath-control. *Prāṇa* is wind (*vāyu*) produced in one's own body. Control (*āyāma*) is its restraint. (31) Because it may be highest, lowest or middling, it is explained as threefold. It is [also] taught to be twofold: full (*sagarbha*) and empty (*agarbha*). (32) The lowest has [a

duration of] twelve measures, the middling breath-restraint, twenty-four measures, [and] the highest, thirty-six measures. (33) The lowest, middling and highest produce perspiration, trembling and levitation respectively, [and] bliss increases from one to the next. (34) The wise teach that [breath-control] with mantra-repetition is full and without mantra-repetition is empty. This indeed is the definition of breath-control taught for yogis. (35) One should recite three times the Gāyatrī, the utterances, *oṃ* and the Śiras, with the breath controlled. This is said to be breath-control.[44] (36) In all texts, yogis who have restrained their minds teach breath-control to be exhalation, inhalation and breath-retention. (37) Exhalation results from uninterrupted breathing out, inhalation from the restraint of that. Breath-retention is remaining in equilibrium.

4.14 Hemacandra's *Yogaśāstra* 5.1–35, with selections from the *Svopajñavṛtti* auto-commentary. Breath-control:

Breath-control is not useful for attaining liberation or meditation, because it does not bring about a good state of mind. Even so, because it is useful for keeping the body healthy and knowing the signs of death, I am explaining it in this text.

(1) After [posture], some, unable to conquer the mind and breath any other way, resort to breath-control in order to master meditation.

Total restraint, i.e. cessation of the movement, of *prāṇa*, i.e. the breath flowing in the mouth and nose, is breath-control (*prāṇāyāma*). Some, i.e. Patañjali and so forth, have resorted to, i.e. accepted, it as a means of mastering meditation. The text gives the reason for resorting to it: conquering the breath and mind is impossible any other way.

Conquest of the breath might arise from breath-control, but how can conquest of the mind? The text explains:

(2) The breath is where the mind is and the mind is where the breath is. Mixed together like milk and water, they thus act in the same way. (3) When one is stopped, the other is stopped; when one is active, the other is

active. When both are stopped, the senses and intellect are destroyed and as a result there is liberation.

(4) Breath-control is taught to be the interruption of the flow of the in- and out-breaths. It is threefold: exhalation, inhalation and retention. (5) Others say that, with the addition of four varieties – drawing in (*pratyāhāra*), pacified (*śānta*), upper (*uttara*) and lower (*adhara*) – it is sevenfold.

(6) Exhalation is taught to be the forceful expulsion of air from the abdomen through the nose, fontanelle or mouth. (7) Inhalation is the filling [with air] drawn in as far as the *apāna* breath. Steadying [the breath] in the navel lotus and stopping it is restraint. (8) Pulling it upwards from place to place is called drawing in. Stopping it using the apertures of the palate, nose and mouth is called pacified [breath-control].

Pulling the breath upwards from a place such as the navel to a place such as the heart is 'drawing in'.

(9) Holding [the breath] in the heart and so forth after breathing it in and drawing it upwards is called upper [breath-control]. The reverse is lower [breath-control].

Lower [breath-control] takes the form of leading the breath down from a higher place.

If breath-control is said to take the form of an interruption of the flow [of the breath], how can it happen in exhalation, etc.? The answer is that in an exhalation in which air from the chest is exhaled and then held externally there is an interruption of the flows of the in- and out-breaths, and in an inhalation in which the external air is inhaled and held internally there, too, is an interruption of the flows of the in- and out-breaths. The same is true for breath-retention and so forth.

(10) Exhalation brings about removal of diseases of the stomach and of *kapha*, the phlegmatic humour. Inhalation results in nourishment and the destruction of disease. (11) Breath-retention soon makes the heart lotus open and the inner knot unravel, and it clearly produces strength, stamina and growth. (12) From drawing in [there arises]

strength and beauty, and from the pacified [breath-control] the calming of [imbalances of] the humours. From the practice of the upper and lower breath-controls [there arises] steadiness of breath-retention.

Breath-control is not only for the conquest of *prāṇa*, but for the conquest of [all] five breaths. Thus the text says:

(13) One should use breath-control to conquer [the five breaths] *prāṇa*, *apāna*, *samāna*, *udāna* and *vyāna*, knowing [their] locations, colours, functions, purposes and seed-syllables.

(14) *Prāṇa* is green and is located in the tip of the nose, the heart, the navel and the tips of the big toes. It is conquered by the practice of going and coming or by holding. (15) The practice of going and coming [is done] by repeatedly inhaling and exhaling using the nose and other locations, and holding results from breath-retention.

(16) *Apāna* is black and found in the nape of the neck, the back, the bottom and the heels. It is to be conquered by repeated exhalation and inhalation using its locations.

(17) *Samāna* is white and located in the heart, navel and all the joints. It is to be conquered by repeated exhalation and inhalation using its locations.

(18) *Udāna* is red and located in the heart, throat and palate, between the brows and in the head. It is to be controlled by the practice of going and coming.

The text explains the practice of going and coming:

(19) By drawing [*udāna*] through the nose one should fix it in the heart and other [locations]. By forcefully drawing it up and stopping it over and over again one brings it under control.

(20) *Vyāna* is active throughout the skin and looks like a rainbow. It is to be conquered through the practice of breath-retention by means of contraction and expansion.

Now the texts give their seed-syllables, which are to be meditated upon.

(21) In the *prāṇa*, *apāna*, *samāna*, *udāna* and *vyāna* breaths the seed-syllables *yaṃ*, *paiṃ*, *vaṃ*, *roṃ* and *loṃ* are to be meditated upon respectively.[45]

(22) When *prāṇa* is conquered, the digestive fire becomes strong, breathing is steady, the [other] breaths are conquered and the body becomes light. (23) When *samāna* and *apāna* are conquered, wounds, fractures and other injuries are healed, the digestive fire is kindled, faeces diminish and diseases are destroyed. (24) When *udāna* is conquered one can perform yogic suicide (*utkrānti*) and one is not troubled by water, mud and such like. When *vyāna* is conquered one cares not for heat or cold, and beauty and health arise.

(25) A person should continuously hold *prāṇa* and the other breaths wherever they have a painful disease in order to cure it.

(26) After thus constantly practising the conquest of *prāṇa* and the other breaths, one should regularly practise fixation and so forth in order to obtain steadiness of mind.

(27) Sitting in one of the postures that have been taught, [the yogi] should gently expel the breath and then inhale through the left channel, filling [the body] as far as the big toes. (28) First restrain the mind in the big toe and then the sole of the foot, the heel, the ankle, the shank, the knee, the thigh, the bottom, (29) the penis, the navel, the belly, the heart, the throat, the tongue, the palate, the tip of the nose, the eye, the brows, the forehead and the head. (30) Thus stringing together these places by fixing the mind, with the breath, at them in sequence, he should lead [the mind and breath] from one location to another until taking [them] to the aperture of Brahmā, the fontanelle. (31) Then in that same sequence he should take the mind back as far as the big toe, and, having taken the breath into the navel lotus, he should exhale.

(32) The breath is held in sequence at the big toe and so forth [i.e. the heel and ankle], the shank, knee, thigh, anus and penis for speed and strength, (33) at the navel to

get rid of fever and so forth, in the stomach to purify the body, in the heart for knowledge, in the tortoise channel (*kūrmanāḍī*) to stop disease and old age, (34) in the throat to get rid of hunger and thirst, at the tip of the tongue to understand taste, at the tip of the nose to understand smell, in the eyes to understand form, (35) at the forehead to get rid of diseases there and to calm anger and at the aperture of Brahmā to have a direct vision of the adepts.

4.15 *Dattātreyayogaśāstra* 54ab, 58c–69d, 72c–83d. Accompanied and unaccompanied breath-control:

> (54) After that he should practise breath-control regularly, sitting in the lotus position.
>
> After spreading out a seat covered with a fine cloth in the middle of it, (59) the wise [yogi] should sit down in its middle, assuming the lotus position. With his body upright, he should put his hands together and worship his personal deity. (60) Then he should block the right nostril with the thumb of the right hand and gradually inhale through the left nostril (61) without interruption as deeply as he can. Then he should perform breath-retention (*kumbhaka*). Next he should exhale through the right nostril gently, not forcefully. (62) He should inhale again, through the right nostril, and gently fill his abdomen. After holding [his breath] for as long as he can, he should gently exhale through the left nostril. (63) He should inhale in the same manner that he exhales and hold [his breath] without interruption. Sitting down in the morning he should perform twenty breath-retentions in this manner. (64) In the same way he should perform twenty breath-retentions at midday. Similarly, in the evening he should again perform twenty breath-retentions. (65) At midnight, too, he should perform twenty breath-retentions in the very same fashion. He should do them every day together with exhalation and inhalation. (66) It is because it is accompanied by exhalation and inhalation

that it is called 'accompanied' (*sahita*) breath-retention. He should practise tirelessly in this fashion four times a day.

(67–9) If he practises thus for three months, purification of the channels results. When the channels are purified, then perceptible signs appear in the body of the yogi. I shall teach all of them. Nimbleness, radiance, an increase in the digestive fire and leanness of the body are sure to arise.

And [the yogi] should perform his breath practice at the aforementioned times. (73) After that he should have the ability to hold his breath as long as he wishes. 'Unaccompanied' (*kevala*) breath-retention is mastered as a result of holding one's breath for as long as one likes. (74) Once unaccompanied breath-retention, free from exhalation and inhalation, is mastered, there is nothing in the three worlds that is unattainable for [the yogi].

(75) At first sweat appears. [The yogi] should massage [himself] with it. By slowly increasing, step-by-step, the retention of the breath, (76) trembling arises in the body of the yogi while he is seated in his *āsana*. Through further increase [in the duration] of the practice, the frog [power] (*darduri*) is sure to arise. (77) In the same way that a frog hops across the ground, so the yogi seated in the lotus position moves across the ground. (78) And through further increase [in the duration] of the practice levitation arises. Sitting in the lotus position, [the yogi] leaves the ground and remains [in the air] (79) without a support. Then peculiar powers arise. The yogi is not troubled whether he eats a little or a lot. (80) His faeces and urine diminish and he sleeps very little. Worms, rheumy eyes, slobber, sweat, body odour: (81) henceforth these never arise for him. Through further increase [in the duration] of the practice, great strength arises, (82) through which he gets the animal power (*bhūcara-siddhi*), the power to overcome animals. A tiger, a buffalo, a wild gayal, an elephant (83) or a lion: these are

killed by a blow from the hand of the yogi. The yogi looks like the god of love.

4.16 *Gorakṣaśataka* 8–10, 28c–49b. The four breath-retentions:

(8) He is without doubt liberated whose breath goes neither in nor out, neither in the left nostril nor in the right, and neither up nor down. (9) The mind has two impulses: past impressions and the breath. On one of them being destroyed, both are destroyed. (10) Of these two, it is the breath which you must first conquer (on being allowed to do so [by your guru]), in order that you might become a liberated man. [. . .]

Now I shall teach in brief the restraint of the breath.

(29) The vital breath (*prāṇa*) is wind born in the body. [Its] restraint (*āyāma*) is known as breath-retention (*kumbhaka*). Breath-retention is said to be of two kinds: accompanied (*sahita*) and unaccompanied (*kevala*).

(30) [The yogi] should practise accompanied breath-retention until unaccompanied breath-retention is mastered. Solar (*sūryā*), victorious (*ujjāyī*), cool (*śītalī*) and the fourth, bellows (*bhastrī*): (31) when breath-retention has these variations it is accompanied breath-retention. I shall now duly teach in brief [their] characteristics.

[*Sūryā* breath-retention]

(32) In a clean place clear of people and mosquitoes and so forth, as long as a bow and free from cold, fire and water, (33) [and] on a seat which is clean, neither too high nor too low, agreeable and comfortable, [the yogi] should assume the lotus position, stimulate Sarasvatī, (34) gently draw in external air through the right channel, fill himself with as much air as is comfortable and then expel it through the left channel.

(35) Alternatively, the wise man should expel the breath once the skull is purified. This destroys the four diseases of the wind humour and problems with worms. (36)

This [breath-retention], which is called the *sūryā* or solar variety, should be practised repeatedly.

[*Ujjāyī* breath-retention]

[The yogi] should close the mouth and gently draw in air through the two channels (37) so that it comes into contact with [the region] from the throat to the heart, making a sound. In the same way as before he should hold his breath and then expel it through the left channel. (38–9) [This] breath-retention, which is called *ujjāyī* ('the victorious'), should be performed when [the yogi is] walking or at rest. It destroys the fire which arises in the head, it completely removes phlegm from the throat, it increases the fire of the body and it gets rid of oedema in the channels and imbalances in the body's constituent parts.

[*Śītalī* breath-retention]

After holding the breath as before, the sage should draw in air with his tongue before gently exhaling it through his nostrils. Inflammation of the spleen and other diseases are destroyed, as is fever caused by an excess of the *pitta* humour. (41) This breath-retention called *śītalī* ('she who is cool') destroys poisons.

[*Bhastrī* breath-retention]

Then the sage should assume the lotus position and, holding his neck and stomach straight, (42) close his mouth and forcefully exhale through his nostrils in such a way that his breath makes contact with his throat, producing a sound in his skull. (43) He should then quickly draw in a small amount of air as far as his heart lotus. Then he should exhale and inhale as before, repeating the process over and over again. (44) The wise man should pump the air that is in his body in the same way that one might quickly pump blacksmiths' bellows.

(45) When the body becomes tired, he should gently

inhale by way of the sun until the stomach becomes full of air. (46) Holding the middle of the nose firmly, without using the index fingers, he should perform breath-retention as before and then exhale through the left channel.

(47) This adamantine [breath-retention] gets rid of bile that has arisen in the throat; it increases the fire of the body; it awakens Kuṇḍalinī; it gets rid of sin; it is auspicious [and] it is pleasant. (48) It destroys the bolt made of substances such as phlegm, which is situated at the mouth at the end of the Brahmā channel [and] it pierces the three knots that are born from the three strands of existence (*guṇa*s). (49) This breath-retention called *bhastrī* ('the bellows') is to be practised above all others.

4.17 *Lallāvākyāni* 4, 56–7. Knowledge through breath-control:

(4) I forced the breath slowly down the bellows' throat;
I lit a lamp, and what I was came into view;
I winnowed the light inside, scattering it out;
I grabbed the dark, and held it fast.

(56) O Guru, Parameshvar,
Please teach me. You know the inner meaning.
The two are born in the city of the bulb,
why is *hah* cold, and *hāh* hot?

(57) The region of the navel is by nature burning.
Prāṇa rises up to the throat
[and meets] the river flowing from the skull.
That is why *hah* is cold and *hāh* hot.

4.18 *Yogabīja* 76–77, 80–86. *Prāṇa* and *apāna:*

(76) From the union of *prāṇa* and *apāna*, the sun and moon are one. The wise man should bake the body with its seven constituents in fire. (77) His diseases disappear, as do hazards such as being cut or hit, and he remains as an embodied being with the form of the supreme ether.

(80) The mind is not mastered by various kinds of reflection, so the method of conquering it is *prāṇa* and nothing else. (81) *Prāṇa* is not controlled by logic, discourses, the many sacred texts (*śāstras*), deduction (*yukti*) nor curative mantras without the method of the adepts, my dear.

(82) One sets out on the path of yoga after learning the method of [mastering] it [i.e. the breath]. He who has only bits and pieces of knowledge gets into trouble. (83) Those yogis who out of foolishness want [to practise] yoga without having conquered the breath are like those who wish to cross the ocean in an unbaked pot.

(84) The body of the practitioner whose *prāṇa* has dissolved while he is still alive does not fall and his mind is freed from afflictions. (85) When his mind is purified, then knowledge of the self shines forth. Thus, Pārvatī, knowledge comes about through yoga in a single lifetime.

(86) Therefore, the practitioner should at the beginning practise yoga constantly. Those desirous of liberation must conquer the breath in order to attain liberation.

4.19 *Ḥawż al-ḥayāt* Chapter 5. The breath and its control:

(1) He said: Know that the creation of the breath in the microcosm comes from the great heat, whose dwelling place is the stomach. It is like a coiled rope in the shape of a circle, around the navel in the belly. This is how it looks. Both sides of it join in the stomach and it comes from the guts.

(2) [The breath] is divided into three portions: one third rises above for cleansing [the body], one third descends below for cleansing [the body], and one third moves throughout the body for the circulation of the blood. Whatever limb it does not enter is paralysed and is deprived of sensation and motion. In these breaths is the pivot (*madar*) of life, which is generated only from food. When the two external portions [of breath] come together with the other, with deliberation, gentleness and

sympathy, so that nothing escapes from below except what is necessary when excreting, or from above except what cannot be avoided, it becomes the instrument of life and life becomes the instrument of the rational soul. The advance from gross to subtle is attained by the subsistence of the contraries, while negating the contraries.

(3) And if this is what you desire, take only the best and cleanest of foods, such as rice with milk or bulgur wheat, at the time of need. Do not use meats and fats except by necessity and need. Moderate portions prevent [breath] from going out, and it does not go out except at the time of excretion. The first portion of expelling breath is through one of the senses. You will find it rising in exhalation the amount of about twelve fingers, and by the power of inhalation it descends the amount of four fingers. It decreases at every breath by the power of eight fingers. So see how much it decreases every day; that is the decrease of one's life. It is appropriate that you reverse that [decrease] by kindness, sympathy and a gradual approach. That is, you should inhale the breath with power and exhale it with gentleness and mildness, to the point where you inhale twelve fingers and exhale four.

(4) When you have reached this station, and this condition becomes characteristic of you, closely examine three things with thought and discrimination: 1. the embryo, how it breathes while it is in the placenta, although its mother's womb does not respire; 2. the fish, how it breathes in the water and the water does not enter it; 3. and the tree, how it attracts water in its veins and causes it to reach its heights. The embryo is Sheikh Gorakh, who is Khidr (peace be upon him), the fish is Sheikh Minanath [Matsyendranāth], who is Jonah, and the tree is Sheikh Chawrangi, who is Ilyas, and they are the ones who have reached the water of life. When you have realized their [mode of] breathing by knowledge and experience, then take the lamp, which is the previously

mentioned chant (*dhikr*). Plunge into the comprehension of this state continually, until you realize it by action and experience. Then you will have reached the water of life and witnessed the hidden without intermediary. Peace.

4.20 *Haṭhapradīpikā* 2.37–43, 54–6, 68–70. Breath-control and the four additional breath-retentions:

(37) [The yogi] who has got rid of impurities such as corpulence or an imbalance of the phlegmatic humour by means of the six cleansing techniques should then tirelessly practise breath-control until it is mastered. (38) Saying that it is by means of breath-control alone that all the impurities dry up, some teachers do not approve of any other method. (39) Fearing death, even Brahmā and the other gods became intent upon breath-practice, so [the yogi] should also practise on the breath. (40) As long as the breath is restrained in the body the mind is calm. As long as the gaze is between the eyebrows there is no danger of death. (41) When all the channels have been purified by correctly performing restraints of the breath, the wind easily pierces and enters the aperture of the Suṣumnā. (42) When the wind is moving in the centre, steadiness of the mind arises. The condition of perfect steadiness of the mind is the supramental state. (43) In order to achieve that, those who know the methods perform various breath-retentions (*kumbhaka*s). Through the practice of the amazing breath-retentions one may attain amazing power (*siddhi*).

[The whistler (*sītkārī*)]

(54) [The yogi] should make a whistling noise in the mouth [while inhaling] and exhale only through the nose. By practising thus, he becomes a second god of love. (55) He is honoured by a circle of Yoginīs and can bring about creation and destruction. Neither hunger nor thirst nor sleep nor laziness afflict him. (56) His

body can change form at will and he is safe from all calamities. By means of this practice he truly becomes a lord among yogis on earth.

[The buzzer (*bhrāmarī*)]

(68) Inhaling forcefully with the sound of a male bee and exhaling slowly with the sound of a female bee: by practising thus a certain blissful levity arises in the minds of master yogis.

[The swoon (*mūrcchā*)]

(69) At the end of inhalation apply the *jālandhara* lock very tightly and exhale gently. This is called the swoon: [it produces] unconsciousness and brings happiness.

[The floater (*plāvinī*)]

(70) By completely filling the stomach with air that has been moved internally, [the yogi] can easily float like a lotus leaf, even in shallow water.

4.21 *Gheraṇḍasaṃhitā* 5.47–57. Seeded and unseeded breath-control:

(47) Assisted (*sahita*) [breath-retention (*kumbhaka*)] is said to be of two kinds: seeded (*sabīja*) and unseeded (*nirbīja*). When it is seeded, the seed mantra is repeated, when it is unseeded it is without a seed mantra.

(48) I shall teach you the seeded breath-control first. Sitting in a comfortable posture and facing east or north, the yogi should meditate on Brahmā the creator as having the quality of passion (*rajas*), the colour red and the letter *a*. (49) The wise yogi should inhale through the left channel (*iḍā*) for sixteen repetitions. At the end of the inhalation and the start of breath-retention the *uḍḍīyāna* [lock] is to be performed. (50) He should meditate on Viṣṇu as having the quality of goodness (*sattva*), the letter *u* and the colour black. He should hold his breath by means of breath-retention for sixty-four

repetitions. (51) He should meditate on Śiva as having the quality of inertia (*tamas*), the letter *ma* and the colour white, and then exhale through the solar channel for thirty-two repetitions. (52) After then inhaling through the right channel he should hold his breath before proceeding to exhale through the left channel with the seed mantra.

(53) Changing from side to side, he should practise over and over again. At the end of the inhalation until the end of retention both nostrils should be held by the little finger, the ring finger and the thumb, without the index and middle fingers.

(54) The seedless breath-control takes place without a seed mantra. The yogi should place the palm of his left hand above his left knee and move it around in a circle. Inhalation, retention and exhalation start at the first rotation and finish with the hundredth.

(55) Three types of breath-control are taught: the highest has an inhalation of twenty measures, in the middle breath-control it lasts sixteen measures and in the lowest twelve. (56) In the lowest heat is produced, in the middle the spine shakes and in the highest the yogi leaves the ground: the signs of success are threefold.

(57) Through breath-control the yogi gets the ability to move in the ether; through breath-control diseases are destroyed; through breath-control the goddess (*śakti*) is awakened; through breath-control the mind enters the supramental state. Bliss arises in the mind and the practitioner of breath-control becomes happy.

4.22 *Gheraṇḍasaṃhitā* 5.79–91. The Ajapā Gāyatrī:

(79) In a day and a night the breath goes out with the sound *haṃ* and comes back in with the sound *saḥ* 21,600 times. The vital essence (*jīva*) constantly repeats this Gāyatrī called Ajapā ('unuttered'). (80) Just as the Haṃsa is in the Base (*mūlādhāra*), so is it in the lotus in

the heart and the two nostrils. Haṃsa comes together by way of these three places.[46]

(81) The body is formed by its actions and measures ninety-six fingers. In the natural state, when air goes out of the body it travels twelve fingers. (82) When one sings it travels sixteen fingers and when one eats, twenty. When one walks it travels twenty-four fingers; in sleep, thirty fingers. During sex it is said to travel thirty-six fingers and during exercise it goes further still. (83) When its natural range decreases, then life is lengthened. Life is said to shorten when the air coming from within travels further.

(84) Thus when the breath is in the body death cannot occur. When air is confined in the body there is unaccompanied breath-retention (*kevala kumbhaka*). (85) While he is alive the yogi should recite the mantra. Unaccompanied breath-retention has the frequency of Ajapā. When unaccompanied breath-retention is performed, +if it is held for too long the rate is disrupted+. (86) For this reason alone should men perform the unaccompanied breath-retention. Unaccompanied breath-retention is at the Ajapā frequency; the supramental state (*manonmanī*) is twice that.

(87) The yogi should draw in air through the nostrils and perform unaccompanied breath-retention. On the first day he should hold it from one to sixty-four times. (88) He should do it eight times a day, every three hours, or he should do it five times a day in the manner that I shall tell you. (89) He should do it in the morning, at noon, in the evening, at midnight and in the fourth watch of the night. Otherwise he should do it at the three junctures in equal intervals every day.[47] (90) The length of Ajapā should be increased every day from one to five times until success arises. (91) The knower of yoga then calls breath-control 'unaccompanied'. When unaccompanied breath-retention is perfected there is nothing on earth that cannot be accomplished.

4.23 *Jogpradīpakā* 393–432. Breath-control:

(393) Breath-control is said to be of three kinds and it can also be accompanied with mantras. Jayatarāma has practised [it and] it resides easily in his mind.

(394) Listen to a discourse on the three kinds of breath-control. They are said to be highest, middling and lowest. Learn their differences from a guru. (395) The name breath-control (*prāṇāyāma*) is used for when one inhales, holds and exhales [the breath]. When it is accompanied by a mantra it is called full (*sagarbha*); when it does not have any mantra it is empty (*agarbha*). (396) Know the lowest breath-control to last twelve measures, the middling, twenty-four, and that which is called the highest, thirty-six.

Now the breath-control taught in the Vedas:

(397) First repeat the mantra of the guru, [then,] holding the image of the guru in your heart, practise breath-control repeatedly while sitting in a hut, engaged in yoga. (398) In cold weather practise this solar variety of breath-retention while keeping the mind focused. After lightly inhaling and exhaling, hold the breath and burn away the cold. (399) In hot weather practise various kinds of breath-retention and get rid of the heat.

Learn the two types of breath-control: that taught in the Vedas and that taught in the tantras. (400) Kṣatriyas and Brahmans practise Vedic (breath-control) and Vaishyas and Shudras that which is taught in the tantras. If Vaishyas or Shudras do the Vedic (breath-control) it is a hindrance [so] that practice is not taught. (401) Vaishyas and Shudras are not entitled to [use] Vedic mantras, which is why they cannot practise [the Vedic breath-control]. When it comes under the control of a sacred mantra the mind masters [this] excellent technique.

(402) First I shall teach the breath-control taught in the Vedas and describe its varieties. One should meditate on Prajāpati at the head, then put the hands together and

bow. (403) When one raises *prāṇa* up the Iḍā channel, one should visualize a half-moon. Know it to be extremely pure and made of the nectar of immortality. Fix the meditation in *trikuṭī* ('between the eyebrows'). (404) After making the breath flow in the solar channel, one should meditate on the sun in the navel, with tens of millions of rays, shining forth there in the navel extremely brightly. (405) Meditate thus on the heart and practise on the Iḍā and Piṅgalā (channels). No obstructions come near them and *prāṇa* and *apāna* become steady. (406) The four castes (*varṇa*s) know this to be correct; they believe the teachings of the Vedas to be true. Such people quickly enter deep *samādhi*; if one does otherwise, disease arises. (407) And those who are beyond caste division [and] always think of devotion to Viṣṇu should obtain the instruction of a true guru, study the mantra and control the breath.

Now the first [and] lowest breath-control, which lasts twelve measures (*mātrā*s), is taught.

(408) Inhale for four measures,[48] hold the breath firmly for five measures [and] exhale for three measures: that is called the lowest [breath-control].

Now the middling breath-control, which is taught to be of twenty-four measures.

(409) Inhale for seven measures, firmly hold the breath for twelve measures and exhale for five measures. That is the middling breath-control.

Now the highest breath-control, which is taught to be of thirty-six measures.

(410) Inhale for eight measures, hold the breath for nineteen measures and exhale for nine measures. That is called the highest [breath-control].

Now the results of breath-control.

(411) In the lowest [breath-control] a lot of sweat is produced. In the middling [breath-control] one trembles. In the highest [breath-control] one rises up. This is a practice whose method is to be [learnt] from the guru's

mouth. (412) Through the lowest [breath-control] one reaches heaven, middling [breath-control] gets one to the Satya Loka [and] the highest [breath-control] bestows liberation; again that is mastered according to the teachings of the guru and it [bestows] *samādhi*.

(413) Through breath-control like this all of yoga is easily obtained. Thanks to the compassion of the guru, Jayatarāma gets rid of death, the disease of existence.

Now the breath-control taught in the tantras is told.

(414) I shall teach the [mantra] pronunciation taught in the tantras, which the four castes (*varṇa*s) are entitled to practise. Kshatriyas and Brahmans, in particular, practise it in the same way that Shudras master it. (415) The practitioner should perform the practice step-by-step, progressing slowly. Inhale for four measures (*mātrā*s), hold the breath steady for eight measures, (416) exhale for four measures: one practises the first breath-control thus. In this way become absorbed, then keep the mind steady before and after. (417) Next inhale for eight [measures], hold the breath firmly for sixteen and exhale for eight; the breath rises fore and aft. (418) One should increase the practice progressively, stopping it at fifty measures. That is called the full breath-retention; understand it to be forwards, backwards and reverse (*loma*, *viloma* and *pratiloma*). (419) I shall teach creation, preservation and destruction: hear their detailed description. In these [processes] Brahmā, Viṣṇu and Rudra [respectively] are known to be the gods; one should worship and serve them. (420) The practitioner who is intent on liberation should practise breath-control. He runs ahead of the three worlds, reaches liberation and becomes absorbed in it.

Now the process of creation is taught:

(421) [Mentally] say the letters from *a* to *aḥ* [*a*, *ā*, *i*, *ī*, *u*, *ū*, *r*, *ṝ*, *l*, *ḹ*, *e*, *ai*, *o*, *au*, *aṃ*, *aḥ*], while inhaling air into the chest. While holding the breath [mentally say] the letters from *ka* to *ma* [*ka*, *kha*, *ga*, *gha*, *ṅa*, *ca*, *cha*, *ja*, *jha*, *ña*, *ṭa*, *ṭha*, *ḍa*, *ḍha*, *ṇa*, *ta*, *tha*, *da*, *dha*, *na*, *pa*, *pha*, *ba*, *bha*,

ma]. (422) Mentally say the letters from *ya* to *kṣa* [*ya*, *ra*, *la*, *va*, *śa*, *ṣa*, *sa*, *ha*, *kṣa*], while exhaling.

Now the process of preservation is taught:

Mentally say the letters from *da* to *ma* [*da*, *dha*, *na*, *pa*, *pha*, *ba*, *bha*, *ma*], while inhaling. [Mentally] say the letters from *ya* to *aḥ* [*ya*, *ra*, *la*, *va*, *śa*, *ṣa*, *sa*, *ha*, *kṣa*, *a*, *ā*, *i*, *ī*, *u*, *ū*, *ṛ*, *ṝ*, *ḷ*, *ḹ*, *e*, *ai*, *o*, *au*, *aṃ*, *aḥ*], while holding the breath. [Mentally] say the letters from *ka* to *tha* [*ka*, *kha*, *ga*, *gha*, *ṅa*, *ca*, *cha*, *ja*, *jha*, *ña*, *ṭa*, *ṭha*, *ḍa*, *ḍha*, *ṇa*, *ta*, *tha*], while exhaling.

Now the process of destruction is taught:

(423) Inhale, while [mentally] saying the letters from *kṣa* [back] to *ya* [*kṣa*, *ha*, *sa*, *ṣa*, *śa*, *va*, *la*, *ra*, *ya*]. Hold the breath firmly, while saying [mentally] the letters from *ma* [back] to *ka* [*ma*, *bha*, *ba*, *pha*, *pa*, *na*, *dha*, *da*, *tha*, *ta*, *ṇa*, *ḍha*, *ḍa*, *ṭha*, *ṭa*, *ña*, *jha*, *ja*, *cha*, *ca*, *ṅa*, *gha*, *ga*, *kha*, *ka*]. (424) Exhale, while [mentally] saying the letters *aḥ* [back] to *a* [*aḥ*, *aṃ*, *au*, *o*, *ai*, *e*, *ḹ*, *ḷ*, *ṝ*, *ṛ*, *ū*, *u*, *ī*, *i*, *ā*, *a*]. People who practise the forwards, backwards and reverse [breath-control] understand the way of yoga. (425) Whoever practises breath-control should do it forwards and backwards. That breath-control is of three parts: exhalation, inhalation and breath-retention. (426) One should practise when [the breath] is flowing through the moon: inhale fully through the moon and hold the breath in the chest. Sit in the auspicious posture (*svastikāsana*), put the left hand in the lap, (427) hold the right hand at the nose and use it to control inhalation and exhalation. Inhale through the Iḍā channel and exhale through the Piṅgalā channel. (428) Inhale again, making a noise, then firmly hold the breath and exhale. By practising this repeatedly with a straight body one masters the technique. (429) While inhaling one should clench the anus, while holding the breath one should keep it clenched and while exhaling one should release it. Know that the three parts of breath-retention should be performed thus. (430) The resolute [yogi] should apply the four locks, make his body look like a snake

and remain thus. He should put his heel at his anus and his navel against his backbone. (431) He should practise like this progressively [and] know inhalation, breath-retention and exhalation [to be thus]. He should fix it at a limit of fifty measures; that is said to be the full breath-control. (432) The way to practise breath-control has been taught in detail. Mastering it, Jayatarāma entered into dissolution and remained there.

FIVE

The Yogic Body

One of the primary conceptual frameworks for the body of the yoga practitioner in today's modern, globalized yoga is the empirical, anatomical, biological and bio-medical body.[1] The predominance of scientific and medical realism in popular yoga discourse has tended to obscure or displace more traditional visions of the body, and has thereby, *mutatis mutandis*, reshaped the perceived function of the yoga practices themselves. This is true also (and perhaps especially) when terms from yogic physiology are imported into modern practices of yoga and reinterpreted within cultural and hermeneutic parameters far removed from pre-modern ones.

Prior to the modern period, the body of the yogi was commonly conceived of as a network of psychophysical centres (*cakra*s, *granthi*s, *ādhāra*s, etc.) linked by conduits (*nāḍī*s) for the movement of various endogenous airs and vital forces (*vāyu*s, *bindu*, Kuṇḍalinī, etc.). These nexuses, conduits and substances have varying levels of empirical existence: some are visualized in meditation and others are manipulated by means of physical techniques. Some, such as Kuṇḍalinī and the *cakra*s, are to be visualized in their earliest teachings, but become increasingly corporeal and thus subject to physical manipulation. The yogic body is visualized or manipulated in order to attain special powers (*vibhūti*, *siddhi*) or to reach liberation from embodied rebirth (*mokṣa*, *mukti*, *kaivalya*, *nirvāṇa*). The body was also often conceived as a microcosm of the macrocosmic universe, complete with hells, heavens, planets, gods, etc.

Some appreciation of the predominant features and principles of such yogic bodies is therefore desirable if one wishes to understand the way yoga has been theorized and practised within the Indian traditions, particularly since the end of the first millennium CE. This is, however, not a straightforward task, even leaving to one side the hermeneutic challenges and cognitive dissonances that sometimes characterize yoga's encounter with modernity. The yogic body is a vast subject and here, as elsewhere in the history of yoga's development, there is considerable variation through time and across traditions. Different traditions present different yogic bodies, some of which are complementary and commensurable, and some of which are not (to say nothing of the vast variety of bodies in other branches of pre-modern Indian thought and praxis, such as Āyurveda).[2] This is in part because yogic bodies arise according to the particular ritual, philosophical or doctrinal requirements of the tradition at hand, and because they are expressions of these requirements, rather than descriptions of self-evident, empirical bodies common to all humans. In other words, the goals of a particular system determine the way the body is imagined and used within its yoga practices. The yogic body was – and continues to be in traditional practitioner circles – one that is constructed or 'written' on and in the body of the practitioner by the tradition itself.[3]

Furthermore, scholarship on the yogic body is as yet undeveloped. In particular, there has been no comprehensive study of the multiple conceptions of the body taught in tantric texts, which form the basis of treatments of the subject in subsequent teachings on yoga. Nevertheless, our preliminary survey of the bewildering array of textual descriptions of the yogic body does reveal significant commonalities, patterns of development and, in later texts, a widespread consensus as to some of the basic features of this body. This is particularly true for systems influenced by the theory and practice of *haṭhayoga* (post-fifteenth century), which, notwithstanding some conflicting interpretations of practices of the yogic body,[4] nonetheless offered a model which was widely accepted.

Channels, Winds and the Vital Principle

A network of channels (*nāḍīs*) within the body is fundamental to many systems of yoga. Such notions appear first in early Upaniṣadic sources, such as the *Bṛhadāraṇyaka Upaniṣad*, which mentions 72,000 channels, originating in the heart (2.1.19).[5] The

Kaṭha Upaniṣad refers to 101 channels which spread out in all directions from the heart, and singles out the channel ascending to the head as the conduit by which one can reach immortality (5.1.1), an idea which may prefigure later models of *utkrānti* ('yogic suicide') and the ascent of Kuṇḍalinī (see below, p. 178). In perhaps the earliest extant tantric text, the fifth- or sixth-century CE *Niśvāsatattvasaṃhitā*, we find a very simple model of the yogic body in which there are just two channels, Suṣumnā and Iḍā (5.1.3). Unlike later models, where Suṣumnā is the name of the central channel, here it is the northern channel and collateral with Iḍā, the southern channel, and the yogi's life-breath circulates in the space between the two, rather than in some third, central channel.[6] In vv. 140–46 of the *Vīṇāśikhatantra*, which may be as old as the *Niśvāsatattvasaṃhitā*, Suṣumnā is the familiar central channel, flanked by Iḍā and Piṅgalā. This is the schema which, with variations, would subsequently become the predominant basic model for the yogic body.[7] However, precisely what moves along the channels may differ across texts and traditions.[8]

The *Sārdhatriśatikālottara*'s tenth chapter describes a wheel (*cakra*) of ten primary channels in the navel. These are among 72,000 channels which emerge as shoots from a bulb (*kanda*) situated at the bottom of the navel region and this notion of a bulb as the source of the channels is widespread in later yoga texts (e.g. the passage from the *Vasiṣṭhasaṃhitā*, found at 5.1.9).

Notions of winds (*vāyus*) which circulate through the body are also ancient. *Prāṇa* is mentioned in the *Ṛg Veda* (1.65.10.2); the *Atharva Veda* lists four more bodily winds: *apāna*, *vyāna*, *samāna* and *udāna* (10.2.13). In the *Aitareya Brāhmaṇa* there are various systems of winds, numbering three, nine or ten (e.g. 2.1, 6.4, 29.3), and the *Jaiminīya Upaniṣad Brāhmaṇa* gives a system of six, adding *avāna* to those mentioned above (2.6.6). But it is the five first mentioned in the Vedic Saṃhitās that come to be accepted as the most important. They are taught together in the *Taittirīya Āraṇyaka* (10.33.1–5), the *Bṛhadāraṇyaka Upaniṣad* (e.g. 3.4.1), the *Chāndogya Upaniṣad* (e.g. 3.13), the *Carakasaṃhitā* (*Cikitsāsthāna* 28.5–11), the *Mahābhārata* (12.178)[9] and the *Pātañjalayogaśāstra* (5.1.7). It is in the last that they are first taught in the context of yogic practice.

Note that *prāṇa* is both a generic name for these winds and the first of this primary set of five. In the *Niśvāsatattvasaṃhitā Nayasūtra* (5.1.8) to this primary set is added a set of five subsidiary winds, of which only three are named: *nāga*, *dhanaṃjaya* and *kūrma*. The *Skandapurāṇa* (*adhyāya* 181, e.g. v. 46) and *Śivapurāṇa Vāyavīyasaṃhitā* (37.36) name the other two as *devadatta* and *kṛtaka*, and this system of ten winds became widespread in subsequent yoga texts.

The winds each have a habitual directional flow and location in the body (see, for example, the *Vasiṣṭhasaṃhitā* (5.1.9)). Yoga practices may manipulate or reverse the movement and direction of these breaths, usually with a view to inducting the primary breath into the central channel and raising it (breath-control practices are dealt with in detail in Chapter 4), but some practices also involve stopping the breath in particular locations. The *Vimānārcanākalpa* (5.1.6), for example, teaches a method of 'withdrawal' (*pratyāhāra*) in which the breath is raised through a sequence of eighteen *marman*s or 'vital points'. The winds are said to take the form of the *jīva* or vital principle of the body, which is controlled by *prāṇa* and *apāna* in particular (e.g. 5.1.4), as well as the yogi's good and bad deeds (5.1.9).

The Body as Microcosm

The body of the practitioner is often understood as a microcosmic manifestation of the macrocosmic universe, containing homologous rivers, mountains, planets and so on. Many of the systems of yoga in this book are based on such models of the body, which is not empirical or biological, but ritually and doctrinally constructed. For example, the *Parākhyatantra* (5.2.1) elaborates the movement of the *prāṇa* through the corporeally located realms of various deities. The *Amṛtasiddhi* (5.2.2) declares that all the elements of the three worlds are in the body, including planets, seers, sages and gods; and the *Siddhasiddhāntapaddhati* (5.2.3) offers a detailed mapping of the realms of the cosmos on to the body of the yogi.

Cakras, Supports and Knots: Locations in the Yogic Body

The *cakras* ('wheels'), which are also known as *padmas* ('lotuses'), are subtle focuses for meditation distributed along the central channel of the body. In yoga traditions from the twelfth century CE onwards there is a widespread consensus that the *cakras* are six in number,[10] although other numerical variations are also common. The *cakras* have become a mainstay of global yoga discourse over the past century, albeit sometimes radically reshaped according to their new hermeneutical environments (such as New Age religiosity and Jungian psychology).[11] However, as we shall see, the *cakras* were not always such a ubiquitous feature of yoga traditions and alternative or complementary schemata are common, such as supports for meditation (*ādhāras*, sixteen of which are enumerated in *Siddhasiddhāntapaddhati* 2.10–25 (5.3.10)), and knots which must be pierced (*granthis*, usually three in number, e.g. *Yogabīja* 97–8 (5.4.4) and *Gorakṣaśataka* 74–86 (5.4.3), but other schemata are found, such as a twelvefold list of knots at *Netratantra* 7.10–25).

As Sanderson puts it, surveying treatments of the yogic body in different tantric traditions: 'There are six "seasons", five "knots", five voids (*vyomas*), nine wheels, eleven wheels, twelve knots, at least three sets of sixteen loci, sixteen knots, twenty-eight vital points (*marmans*), etc.' (1986: 164). Even within single traditions, the array of locations within the yogic body can be highly complex, such as that taught in the *Netratantra* (5.3.1). What is more, unlike the *cakras*, some of these points (such as *marmans* and *ādhāras*) are not on the body's central axis (e.g. *Vimānārcanākalpa* 97 (5.1.6), *Siddhasiddhāntapaddhati* 2.11 (5.3.10)), and *cakras* themselves may even be located outside the physical body (such as the *dvādaśānta*, on which see below, pp. 178, 301). This, once again, is because certain elements of yogic physiology, in particular the *cakras* and *ādhāras*, are not a result of the yogi's empirical observation, but rather parts of a visualized installation on the body of tradition-specific metaphysics and ritual schemata.[12] In this regard, it is also interesting to note that in the *Ṣaṭsāhasrasaṃhitā* (165–76) a person who is not capable of the internal meditation on the (five) *cakras* may undertake an external *pūjā* (ritual of worship) instead (Heiligjers-Seelen 1994: 32), an alternative which may suggest that – at least in this system – the actual physical location of the *cakra*s is relatively unimportant. The variety of different schemata of places in the yogic body can appear bewildering, and indeed it may be that the redactors of some tantric texts did not themselves have substantial, specialized knowledge of the subject, thereby compounding our confusion.[13] A range of differing systems appears in our text selections for this chapter: for example, the eleven-*cakra* system found in the *c.* tenth-century *Kaulajñānanirṇaya* (5.3.5); the four-*cakra* system in the tenth-century Buddhist *Hevajratantra* (5.3.6);[14] and the nine-*cakra* system in the *c.* eighteenth-century *Siddhasiddhāntapaddhati* (5.3.9). However, we will restrict ourselves here to a brief outline of the development of what would become the predominant model of the *cakra*s for later yoga-practising traditions.

There are several precursors to the later ubiquitous six-*cakra* system. The *Mahābhārata* (12.187.51) mentions a knot (*granthi*) at the heart, the untying of which brings happiness. A navel *cakra* and heart lotus (*puṇḍarīka*) are mentioned in the *Pātañjalayogaśāstra* (1.36, 3.1, 3.29, 3.34) as focuses for meditation and several early tantras also mention *cakra*s or lotuses at the heart and navel (*Vīṇāśikhatantra* 141, 364, *Svacchandatantra* 7.20, *Sārdhatriśatikālottara* 8.32, 10.18, 11.15, 11.17). The *Svacchandatantra* (7.8) describes a nexus of channels (*nāḍī*s) configured 'like [the spokes of] a wheel' (*cakravat*), which the eleventh-century Kashmiri commentator Kṣemarāja locates in the navel and, as mentioned above, the *Sārdhatriśatikālottara*'s tenth chapter also describes a wheel of ten primary channels in the navel.

An early systematization of locations along the body's central axis is taught in the seventh- to eighth-century *Brahmayāmala* (5.3.2).[15] These nine locations, which in the passage cited are referred to as lotuses (*padma*s) and some of which are elsewhere in the text called *cakra*s, are sites for the installation of mantra-deities. The *Netratantra*, which dates to 800–850 CE, is the earliest known work to teach a system of six points all called *cakra*s (5.3.1), which the meditating yogi is to pierce 'with the spear of knowledge'. A non-tantric work, the *c.* 900 CE *Bhāgavatapurāṇa*, instructs the sage to raise his breath through six *sthāna*s or 'locations' (5.3.3). These locations correspond closely to those of the six *cakras* taught in the *c.* tenth-century *Kubjikāmatatantra* (5.3.4), which is the first text to teach the *cakra* system that became far and away the most widespread blueprint for the yogic body: (Mūl)ādhāra at the perineum, Svādhiṣṭhāna at the genitals, Maṇipūra(ka) at the navel, Anāhata at the heart, Viśuddhi in the region of the throat and Ājñā between the eyes.[16]

The *Kubjikāmatatantra* is a text of the Western Transmission (*paścimāmnāya*) of Kaula Śaivism associated with the Śākta cult of the goddess Kubjikā.[17] Its six-*cakra* system is subsequently found in texts of the Southern Transmission (*dakṣināmnāya*) of Kaula Śaivism associated with the cult of the goddess Tripurasundarī, which later came to be known as Śrīvidyā. The Śrīvidyā *Śivasaṃhitā* provides very long and detailed descriptions of the lotuses, the first of which, the Base (*ādhāra*) lotus, is given in this chapter (5.3.8). These connections enabled the subsequent popularization of the *Kubjikāmatatantra*'s system, because India's two best-known ascetic yogi lineages, those of the Nāths and Saṃnyāsīs, inherited the yoga traditions of the Western and Southern Transmissions respectively. The popularity of the *Kubjikāmatatantra*'s six-*cakra* system was subsequently reinforced by its ubiquity in modern representations of tantric and yogic esoteric anatomy, beginning perhaps with Arthur Avalon's 1919 English edition of the sixteenth-century *Ṣaṭcakranirūpaṇa* ('The Description of the Six *Cakras*'), a text in the tradition of the Southern Transmission of Kaula Śaivism (Avalon 1919; see also Taylor 2001), whose detailed descriptions of the *cakras* resemble those of the *Śivasaṃhitā*.

Included in this section is a passage from a thirteenth-century musicological text, the *Saṃgītaratnākara*, on the various emotional states which result from situating the self in the petals of the *cakras* (2.120–45, (5.3.7)). Similar (if simpler) representations are common in popular, modern conceptions of the *cakras*.[18]

In some systems, such as those of the *Śivasaṃhitā* and *Tirumandiram*, but not in those of the Paścimāmnāya and Nāth traditions, a seventh *cakra*, the Sahasrāra ('thousand-spoked'), is added to the six first taught in the *Kubjikāmatatantra*. The Sahasrāra is sometimes said to be located at the *brahmarandhra* ('the aperture of Brahmā/Brahman'), the fontanelle on the top of the skull through which the yogi's self or vital principle exits at death. This location is also called the *daśamadvāra* or 'tenth door', and is said to be the top of the Suṣumnā channel (Mallinson 2007a: 205 n.240). The Sahasrāra is also sometimes said to be beyond the body (e.g. *Śivasaṃhitā* 5.191–2). Similarly, several Śaiva texts mention a location called the Dvādaśānta ('at the end of twelve [finger-widths]'), which is a focus for meditation twelve finger-widths beyond the tip of the nose or above the *brahmarandhra*.

Kuṇḍalinī

Kuṇḍalinī (also Kuṇḍalī), meaning 'she who is coiled', signifies the power of the divine feminine (*śakti*) residing within the body of the yogi, which can be stimulated by means of yoga practices in order to actualize spiritual potential. The goddess Kuṇḍalinī is often symbolically represented as a serpent lying coiled and dormant at the base of the spine, with her head blocking the entrance to the central channel. By means of yoga practices such as visualization, breath-restraint, haṭhayogic seals, mantras and so on, the vital air (*prāṇa*) is forced out of its habitual location in the principle collateral channels (Iḍā and Piṅgalā) and into the central channel. When this occurs, Kuṇḍalinī – who resides at the entrance to the central channel (Suṣumnā), which in later sources is located at the base of the spine, but in earlier texts is sometimes said to be in the *cakra*s of the heart or the navel, or in the *kanda*, a 'bulb' located somewhere below the navel – awakens, straightens and rises up through the central axis of the body, passing through the various *cakra*s or piercing the 'knots' (*granthi*s) which lie along it (e.g. *Yogabīja* 93–9 (5.4.4)). This process gives rise to special powers (*siddhi*s) and, ultimately – when Kuṇḍalinī reaches the seat of the deity in the head, or twelve fingers beyond the head (the *dvādaśānta*) – to liberation (*mokṣa*) or immortality. Liberation is effected by her dissolution (*laya*) into Śiva at the top of the central channel (e.g. *Gorakṣaśataka* 74–86 (5.4.3)); immortality by her accessing the nectar of immortality situated in the head and flooding the body with it during her return to the base of the central channel (e.g. *Khecarīvidyā* 3.8c–14d (5.4.2)).

Kuṇḍalinī is not mentioned in the *Pātañjalayogaśāstra*; her first descriptions are in texts of tantric Śaivism. Perhaps the earliest is in the *Sārdhatriśatikālottaratantra* (12.1–2), which mentions a 'primordial coil' (*ādyā kuṇḍalinī*) in the heart. One of the first texts to describe the Kuṇḍalinī *śakti* in a yogic context is the eighth-century *Tantrasadbhāva* (15.128–30), which may also be the first to say that she takes the form of a serpent. Kuṇḍalinī is a central feature of the yoga system of the *Kubjikāmatatantra* of the Paścimāmnāya or Western Transmission of Kaula Śaivism, in which she is equated with Kubjikā, the Western Transmission's most important goddess. Like its *cakra* system, in which Kuṇḍalinī has an important role to play, the teachings on Kuṇḍalinī in the *Kubjikāmatatantra* were influential in shaping the yogic body as conceived within *haṭhayoga*.

In many Śaiva traditions Kuṇḍalinī is also the goddess of creation, the supreme energy which makes manifest the elemental principles (*tattva*s) and effects the evolution of sound. Her different functions result in her being analysed into types: Abhinavagupta talks of the *prāṇakuṇḍalinī*, the *śaktikuṇḍalinī* and *parākuṇḍalinī*, the life force, the power of creation and the supreme goddess, respectively (*Tantrāloka* 3.139c–140b). A small number of texts echo this threefold cosmogonic[19] Kuṇḍalinī by locating three Kuṇḍalinīs – lower, middle and higher – in the yogic body (see *Siddhasiddhāntapaddhati* 4.17 (5.4.5)). In the most common formulations, the ascent of a single Kuṇḍalinī reverses her cosmogonic role. As she rises through *cakra*s associated with increasingly subtle elements, creation is resorbed until finally she goes to dissolution (*laya*) by uniting with Śiva, the supreme element (on dissolution, see Chapter 9).

Although ascent through the central channel is a shared feature across yoga traditions, there is, in practice, considerable diversity in conceptions of what ascends: 'the soul or self' – designated *jīva* ('life essence') or *haṃsa* ('the gander') – vital air (*prāṇa*), seed or seminal essence (*bindu*), mantric resonance, Kuṇḍalinī, or, in Buddhist tantric systems of yoga, the fiery energy known as Caṇḍālī.[20] In the *c.* tenth-century *Pādmasaṃhitā*, Kuṇḍalinī is not represented as a dynamic, piercing force, but as a coiled obstruction that must be straightened out with heat in order to allow breath to rise up the central channel (5.4.1; cf. *Netratantra* 7.21 which mentions a blockage called Kuṇḍalā). This is noteworthy in terms of modern yoga theory and practice, as it also seems to have been how the renowned twentieth-century yogi T. Krishnamacharya (and subsequently his son, T. K. V. Desikachar) understood the nature and function of Kuṇḍalinī.[21]

Bindu

As we have seen, the Kuṇḍalinī model of the yogic body originates in early tantric traditions, and subsequently becomes assimilated into *haṭhayoga*, which in turn becomes the dominant method of yoga practice in India from the sixteenth century onwards. However, in the earliest expressions of *haṭhayoga* another, quite distinct, conception of the yogic body predominates. In this model, semen, known as *bindu* (lit. 'drop' or 'point'),[22] is returned to, and prevented from dripping from, its store in the head. Although its workings are not explained in texts prior to those of the *haṭha* corpus, this model has a clear antecedent in the ancient ascetic tradition of the *ūrdhvaretāḥ tapasvī* ('the ascetic whose seed is [turned] upwards'), who is closely associated with the practice of yoga in texts like the *Mahābhārata*, and by whom the loss of semen is to be prevented at all costs. In the bodies of ordinary men, semen continually drips from its lunar home in the head and is ejaculated or burnt up in the digestive fire. This process results in the ageing of the body and, ultimately, death. However, the (*haṭha-*) yogi can reverse this flow, impelling *bindu* upwards through the central channel and into the head by means of various *mudrā*s (on *mudrā*s, see Chapter 6), thereby attaining immortality.[23] Other *mudrā*s, such as *viparītakaraṇī* (lit. 'the inverter'), in which the body is inverted with the head down and the feet up, function to preserve *bindu* in the head and prevent its fall. This model is evident in early *haṭha* texts like the *Amṛtasiddhi* (**5.5.1**), the *Dattātreyayogaśāstra* and the *Vivekamārtaṇḍa* (**5.5.2**).

It is only with the *Amṛtasiddhi* that the notions of the accumulation of *bindu* in the head and the dripping of *bindu* from the moon (*candra*) into the sun (which is equated with the digestive fire) are first mentioned in texts. The central place of *bindu* within early *haṭhayoga* is attested to by the *c.* fourteenth-century *Amaraughaprabodha*, which in its brief description of four types of yoga explicitly identifies *haṭha* as involving techniques which use the breath and *bindu* (see 1.3.1).

Like the breath and the mind, the *bindu* of ordinary people is said to be always moving. The breath, *bindu* and mind are in fact connected, and yogic techniques which hold in check *bindu* also restrain the breath (and vice versa), and the mind is stilled as a result (*Amṛtasiddhi* 7.16–20 (5.5.1)).

In *haṭhayoga* texts from the *Vivekamārtaṇḍa* onwards, the older, *tapas*-oriented *bindu* scheme is overlaid with the tantric Kuṇḍalinī model of *layayoga*, complete with its associated *cakra* systems, which are not found in the earliest teachings on *bindu*-oriented *haṭhayoga*. As we have seen, in the tantric Paścimāmnāya tradition Kuṇḍalinī rises through the central channel and, upon reaching the store of *amṛta* ('nectar of immortality') in the head, floods the body with this liquid, thus making it immortal (*Khecarīvidyā* (5.4.2)). *Bindu*-oriented practices, on the other hand, aim to accumulate and preserve the *bindu* in the head. The merger of these two paradigms and the resultant identification of *bindu* and *amṛta* sometimes result in inconsistencies with regard to the function and goal of yoga practice. To take but one example, in the *Vivekamārtaṇḍa*, the earliest text to synthesize the two paradigms, *khecarīmudrā* is initially said to prevent *bindu* from falling (v. 51, *bindu* model), but later an identical technique is said to result in the body being flooded with *amṛta* (vv. 127–31, Kuṇḍalinī model) (5.5.2). These apparently contradictory verses are subsequently both incorporated into the description of *khecarī* in the fifteenth-century locus classicus of *haṭha*, the *Haṭhapradīpikā* (3.31–53 and 4.43–53). The *Haṭhapradīpikā*, moreover, in spite of being in large measure a compendium of earlier sources on *haṭha*, states that the purpose of *mudrā*s is to raise Kuṇḍalinī (3.5) rather than *bindu* (as was originally intended in early *haṭha* texts). Similarly, of the ten *mudrā*s of the *Śivasaṃhitā*, some work on *bindu*, some on Kuṇḍalinī, and some on both, but the text explicitly states that the purpose of *mudrā*s is the raising of Kuṇḍalinī (4.22).

The Ontological Status of the Yogic Body

The conflation of the *bindu* and Kuṇḍalinī/*cakra* models of the yogic body also results in an ontological clash. *Bindu* is a real physical substance, whereas Kuṇḍalinī and the *cakra*s – in all their early teachings and many of their later ones – are to be mentally created by the yogi. Thus in texts from the early ninth-century *Netratantra* to the early modern *Yogamārgaprakāśikā* the *cakra*s are described in passages on meditation and the yogi is instructed to visualize or imagine them. In Śaiva texts, *cakra*s may also be circular configurations of mantra-deities external to the body, to be meditated upon, and those Śaiva texts such as the *Brahmayāmala* and *Kubjikāmata* which teach internal *cakra*s also teach external *cakra*s, sometimes homologizing the two (e.g. *Brahmayāmala* 84.140).

As objects for internal meditation, the *cakra*s came to replace or appropriate the *tattva*s ('elemental levels'), which are the focuses of much tantric meditation. Thus, each *cakra* is often associated with an element and is to be visualized with that element's attributes, in a manner very similar to the elemental fixations (*dhāraṇā*s, on which see Chapter 8). But the disconnect between the physical body and Kuṇḍalinī and the *cakra*s was not absolute: in early teachings the yogi is instructed, as part of his meditation, to fix his breath at the locations of the *cakra*s when visualizing them (e.g. *Parākhyatantra* 14.81–3) or to use the breath to stimulate Kuṇḍalinī (e.g. *Pādmasaṃhitā* 2.13c–17b (**5.4.1**).[24] With the development of the *haṭhayoga* corpus, the connections between the gross body and Kuṇḍalinī and the *cakra*s became stronger. Thus, in *Gorakṣaśataka* 16–28 pulling on the tongue awakens Kuṇḍalinī (cf. **6.2.3**; in *Haṭharatnāvalī* 1.61 the haṭhayogic methods for cleaning the body are said to purify the *cakra*s (cf. **2.5.3**)).[25]

Baking and Mortification of the Body

Further reflecting the different origins of the yoga methods that work on *bindu* and Kuṇḍalinī is the sharp distinction between Kuṇḍalinī practices by means of which the body is flooded with cooling, rejuvenating *amṛta* ('the nectar of immortality'), and an important current of practice which aims to dry up or bake the body. For example, in two of the earliest texts to teach haṭhayogic methods of raising Kuṇḍalinī, the *Gorakṣaśataka* and the *Jñāneśvarī* (5.6.1), bodily secretions are dried up as Kuṇḍalinī rises through the body, after which the moon itself is also dried up and Kuṇḍalinī embraces Śiva and disappears: she does not subsequently re-descend, nor does the body get drenched in *amṛta*. In the *Yogabīja* the constituents of the body (*dhātus*) are burnt up (*dagdha*) by the fire of yoga (vv. 51 and 76; cf. 5.6.2), and the body is said to become baked (*pakva*) by means of yoga (v. 34; see also *Gorakh Sabdī* 156–7). And in the *Vivekamārtaṇḍa* (v. 58) the practice of *mahāmudrā* is said to dry up the juices of the body. These texts represent an ascetic orientation in which the body is to be mortified through *tapas*, in contrast to tantric-oriented practices, which affirm and cultivate the body. It is also, unsurprisingly, in evidence in Brahmanical yoga texts like the *Yogayājñavalkya*, in which fasting according to the phases of the moon (*cāndrāyaṇa vrata*) is said by practitioners of *tapas* to be the best way to dry up the body (2.2c–3b).[26]

Drying out the body with Kuṇḍalinī or by means of yogic practices like *mudrā* and *prāṇāyāma*[27] (which may or may not involve Kuṇḍalinī) can be considered as part of a wider, pervasive ascetic world view in which the body is an obstacle – or a mere irrelevance – within the broader soteriological framework of liberation from cyclic existence. The prevalence of this ascetic current in yoga traditions may be surprising to some contemporary practitioners of globalized yoga systems, for whom yoga is understood as intrinsically body-affirming (perhaps in contrast to perceived body-denying currents within, say, Christianity). But it is in fact this modality which predominates in renunciatory Hinduism, as well as in ascetic (i.e. non-householder) Buddhism, Jainism and so on. It can also be clearly discerned in the classical yoga of the *Pātañjalayogaśāstra* (2.40), in which the yogi cultivates a disgust for the body through the observance (*niyama*) of purity (*śauca*) (see **2.6.2**).

A Note on the *Kośa*s

Within some streams of popular modern yoga, the body is said to be composed of five 'sheaths' (*kośa*s), ascending in subtlety from the gross 'food sheath' (*annamayakośa*) through sheaths constituted of (*-maya-*) *prāṇa*, mind (*manas*), discernment (*vijñāna*) and bliss (*ānanda*).[28] This scheme is first outlined in the *Taittirīya Upaniṣad* (2.1–5), but it is not found in any pre-seventeenth century texts on yoga, suggesting that it is a later addition to yoga theory. Perhaps its earliest mention is in the 1623 CE *Yuktabhavadeva*, an otherwise lengthy and comprehensive text on yoga, which devotes just one line (3.6) to the *kośa*s. The only other mentions of the *kośa*s occur in the post-*Haṭhapradīpikā* 'Yoga Upaniṣads', the *Triśikhībrāhmaṇopaniṣad* (12–13) and the *Tejobindūpaniṣad* (4.74–5 and 6.56), where again they are presented without any detail or explanation. More research is required, but it may be the case that as Vedānta became the dominant philosophy in India, and as *haṭhayoga* became widely assimilated across traditions, this Upaniṣadic model of the body was grafted on to – or displaced – other, more commonly accepted conceptions of the yogic body. Until the modern age, however, the *kośa* model of the yogic body is insignificant in comparison to the schemata outlined above.

Chapter Contents

5.1 Channels and Winds

5.1.1 *Kaṭha upaniṣad* 6.16. The channels.

5.1.2 *Mahābhārata* 12.178.15a–16b. The channels and breaths.

5.1.3 *Niśvāsatattvasaṃhitā Uttarasūtra* 5.37a–39b. The channels.

5.1.4 *Parākhyatantra* 14.51–61. The channels and winds.

5.1.5 *Hevajratantra* 1.13–20. The channels.

5.1.6 *Vimānārcanākalpa* 97. Raising the breath through the eighteen *marmans*.

5.1.7 *Pātañjalayogaśāstra* 3.39. The five winds.

5.1.8 *Niśvāsatattvasaṃhitā Nayasūtra* 4.119–33. The breaths.

5.1.9 *Vasiṣṭhasaṃhitā* 2.1–55. The purification of the channels (*nāḍīśuddhi*) and the location of the breaths.

5.1.10 *Haṭharatnāvalī* 4.33–40. The channels.

5.1.11 *Vivekamārtaṇḍa* 23c–27d. The vital principle.

5.2 The Body as Microcosm

5.2.1 *Parākhyatantra* 14.69–72. Winds and channels in the body.

5.2.2 *Amṛtasiddhi* 1.15–21, 2.1–8. The universe in the body and the Goddess of the Centre.

5.2.3 *Siddhasiddhāntapaddhati* 3.1–5. The realms within the body.

5.2.4 *Śivasaṃhitā* 2.13–20. The channels.

5.3 *Cakra*s, Supports and Knots

5.3.1 *Netratantra* 7.1–5, 28c–30d. Subtle meditation using the yogic body and the six *cakra*s.

5.3.2 *Brahmayāmala* 12.60c–62d. The sites of *nyāsa* ('mantra-installation').

5.3.3 *Bhāgavatapurāṇa* 2.2.19–21. The six places to fix the breath.

5.3.4 *Kubjikāmatatantra* 11.34c–37d. The six *cakra*s.

5.3.5 *Kaulajñānanirṇaya* 5.21cd–32. The eleven *cakra*s.

5.3.6 *Hevajratantra* 1.21–31. The four *cakra*s.

5.3.7 *Saṃgītaratnākara* 2.120–39. The emotional states resulting from situating the self in the petals of the *cakra*s.

5.3.8 *Śivasaṃhitā* 5.77–103. The Base (*ādhāra*) lotus.

5.3.9 *Siddhasiddhāntapaddhati* 2.1–9. The nine *cakra*s.

5.3.10 *Siddhasiddhāntapaddhati* 2.10–25. The sixteen supports (*ādhāra*s).

5.4 Kuṇḍalinī

5.4.1 *Pādmasaṃhitā* 2.13c–17b. Kuṇḍalī.

5.4.2 *Khecarīvidyā* 3.8c–14d. Kuṇḍalinī.

5.4.3 *Gorakṣaśataka* 74–86. Kuṇḍalinī.

5.4.4 *Yogabīja* 93–9. Kuṇḍalinī and piercing the knots.

5.4.5 *Siddhasiddhāntapaddhati* 4.14–27. Kuṇḍalinī.

5.5 Nectar, *Bindu*, Moon

5.5.1 *Amṛtasiddhi* Chapters 3, 4, 5 and 7. The moon, sun and fire, and the restraint of *bindu*.

5.5.2 *Vivekamārtaṇḍa* 126–31. Keeping the body full of *amṛta* and so immortal.

5.5.3 *Jñāneśvarī* 6.247–70. The transformation of the body with the nectar of immortality.

5.5.4 *Lallāvākyāni* 22. The moon.

5.5.5 *Gorakṣa Bijaẏ* 1, 4–8. The practice of the moons.

5.6 Baking and Mortification of the Body

5.6.1 *Jñāneśvarī* 6.228–40. Kuṇḍalinī's awakening.

5.6.2 *Yogabīja* 49–53. Baking the body's constituents in the fire of yoga.

5.1

Channels and Winds

5.1.1 *Kaṭha Upaniṣad* 6.16. The channels:

There are 101 channels (*nāḍīs*) of the heart. One of them flows to the head. Going upwards by means of it, one reaches immortality. The others spread up and out in all directions.

5.1.2 *Mahābhārata* 12.178.15a–16b. The channels and breaths:

(15) Issuing from the heart, the ten channels all carry the nourishing essence of food sideways, upwards and downwards, driven by the breaths. (16) And this is the way of the yogis, by which they go to the supreme state (*tatpadam*).

5.1.3 *Niśvāsatattvasaṃhitā Uttarasūtra* 5.37a–39b.[29] The channels:

(37) The upward breath is taught to be 'day' and the downward breath is 'night'. [The tube called] Suṣumnā should be known to be the northward [movement of the sun]; Iḍā is the southern movement. (38–39b) When the [life-breath that in some sense carries and is therefore identified with the] 'soul' is in the centre [between the two above-mentioned tubes], then the wise know this to be 'equinox'. When the 'soul' comes and goes [from or] into the centre, then this is taught to be 'transition'. Hear from me also about *śakti*.

5.1.4 *Parākhyatantra* 14.51–61. The channels and winds:[30]

(51) Having [thus] achieved the conquest of the fixations (*dhāraṇās*), [and being thereby] successful in achieving the rewards that are the strengths of those [fixations], the yogi should engage in yoga[-meditation] upon the

cage that is [the earthly] body, [and which is for his practice of yoga] the most important element.

(52) Even yoga cannot accomplish its fruits if it is devoid of a support. Its support is the body, which is covered with a network of tubular vessels (*sirās*). (53) Some among these are gross vessels; others are subtle and extremely subtle. They are called channels (*nāḍīs*); in those take place the movements of the wind in this body.

(54) The wind in the vessels kindles the fire in the belly. +That [fire in turn] troubles the eater, and therefore that is brought into equilibrium by [the wind called] *samāna* +. (55–56b) It flows in the form of nourishing fluid into the openings of the channels. It constantly causes the increase of the group of substances semen, marrow and bone, and also of blood, flesh and phlegm, as well as of its tubes. (56c–57) The tubes that are located in the navel reach below that to the bulb above the testicles. The tubes that are located in [the bulb] spread outwards in all directions: sideways, upwards, downwards. Among these there are eight principal ones that go to the extremities of the petals of the lotus of the man's heart.

(58) Aindrī, that in [the direction of] Agni, Yāmyā, Nairṛtyā, Āpyā, that in [the direction of] the wind, Kauberī, and the tube Śāṅkarī; they are the locuses of the deities of the directions.

(59–60) In these [tubes] the soul (*kṣetrin*), [usually] situated in the central receptacle[31] [of the lotus of the heart] moves about from petal to petal. Whatever be the nature of the deity of the direction, he then [i.e. upon moving into that direction] becomes of the nature of that [deity]. By moving into the gaps between those petals the bound soul becomes empty-natured: he thinks himself to be as it were empty because he appears to be qualified by the adventitious quality of emptiness.

(61) Thus, located in the centre of the lotus of the heart, the vital principle (*jīva*) 'moves about' in all directions,

since, when situated there, the individual (*pudgala*) observes everything. For when it is situated there, [the soul] is said to be especially all-pervading.

5.1.5 *Hevajratantra* 1.13–20. The channels:

Vajragarbha said:

(13) O Lord, how many channels are in the *vajra* body?

The Lord said:

Thirty-two channels. Thirty-two flow in the place of great happiness, carrying semen (*bodhicitta*). In their middle are the three most important channels: Lalanā, Rasanā and Avadhūtī.

(14) Lalanā has Wisdom (*prajñā*) as its nature; Rasanā consists in Means (*upāya*) [and] Avadhūtī is in the area in between, devoid of the perceived and the perceiver. (15) Lalanā carries semen, Rasanā carries blood [and] she who is called the carrier of blood and semen is known as Avadhūtī.

(16) [The thirty-two channels are] Abhedyā, Sūkṣmarūpā, Divyā, Vāmā, Vāminī, Kūrmajā, Bhāvakī, Sekā, Doṣā, Viṣṭā, Mātarī, Śavarī, Śītadā, Uṣmā, Lalanā, Avadhūtī, Rasanā, (17) Pravaṇā, Kṛṣṇavarṇā, Surūpiṇī, Sāmānyā, Hetudāyikā, (18) Viyogā, Premaṇī, Siddhā, Pāvakī, Sumanāḥ, Traivṛttā, Kāminī, Gehā, Caṇḍikā [and] Māradārikā.

Vajragarbha said:

(19) What are these thirty-two channels like, O Lord?

The Lord said:

(20) They are all transformations of the three modes of being, devoid of the perceived and of the perceiver. Alternatively, as means they are all conceived with the characteristics of objective phenomena.

5.1.6 *Vimānārcanākalpa* 97. Raising the breath through the eighteen *marmans*:[32]

The eighteen vital points (*marmans*) [and] their characteristics.

Big toe, ankle, middle of the shank, root of the shin (*citimūla*),[33] knee, middle of the thigh, anus, middle of the body, penis, navel, heart, throat, root of the palate, bridge of the nose, the region of the eyes, the space between the eyebrows, forehead [and] crown: these are the eighteen locations.

Their measurements [are as follows]: the size of the foot is four and a half fingers. Then the ankle is one finger. Then the middle of the shank is ten fingers. Then the root of the shin is ten fingers. Then the knee is two fingers. Then the middle of the thigh is nine fingers. The region of the anus is nine fingers. Then the middle of the body is three and a half fingers. Then the root of the penis is two and a half fingers. The navel is four fingers. Then the middle of the chest is eleven fingers. Then the Adam's apple (*kaṇṭhakūbara*)[34] is twelve fingers. The root of the palate is six fingers. Then the bridge of the nose is four fingers. The region of the eyes is two fingers. The space between the eyebrows is two fingers. Then the top of the forehead is two fingers. The crown is three fingers.

After raising the breath through these locations by means of the mind, one should draw it upwards or downwards from [each] location in sequence and hold the breath [there]. After raising the breath through the Iḍā and Piṅgalā channels on both sides of she who is coiled (*kuṇḍalī*) one should inhale, then raise the breath that is in the abdomen through the nostrils and inhale, then raise the two [?] (*kurcau*) into the space between the eyebrows and hold them there. One should regularly practise in this way. It is known that after raising the breath of the self up to the space between the eyebrows by way of the Suṣumnā channel one should restrain [it] until the rising of the orb (? *maṇḍalodaya*).

5.1.7 *Pātañjalayogaśāstra* 3.39. The five winds:

> By mastering the *udāna* wind, water, mud and thorns do not stick [to the yogi] and [he is able to perform] yogic suicide (*utkrānti*).

Life is activity of all the sense organs, characterized by [the flow of] *prāṇa* and the other [winds]. Life's actions are fivefold. *Prāṇa* flows through the mouth and nose [and] is active as far as the heart. *Samāna* [is so called] because it carries [nourishment] equally [through the body]; it is active as far as the navel. *Apāna* [is so called] because it carries away [food, drink, faeces, urine and semen]; it is active as far as the soles of the feet. *Udāna* [is so called] because it carries [bodily fluids] upwards; it is active up to the head. *Vyāna* is so called because it pervades [the body]. The most important of these is *prāṇa*.

5.1.8 *Niśvāsatattvasaṃhitā Nayasūtra* 4.119–33. The breaths:[35]

> (119) These [five breaths] beginning with *prāṇa* are situated [respectively] in the heart (*prāṇa*), anus (*apāna*), navel (*samāna*), throat (*udāna*) and all joints (*vyāna*). Hear from me [their] colour[s] and sound[s]. (120–21) Having the appearance of molten silver; yellow; like a firefly; milky; crystalline: this is the definition of the colours of the five [breaths]. Bell; gong; sweet; elephant-trumpeting; many/much sounds: this is said to be the [group of] sound[s] of the five beginning with *prāṇa*.
>
> (122–5) Talking, laughing, singing, dancing, fighting, the arts (?), craft, all tasks: these are the activities of *prāṇa*. The downward breath (*apāna*) allows food and drink to enter the body; it causes human waste to flow down [out from the body]; it will also cause blindness and ear disease. *Samāna* homogenizes what is eaten, licked, drunk. The function[s] of the rising breath (*udāna*) are sneezing, hiccoughs, vomiting and coughing. These are the functions of *vyāna*: horripilation, sweating; it causes [stomach-]pain; it causes the limbs to bend, and it knows the sense of touch.
>
> (126–8) In the big toes, the knees, the heart, the eyes and

the head are the [five subsidiary breaths] beginning with *nāga*, which have various forms; hear from me their function[s]. [The first four] produce pleasure, excitement, drying, terror. The other, *dhanaṃjaya*, who joins [the soul to its next embodiment], produces sleep and weariness. (129) The *kūrma* alone remains [at death] and does not leave by exiting [the body]. The *kūrma* causes the corpse to contract and dries it out.

(130) It is *prāṇa* that he should conquer first; once *prāṇa* is conquered, the mind is conquered; once the mind is conquered the soul is calmed. (131) *Prāṇa* together with *apāna* one should visualize in the anus; *prāṇa* together with *samāna* in the navel; *prāṇa* together with *udāna* in the throat; *prāṇa* together with *vyāna* [one should visualize] everywhere [in the body].

(132–3) He should restrain *nāga* and the other [five breaths, [each] together with *prāṇa* in their proper places. I will teach [you] the time for [which] each one [should be] restrained: listen. [Each breath] should be held for [a period] from one *tāla* going up to 500 [*tāla*s]. In this way breath will be conquered; [it will be capable of] performing the functions of migration [into another living being's body] and [yogic suicide by] exiting [the body].

[Hereafter, (134–44) describe the joining of the breaths in different parts of the body, the application of mantras and the experiences that arise as a result, e.g. by joining *prāṇa* and *apāna* in the navel, trembling arises (137); by joining them in the heart, the yogi faints (138); by blocking *prāṇa* in the centre of the eyebrows, he will fall into a deep sleep and instantly awaken (140). Finally, he attains the special power (*siddhi*) of omniscience (143–44b).]

5.1.9 *Vasiṣṭhasaṃhitā* 2.1–55. The purification of the channels (*nāḍīśuddhi*) and the location of the breaths:

[Śakti said:]

(1) Blessed lord, teach me the purification of the channels according to the rules: by what method are the channels of all embodied beings purified? (2) And [teach me] the origin of the channels and their correct maintenance. What is the bulb (*kanda*) said to be like? How many breaths are there? (3) And [I] must know the locations of the breaths and their various separate functions in the body, O best of embodied beings. Please teach [them] as they truly are; no one other than you knows.

(4) Having been spoken to thus by Śakti, the yogi [Vasiṣṭha], his mind duly focused on that [subject], looked at his son with compassion and explained everything.

Vasiṣṭha said:

(5) First, O Brahman, you should know this: the body of all creatures is ninety-six fingers [long] when measured by its own fingers. (6) In the body there are thirty-two bones on either side of the spine and 72,000 channels are fixed [in it], too. (7) *Prāṇa* measures twelve fingers more than the body. The breath (*vāyu*) causes activity (*prayāṇa*), which is why it is called *prāṇa*. (8) In the middle of the body is the place of fire, which resembles molten gold. In humans it is triangular, in four-footed animals square and in birds it is circular. I am telling you what is true. (9) In the middle of that a slender flame constantly burns.

If you want to hear where the middle of the body (*dehamadhya*) is, listen. (10) The region [measuring] one finger [wide] in the middle of the area two fingers above the anus and two fingers below the penis is called the middle of the body. (11) There is a bulb in this body nine fingers from the middle of the body. It is four fingers wide and four fingers high. (12) It resembles an egg in shape and is surrounded by skin and bone. Its middle is called the navel (*nābhi*) and from that a wheel (*cakra*) arises. (13) The wheel has twelve spokes and it is the foundation of the body. The vital principle (*jīva*) wanders in this wheel, driven on by the effects of its good and bad deeds. (14) In the same way that a spider wanders about in its web, so the *prāṇa* of the vital principle moves lower down in the wheel at the base (*mūlacakra*). (15) The vital principle in all bodies can become constantly steady by means of *prāṇa*.

Above that [*cakra*], above, below and to the side of the navel, is the place of Kuṇḍalinī. (16) She who has the form of the eight constituents of matter (*aṣṭaprakṛti*), and [so] is coiled eight times, [and] who starts with *a* and ends with *kṣa*[36] is called Kuṇḍalinī. She constantly checks the proper flow of the breath, (17) covering the mouth of the aperture of Brahman with her mouth. But at the time of yoga she is woken by the *apāna* breath together with fire. (18) Flashing forth from the space in the heart in the form of a blazing snake, always dancing in the middle of the space in the heart of yogis, +she then, together with the breath,+ goes by way of the Suṣumnā.

(19) The channel located in the middle of the bulb is called Suṣumnā. All those which are called channels in this wheel are located around it. (20) Of all the channels, fourteen are pre-eminent, my son. (21) Suṣumnā, Iḍā, Piṅgalā and Sarasvatī; (22) Kuhū, Varaṇā and the seventh, Yaśasvinī; Pūṣā, Payasvinī and Śaṅkhinī, the tenth; (23) Gāndhārī, Hastijihvā, Viśvodarā and Alambuṣā: of all [channels] these fourteen are pre-eminent.

(24) Among them three are especially important, and among those three one is considered to be the best on the path to liberation. She is the blazing Suṣumnā, who supports the universe. (25) The Suṣumnā is firmly fixed in the middle of the bulb, my son. Together with the backbone, she is [also] permanently located in the head. (26) As the path to liberation in the aperture of Brahman, she is known as Suṣumnā. When unmanifest and subtle she is to be known as Vaiṣṇavī.

(27) Iḍā and Piṅgalā are on her left and right. Iḍā is situated to her left and Piṅgalā on the right. (28) The moon and sun move in Iḍā and Piṅgalā. Know the moon to be in Iḍā; the sun is said to be in Piṅgalā. (29) The moon is said to have a predominance of the *tamas guṇa*, and the sun of *rajas*; it is these two that cause time, with its days and nights. (30) Suṣumnā consumes time: this that has been taught is a secret.

(31) Sarasvatī and Kuhū are situated on either side of Suṣumnā. Gāndhārī and Hastijihvā are behind and in front of Iḍā. Pūṣā and Yaśasvinī are behind and in front of Piṅgalā. (32) Viśvodarā is situated between Kuhū and Hastijihvā, and Varaṇā is fixed between Yaśasvinī and Kuhū. (33) Payasvinī is situated between Pūṣā and Sarasvatī, and Śaṅkhinī is situated between Gāndhārī and Sarasvatī. (34) And, O best of Brahmans, Alambuṣā is situated below the middle of the bulb. Kuhū is situated on the front part of the Suṣumnā and extends as far as the end of the penis. (35) Know Varaṇā to pervade the body, below and above. And Yaśasvinī extends as far as the big toe of the right foot. (36) And know Piṅgalā, my son, to go upwards on the right as far as the nose, and Pūṣā to be on the right, behind Piṅgalā, as far as the eye. (37) And Payasvinī, O best of Brahmans, is on the right, extending as far as the ear, and Sarasvatī is in the upper part [of the body] as far as the tongue. (38) O Brahman sage, Śaṅkhinī reaches upwards as far as the left ear. Gāndhārī is situated behind Iḍā and ends at the left eye. (39) Iḍā ends at the left nostril; Piṅgalā is taught to be [the same] on the right. Know Pūṣā [also] to be located on the left side, and Hastijihvā extends as far as the left big toe. (40) Viśvodarā is the channel which goes everywhere on the left side. Alambuṣā is on the left side, below the anus. (41) The other channels originate in these ones, and others in them too. Know [the channels arising in] all channels to be like [the veins] in a fig leaf (*aśvatthadala*).

(42) *Prāṇa*, *apāna*, *samāna*, *udāna*, *vyāna*, *nāga*, *kūrma*, *kṛkara*, *devadatta*, *dhanaṃjaya*: (43) these ten breaths flow through all the channels. Among these, the five breaths beginning with *prāṇa* are considered pre-eminent. (44) Of them the most important is *prāṇa*, which has its base below the bulb. It moves in the mouth, the nostrils, the heart, the navel region and the big toe, and stops in these places. (45) *Apāna* is in the penis and anus, in the thighs, testicles and knees, and in the shanks and belly, and in the waist and in the root of the navel. (46) *Vyāna* is between the ears and eyes, in the neck and the ankles, in the nose, the throat and the region of the eyes, and it stops in these locations. (47) *Udāna* is in all the joints and the feet and hands too. (48) *Samāna* is always in the body, pervading it. Together with the fire, it carries all the fluid produced by digestion to every part of the body. (49) Moving through the 72,000 channels, the *samāna* breath is the only one that pervades the body. (50) The five breaths beginning with *nāga* are located in the skin and bones and so forth. (51) The functions of *prāṇa* are inhalation, exhalation, coughing and so forth. The function of the *apāna* breath is the expulsion of faeces, urine and so forth. The functions of *vyāna* are said to be activities such as letting go of and taking things. (52) The functions of *udāna* are said to be those such as raising the body. The functions of *samāna* are those such as nourishment of the body. (53) The functions of *nāga* are vomiting and so forth. Of *kūrma* they are actions such as blinking and of *kṛkara*, sneezing and so forth. (54) The function of *devadatta*, O lord of Brahmans, is to create fatigue. Of *dhanaṃjaya*, the functions are desiccation and so forth.

All the functions [of the channels] have been proclaimed.

(55) Having carefully learnt thus the system of the channels and the locations of the breaths, [the yogi] should practise purification of the channels according to the instructions.[37]

5.1.10 *Haṭharatnāvalī* 4.33–40. The channels:

(33) The *cakra* which is located at the root *ādhāra* and which resembles a hen's egg is known as the Channel (*nāḍī*) *cakra*. All the channels meet there.

(34–5) Among all the channels, there are fourteen principle ones: Suṣumnā, Piṅgalā, Sarasvatī, Kuhu, Yaśasvinī, Vāruṇī, Gāndhārī, Śaṅkhinī, Pūṣā, Viśvodarī, Jihvā, Alambuṣā, Haṃsinī and Iḍā. These fourteen are the most important.

(36) Of these (fourteen) three are primary and, out of those three, one is the best. Moon (*soma*) and sun (*sūrya*) reside within Iḍā and Piṅgalā.

(37) Their predominant characteristics are inertia and passion, [and] they are situated on the left and right. Understand Iḍā to be the moon, the maker of night, and Piṅgalā to have the form of the sun.

(38) The spine (*vīṇādaṇḍa*)[38] is Mount Meru [and] the bones are the major mountains. Iḍā is said to be the river Gaṅgā, Piṅgalā is the river Yamunā, [and] Suṣumnā is the river Sarasvatī. (39) The other channels are the rivers. The seven bodily constituents are the islands, with sweat, saliva and so forth their waves.

(40) The Fire of Time (*kālāgni*) is at the root (*mūla*). The disc of the moon is at the skull. Other heavenly bodies are said to exist like this [in the body]. The wise should practise yoga on them.

5.1.11 *Vivekamārtaṇḍa* 23c–27d. The vital principle:

These [breaths] exist in the thousands of channels in the form of the vital principle (*jīva*). (24) Under the control of *prāṇa* and *apāna* the vital principle rushes up and down. Because it is so flighty it is not seen in the left and right paths. (25) In the same way that a ball jumps when hit by a stick, so the vital principle, tossed about by *prāṇa* and *apāna*, does not rest. (26) In the same way that a hawk tied by a rope is pulled back when it moves away, so the vital principle, bound by the *guṇas*,[39] is pulled by *prāṇa* and *apāna*. (27) *Apāna* pulls *prāṇa* and *prāṇa* pulls *apāna*, like the bird and the rope. He who knows this knows yoga.

5.2

The Body as Microcosm

5.2.1 *Parākhyatantra* 14.69–72. Winds and channels in the body:[40]

(69–70b) The breath is called the vital principle (*prāṇajīva*); because of its movement we speak figuratively of movement [of the soul], since without it we say that [a body is] dead. The manifestation of consciousness has that [breath] as its locus; where [the breath] goes, there it [viz. the manifestation of consciousness] will be.

(70c–71) Above the lotus of the heart there are two principal channels to the left and right of it. That which passes on the left is mild [and] belongs to the moon; that which passes on the right is fiery [and] belongs to the sun. Adorned with the moon and the sun is the central channel (*madhyā*), which is foremost among all the channels.

(72) That [breath] moves – by the middle course or by the right [or] by the left – to the heart, the throat, then the palate, the middle of the brows, the tip of the nose. (73–4) From there it travels up twelve digits and returns from that place. Brahmā is in the heart, Viṣṇu in the throat, Rudra in the palate, and Īśvara is between the brows, and at the tip of the nose is Sadāśiva. [Thus] the various places are taught in accordance with [their] various deities, for the purpose of [gradual] reabsorption.

5.2.2 *Amṛtasiddhi* 1.15–21, 2.1–8. The universe in the body and the Goddess of the Centre:

(15) [Mount Meru] exists in the body, with seven islands, three worlds and fourteen levels. (16) In it are oceans, rivers, regions [and] guardians of the regions; gathering places (*chandohas*), sacred sites, seats [of deities and] the deities of the seats; (17) lunar mansions, all the planets, sages and holy men; the moon and the sun, moving about causing creation and destruction; (18) the sky, the wind and fire; water and earth; Viṣṇu divided and undivided, [Śiva] the lord of beings (*bhūtanātha*) [and] Prajāpati. (19) The elements which [exist] in the three worlds are all [found] in the body [and] the elements which are in the body [also] exist elsewhere.

(20) A human birth is attained through great merit and good fortune. When the teaching of the guru is established, one does not go to +the sole destination+. (21) Having verified [him], prostrate yourself at the feet of the true guru so that the sorrows of transmigration, even if they are great, are dissolved.

Thus ends [Chapter 1 of the *Amṛtasiddhi*,] the Inquiry into the Body.

[Chapter 2, the General Inquiry into the Goddess of the Centre (Madhyamā)]

(1) Activity takes place all around [Mount] Meru, but in the middle is a pathway without peer. It is situated around [Mount] Meru. (2) It has two sacred openings in it, at its top and bottom. The splitting of the lower door occurs spontaneously at birth and death. (3) Those fortunate mortals who have knowledge, vigour and great strength enter by way of the door of creation and go to the door of liberation. (4) This goddess, the great knowledge (*mahāvidyā*), is hard for even the gods to reach. She is said to be the creator of all [beings] [and] the destroyer of ignorance. (5) All her mighty goddesses are located at the door of creation. The lord, with parts and whole, is situated at the door of liberation. (6) Some

call [her] the place of Avadhūtī, the cremation ground [and] the great pathway; some call her the substrate, Suṣumnā and Sarasvatī. (7) In different doctrines she has different names, [but] she is always one to those who have the eye of knowledge. Dependent on her the elements reside in the body of man. (8) She flows between Gaṅgā and Yamunā alone, endowed with bliss. After bathing in the confluence of those [three channels] the fortunate ones go to the supreme destination.

5.2.3 *Siddhasiddhāntapaddhati* 3.1–5. The realms within the body:

Now the understanding of the body is taught:

(1) The yogi who knows all things in the body, movable and immovable, gets understanding of the body.

(2) The turtle resides in the sole of the foot. [The subterranean realm called] Pātāla is in the big toe. [The underworld called] Talātala is in the tip of the big toe. [That called] Mahātala is in the top of the foot. [That called] Rasātala is in the ankle. [That called] Sutala is in the lower leg. [That called] Vitala is in the knees. [That called] Atala is in the thighs.

The seven lower realms are located thus under the sovereignty of the god Rudra. In the midst of the body is the emotion whose form is anger. It is Rudra as the fire of time (*kālāgnirudra*).

(3) The earth realm is at the anus. The realm of the atmosphere is at the penis. The heavenly realm is at the navel.

Indra is the deity in these three realms. Indeed, it is Indra who governs all the sense faculties within the body.

(4) The Mahar realm is at the coccyx. The Jana realm is in the hollow of the spine. The Tapas realm is in the spinal cord. The Satya realm is in the root lotus.

Brahmā is the deity in these four realms. He resides within the body in his manifold forms of pride and conceit.

(5) The realm of Viṣṇu is at the belly. Viṣṇu is the deity there and he carries out various functions within the body.

The realm of Rudra is at the heart. Rudra is the deity there. He resides within the body in his fierce form.

The realm of Īśvara is at the chest. Īśvara is the deity there and he takes the form of satisfaction within the body.

The realm of Sadāśiva is at the base of throat. Sadāśiva is the deity there. He resides within the body in his gentle form.

The realm of Nīlakaṇṭha ('Blue-throated [Śiva]') is in the middle of the throat. Nīlakaṇṭha is the deity there. He resides within the body in his form as [the granter of] safety.

The realm of Śiva is at the opening of the palate. Śiva is the deity there. He resides within the body in his peerless form.

The realm of Bhairava is at the root of the uvula. Bhairava is the deity there. He resides within the body in the best of all forms.

The realm of the Great Adept (*mahāsiddha*) is in there [i.e. the realm of Bhairava]. The Great Adept is the deity there. He resides within the body in his form as awakening.

The realm of the Beginningless (*anādi*) is in the forehead. The Beginningless is the deity there. He resides within the body in the form of ego intent on bliss.

The realm of the Kula is at the *śṛṅgāṭa*.[41]

The Lord of the Kula (Kuleśvara) is the deity there. He resides within the body in his bliss form.

The realm of the Lord of the not-Kula (Akuleśa) is in the lotus at the temple. The deity Akuleśa resides there within the body, as the state of having no pride.

The realm of the supreme Brahman is at the aperture of Brahman (*brahmarandhra*).[42] The deity there is the supreme Brahman. He dwells within the body as the state of completeness.

The realm of Parāpara is at the upper lotus. The

supreme Lord (Parameśvara) is the deity there. He resides within the body as the state of *parāpara* ('beyond and not beyond').

The realm of the goddess (*śakti*) is at the place of the three peaks (*trikūṭa*). The supreme goddess (*parāśakti*) is the deity there. She dwells within the body as the states of existence and omnipotence found in all [goddesses].

Thus [concludes] the discussion of the twenty-one locations in the egg of Brahmā [that is] the body, together with the seven underworlds.

5.2.4 *Śivasaṃhitā* 2.13–20. The channels:

(13) There are 350,000 channels in the human body. Of these, fourteen are the most important: (14) Suṣumnā, Iḍā, Piṅgalā, Gāndhārī, Hastijihvikā, Kuhā, Sarasvatī, Pūṣā, Śaṅkhinī, Payasvinī, (15) Vāruṇī, Alambuṣā, Viśvodarī and Yaśasvinī.

Of these, three are pre-eminent: Piṅgalā, Iḍā and Suṣumnā. (16) Of the three, Suṣumnā is the most important, the sweetheart of the master yogis. The other channels in embodied beings are connected to her. (17) The three channels face downwards and resemble lotus fibres. They are joined to the spinal column and take the form of the moon, the sun and fire. (18) In their middle is the Citrā channel. She is beloved of me. In her is the aperture of Brahman (*brahmarandhra*), which is considered to be extremely subtle. (19) Resplendent in five colours, she is pure, goes through the middle of Suṣumnā, is the substrate of the body and has a different appearance from Suṣumnā. (20) This divine path is said to bestow immortality and bliss. Merely by meditating on it the master yogi destroys all his sins.

5.3

Cakras, Supports and Knots

5.3.1 *Netratantra* 7.1–5, 28c–30d. Subtle meditation using the yogic body and the six *cakras*:

(1) Next I shall teach the peerless subtle meditation. Possessing six *cakras*, sixteen supports (*ādhāras*), three focuses (*lakṣyas*), five voids (*vyomas*), (2) twelve knots (*granthis*), three powers (*śaktis*), a pathway to the three abodes [and] three [main] channels: (3–5) knowing the beautiful body to be thus, but [finding it] filled with the pathways of ten [other main] channels, overrun with a mass of [yet more] channels, 35,072,000 of them, filthy and rife with diseases, the yogi nourishes either his body or someone else's with the nectar of immortality that has arisen from the great subtle meditation [and] gets a divine body free from all diseases. [. . .]

In the [place] called [the organ of] generation (*janma*) is the Nāḍi *cakra*; in the navel the great [*cakra*] called Māyā; (29) the Yogi *cakra* is in the heart; [the *cakra*] at the palate is called Bhedana; at the *bindu* [in the forehead][43] is the Dīpti *cakra*; the *cakra* at *nāda* is called Śānta. (30) [The yogi] should pierce all the [*cakras*] which have just been taught with the spear of knowledge.

5.3.2 *Brahmayāmala* 12.60c–62d. The sites of *nyāsa* ('mantra-installation'):

Having installed the sacred syllable called Bhairava (*hūṃ*) on the crest + . . . + (61) and Raktā on the forehead, he should install Karāla on the mouth. He should install Caṇḍākṣī on the throat lotus [and] Mahocchuṣmā on the heart. (62) Karālī is on the lotus of the navel, Danturā on the lotus of the genitals, Bhīmavaktrā on the knee, Mahābalā on the lotus of the feet.

5.3.3 *Bhāgavatapurāṇa* 2.2.19–21. The six places to fix the breath:

(19) The sage should thus be still, resolute [and] with his mind firmly under control with respect to consciousness, vision and vigour. Pressing his anus with his heel he should then tirelessly raise the breath through the six places (*sthāna*s). (20) The sage should raise [the breath] in the navel to the heart and from there lead it along the path of the *udāna* breath to the chest. Then, having focused [on it] with his mind, the wise man should gently lead it to the root of his palate. (21) From there he should raise it to the place between the eyebrows. Having blocked the seven abodes of life,[44] he should pause for half a moment, indifferent, his gaze on the eternal, and then break open his head and burst forth, gone to the supreme.

5.3.4 *Kubjikāmatatantra* 11.34c–37d. The six *cakra*s:

The anus is called the Base (*ādhāra*). The Svādhiṣṭhāna arises at the penis. (35) Maṇipūraka is in the navel and Anāhata is in the heart. Viśuddhi is in the region of the throat and Ājñā is between the eyes. (36) Viśuddhi has sixteen divisions (*bheda*s), while Anāhata is tenfold. Know Maṇipūraka to have twelve divisions. (37) Svādhiṣṭhāna, meanwhile, is the support of several objects and qualities, and has six parts. The Base, on the other hand, has four parts. It is taught that the Ājñā has two divisions.

5.3.5 *Kaulajñānanirṇaya* 5.21cd–32. The eleven *cakra*s:[45]

O goddess, listen with single-minded attention to something else wondrous. (22) A great lotus having sixteen petals, possessing the radiance of ice, jasmine and the moon – having meditated upon this in each of the respective places [in the body], from the [world of] Śiva to the Avīci [hell], (23) the body becomes filled with the descending stream from Bindu, and by drops [of nectar]; and via one's hair follicles emerges [a liquid] having the colour of cow's milk and ice. (24–25ab) He has no old age or death; there is no disease or illness. Autonomous, and equal to Siva, with activity and movement as he pleases, he is worshipped by the hosts of gods [and] by divine maidens in various ways. (25cd–27) In the loins, navel, heart, throat, mouth, head, inside the crest; O goddess, in the triple-staff in the middle of the back, [extending up to] the juncture of the head [and neck] – O goddess, the *cakra*s are elevenfold and a thousand [?], having five petals, eight petals, ten and twelve petals, sixteen, a hundred petals, or else a hundred thousand petals. (28) With these [petal configurations], practised in the place[s], [they] give manifold results.

[Meditating upon the lotus as] red is always [for] subjugation, O goddess; it bestows great supernal enjoyments. (29) Yellow is [for] stunning, O mistress. Grey is always [for] driving away. White is declared for nurturing, especially [for] causing pacification. (30) White like a stream of cow's milk is taught [as] good for defeating death. Having the colour of molten gold causes the shaking of cities, etc. (31–2) Having meditated thus upon [the plexuses of] *bindu* [between the eyebrows], *nāda* [in the forehead] and *śakti* [in the crown of the skull], each separately, there transpires [accomplishment of the four aims:] *dharma*, material success, pleasure and liberation; the group of eight powers, beginning with miniaturization; [knowledge of] what was and will be; and shapeshifting, no doubt, through practice, for one whose mind is intent.

5.3.6 *Hevajratantra* 1.21–31. The four *cakra*s:

The division of Saṃvara[46] is taught:

(21) The vowels (*āli*) and the consonants (*kāli*); the moon and the sun; wisdom and means; the *dharma*, *saṃbhoga*, *nirmāṇa* and *mahāsukha* bodies; voice; mind.

Thus I have [heard].

(22) By the letter *e* is signified the goddess Locanā; by the letter *vaṃ*, Māmakī; by the letter *ma* Pāṇḍurā and by the letter *yā*, Tāraṇī.

(23) In the Nirmāṇa *cakra* [in the navel][47] is a lotus with sixty-four petals. In the Dharma *cakra* [in the heart is a lotus] with eight petals. In the Saṃbhoga *cakra* [in the throat is a lotus] with sixteen petals. In the Mahāsukha *cakra* [in the head is a lotus] with thirty-two petals.

The arrangement [in these *cakra*s of the following attributes] follows the order of the *cakra*s' enumeration.

(24) The four moments: variegated, fruition, destruction and unmarked.

(25) The four auxiliaries: attendance, worship, propitiation and special propitiation.

(26) The four noble truths: suffering, [its] arising, [its] prevention and the path [to its prevention].

(27) The four realities: self, mantra, deity and knowledge.

(28) The four blisses: bliss, supreme bliss, bliss of cessation, natural bliss.

(29) The four schools: Sthāvarī, Sarvāstivāda, Saṃvidī and Mahāsaṅghika.

(30) Moon, sun, vowels, consonants; the sixteen [celestial] transits; the sixty-four *daṇḍa*s;[48] the thirty-two channels (*nāḍī*s);[49] the four *prahara*s:[50] in this way they are all tetrads.

(31) Caṇḍalī, blazing in the navel, burns up the five Tathāgatas and burns up Locanā and the other [goddesses]. When [the syllable] *haṃ* is burnt the moon flows.

5.3.7 *Saṃgītaratnākara* 2.120–39. The emotional states resulting from situating the self in the petals of the *cakra*s:[51]

(120–21) Between the anus and penis is the *cakra* called the Base (*ādhāra*), which has four petals. The result [of situating the self] on those petals, Aiśāna and the others, [Āgneya, Nairṛta and Vāyavya], is supreme bliss (*paramānanda*), natural bliss (*sahajānanda*), heroic bliss (*vīrānanda*) and yoga bliss (*yogānanda*). In the Base lotus is Kuṇḍalinī, the *śakti* of Brahman. (122) When she straightens as far as the aperture of Brahman she bestows the nectar of immortality.

At the base of the penis is the Svādhiṣṭhāna *cakra*, which has six petals. (123) In its petals, in sequence from the east, are said to be these results: modesty, cruelty, loss of pride, swooning, (124) scorn and mistrust. It is the home of the power of love (*kāmaśakti*).

At the navel is the *cakra* with ten petals called Maṇipūraka. (125–7) In its petals, in sequence from the east, are deep sleep, desire, envy, slander, shame, fear, compassion, stupor, impurity [and] anxiety, and it is the abode of the [*prāṇa* called] sun.

At the heart is the Anāhata *cakra*. It is designated as the site of the worship of Śiva in the form of the syllable *oṃ*. It has twelve petals. The removal of unsteadiness, clear reasoning, remorse, (128–9) hope, openness, worry, longing, equanimity, insincere religiosity, fickleness, discernment and hubris: these, in sequence, are said to be the results for the self when situated in its petals, starting with the east.

In the throat is the place of Bhāratī [the goddess of speech], the Viśuddhi [*cakra*], which has sixteen petals. (130–31) The following sixteen results arise in the self when it is situated in its petals, starting with the east: the syllable *oṃ*, the Udgītha (i.e. the second part of a Vedic Sāman chant), [the offering words] *huṃphaṭ*, *vaṣaṭ*, *svadhā*, *svāhā* [and] *namaḥ*, the nectar of immortality, the seven musical notes beginning with Ṣaḍja [i.e. Ṣaḍja, Ṛṣabha, Gāndhāra, Madhyama, Pañcama, Dhaivata and Niṣāda, and] poison.

At the uvula is the *cakra* called Lalanā, which has twelve petals. (132) Intoxication, pride, affection, sorrow [i.e. suffering whose cause is known], melancholy [i.e. suffering whose cause is not known], excessive greed, discontent, panic, the 'wave' (*ūrmi*) [i.e. hunger and thirst, sorrow and delusion, old age and death], belief, faith [and] courtesy: (133) these are the results [of situating the self] in the petals beginning with the east in the Lalanā *cakra*.

Between the eyebrows is the three-petalled *cakra* called Ājñā. [Its] results are (134) taught to be manifestations of [the *guṇas*] *sattva*, *rajas* and *tamas* in sequence.

Next is the Manas *cakra*, which has six petals. Its results are, (135) in the petals starting with the east: sleep, enjoyment of taste, smell, perception of form, touch and cognition of sound.

(136) Next is the sixteen-petalled *cakra* called Soma. In its sixteen petals are found sixteen parts (*kalā*s). (137) Compassion, patience, rectitude, steadfastness, dispassion, resolve, joy, laughter, horripilation, tears produced by meditation, steadiness, (138) profundity, effort, clarity, generosity and focus: [these] results arise in sequence in a self moving through [its] petals, starting with the east.

(139) In the aperture of Brahman is the nectarean *cakra* with a thousand petals. It nourishes the body with streams of nectar.

5.3.8 *Śivasaṃhitā* 5.77–103. The Base (*ādhāra*) lotus:

(77) Two fingers above the anus and one finger below the penis is a single flat bulb four fingers across. (78) Facing backwards in the space between the anus and the penis is the Yoni. In it is said to be the bulb (*kanda*). Kuṇḍalinī resides there at all times. (79) She is found at the opening of Suṣumnā. She encircles all the channels, is coiled three and a half times and has inserted her tail into her mouth. (80) She is like a sleeping serpent and sparkles with her own light. Made of links like a snake, she is the goddess of speech and is called the seed (*bīja*). (81) Know her to be the power (*śakti*) of Viṣṇu, spotless and brilliantly golden. She is made to expand by the three *guṇa*s, *sattva*, *rajas* and *tamas*.

(82) The seed-syllable of Kāma is said to be there, looking like a *bandhūka* flower.[52] With the addition of [the

seed-syllable called Vāgbhava or] Kalahaṃsa it [partially] takes the form of the syllable that is used. (83) Clinging tightly to Suṣumnā, the precious seed-syllable [called Śakti] is found there, a light resembling the autumn moon. This [i.e. the combination of the Kāmarūpa, Vāgbhava and Śakti seed-syllables] is the foremost triad. (84) As bright as ten million suns and as cool as ten million moons, when this triad comes together it makes the goddess Tripurabhairavī.

(85) Only that great light is said to be called the seed. Joined with the action and consciousness powers it wanders all around. (86) That great light looks like an upright lotus fibre, is subtle, joined with a red flame, and found at the *yoni* and the self-born *liṅga*.

(87) The latter is the Base (*ādhāra*) lotus, at the bulb of which is the *yoni*. It is brilliant, contains the four syllables starting with *va* and ending in *sa* [*va*, *śa*, *ṣa* and *sa*], and has four petals. (88) It is called Kula, is golden and is known as the self-born *liṅga*. In it are the adept Dviraṇḍa and the goddess Ḍākinī. (89) Within that lotus is the *yoni*, where Kuṇḍalinī is found. Above her is a sparkling light taught to be the wandering seed-syllable of Kāma.

(90) The wise man who regularly meditates upon the Base gradually attains *dardurī*, the ability to leave the ground like a frog. (91) His body becomes extremely beautiful and his digestive fire increases. He does not fall ill and his faculties become sharp. (92) He knows what has really happened and what is to happen in the future, and he understands the speech of everyone. He is certain to recite sacred texts which he hasn't even heard, together with their secret doctrines. (93) The goddess Sarasvatī for ever dances with abandon in his mouth. Through repetition he is sure to attain mastery of the mantra.

(94) The word of the guru destroys old age, death and a host of sorrows. This great meditation is to be performed regularly by the practitioner of breath-control.

Merely through meditation the master yogi is sure to be freed from every sin.

(95) When the yogi meditates upon the Base lotus, which is called the self-born *liṅga*, he is sure to destroy all his sins immediately. (96) He obtains whatever reward he desires in his mind. Through constant practice he sees the giver of liberation.

(97) The internal meditation is better than the external and should be carefully cultivated. This is the very best meditation in [this] system (*tantra*). I approve of no other. (98) He who rejects the internal Śiva and worships the external casts aside the food in his hand to wander in search of sustenance. (99) Complete perfection arises for him who tirelessly worships his internal *liṅga* every day. This is not to be doubted.

(100) Through constant practice the yogi attains success within six months. His breath is sure to enter Suṣumnā. (101) He conquers his mind, checks his breath and *bindu*, and attains success both in this world and the next. In this there is no doubt.

(102) And the second lotus, which is found at the base of the penis, contains the six syllables starting with *ba* and ending in *la* [*ba*, *bha*, *ma*, *ya*, *ra* and *la*], and has six shining petals. (103) That lotus is called Svādhiṣṭhāna and is red. The adept called Bāla and the goddess Rākinī reside in it.

[Verses 104–55 describe the remaining *cakra*s.]

5.3.9 *Siddhasiddhāntapaddhati* 2.1–9. The nine *cakra*s:

Now the doctrine of the body is explained:

(1) There are nine *cakra*s in the body. At the base [of the body] is Brahmā *cakra*, which is coiled around three times and has the form of a vulva (*bhagamaṇḍala*). The root bulb (*mūlakanda*) is located there. In that, visualize the goddess in the form of fire. There, indeed, is the seat of Kāma, the god of love, which bestows all desires.

(2) The second is the Svādhiṣṭhāna *cakra*. In its middle, visualize a backwards-facing *liṅga* resembling an outgrowth of coral. There, indeed, is the seat of Uḍḍiyāna, which bestows the power of attracting the world.

(3) The third is the navel (*nābhi*) *cakra*, which is coiled round like a snake five times. In the middle of it visualize the goddess Kuṇḍalinī as being like ten million rising suns. She is the central goddess (*madhyā śakti*), who bestows all the supernatural powers.

(4) The fourth is the heart *cakra*, which is a downward-facing, eight-petalled lotus. In its middle, on the central receptacle, visualize a light in the shape of a *liṅga*. That is the Haṃsakalā. Mastery over all the senses arises.

(5) The fifth is the throat *cakra*, measuring four finger-widths. There on the left side is the moon channel Iḍā. On the right is the sun channel Piṅgalā. Between them, visualize the Suṣumnā. This is the Anāhatakalā, which gives mastery over the unstruck sound (*anāhatasiddhi*).

(6) The sixth is the palate *cakra*, through which the nectar (*amṛta*) flows. [It is also called] the *liṅga* at the uvula, the opening at the base, the royal tooth, the opening of Śaṅkhinī and the tenth door. Meditate on emptiness there. The mind dissolves.

(7) The seventh is the brow *cakra*, which measures the size of a thumb. Visualize the eye of knowledge like a lamp's flame there. This brings mastery of speech.

(8) The eighth is the *nirvāṇa cakra* at the aperture of Brahmā (*brahmarandhra*), and which looks like the tip of a needle. Visualize a crest of smoke there. The seat of Jālandhara, which bestows liberation, is there.

(9) The ninth is the ether *cakra*, an upward-facing, sixteen-petalled lotus. In its central receptacle, visualize its upper power (*ūrdhvaśakti*), which takes the form of three peaks, as the great emptiness. The seat of Pūrṇagiri, which accomplishes all desires, is there.

This concludes the discussion of the nine *cakras*.

5.3.10 *Siddhasiddhāntapaddhati* 2.10–25. The sixteen supports (*ādhāras*):

Now the sixteen supports are taught:

(10) Of them, the first is the big-toe support. Visualize the tip as being made of light. The gaze becomes steady.

(11) The second is the Base support (*mūlādhāra*). Steadily press it with the left heel. This kindles the [digestive] fire.

(12) The third is the rectal support, which one should dilate and squeeze. The *apāna* wind becomes steady.

(13) The fourth is the penis support. When, by contracting the penis one pierces the three knots and comes to rest in the bee cave,[53] then, when [the support] is facing upwards, the semen is stabilized. This is well known as *vajrolī*.

(14) The fifth is the Uḍḍiyāna support, the locking of which brings a reduction in excrement and urine.

(15) The sixth is the navel support. Make the syllable *oṃ* resound in it with a focused mind. This brings about dissolution by means of sound (*nādalaya*).

(16) The seventh is the heart support. Restrain *prāṇa* in it. The lotus blooms.

(17) The eighth is the throat support. Press the chin on it, at the base of the throat. The breath becomes fixed in the Iḍā and Piṅgalā channels.

(18) The ninth is the uvula support. Hold the tip of the tongue on it. The nectar of immortality flows forth.

(19) The tenth is the palate support. Lengthen the tongue by moving it about (with the hands) and milking it, then turn it backwards and insert it into the inner palatal cavity. One becomes like a piece of wood.

(20) The eleventh is the tongue support. Hold the tip of the tongue steady. All diseases are destroyed.

(21) The twelfth is the between-the-brows support. Visualize there the disc of the moon. One becomes cool.

(22) The thirteenth is the nose support. Focus on its tip. The mind becomes steady.

(23) The fourteenth is the doorway support at the bridge of the nose. Direct the gaze there. After six months, one sees a mass of light.

(24) The fifteenth is the forehead support. Focus on a mass of light there. One becomes resplendent.

(25) The sixteenth remains: it is the aperture of Brahmā (*brahmarandhra*) [i.e. the fontanelle], the sky *cakra* (*ākāśa-cakra*). Constantly visualize there the two lotus feet of the blessed guru. One becomes as all-pervasive as the sky.

5.4

Kuṇḍalinī

5.4.1 *Pādmasaṃhitā* 2.13c–17b. Kuṇḍalī:

Above and to the side of [the navel *cakra* in the middle of the bulb] is the place of Kuṇḍalī. (14–15) Taking the form of the eight constituents of matter (*prakṛti*),[54] she is eightfold and coiled. Located all around the edge of the bulb, she constantly blocks the correct movement of the breath and the regular [functioning of] fire and so forth, and thus covers the opening of the aperture of Brahmā with her mouth. (16) And when, during yoga, she has risen because of the breath together with fire, she bursts forth into the void of the heart in the form of a snake, blazing brightly. (17) Then the breath travels through the breath aperture along the Suṣumnā.

5.4.2 *Khecarīvidyā* 3.8c–14d. Kuṇḍalinī:

Between Iḍā and Piṅgalā is the luminous Suṣumnā. (9) There is an undecaying light there, free of the qualities of colour and shape. She who looks like a sleeping serpent is the great Kuṇḍalinī. (10) Gaṅgā and Yamunā are called Iḍā and Piṅgalā. [The yogi] should insert that goddess, in the form of the supreme *amṛta*, between Gaṅgā and Yamunā, (11) as far as the abode of Brahmā, O goddess. Truly he becomes identical with Brahmā and automatically gets an immortal body for ever. (12) The goddess, having reached the abode of Śiva, the place beyond the Supreme Lord, satiated by the pleasure of enjoying that place and filled with supreme bliss, (13) sprinkling the body of the yogi from the soles of his feet to his head with the dewy, unctuous, cool nectar, O supreme goddess, (14) proceeds again by the same path to her own home, O goddess. This is the secret yoga taught [by me], O you who are honoured by the master yogis.

5.4.3 *Gorakṣaśataka* 74–86. Kuṇḍalinī:

(74) The mind is absorbed into the Suṣumnā and the breath does not rush forth. As a result of his secretions being dried up, the yogi's journey is set in motion. (75) He should force the downward moving *apāna* breath to move upwards by means of contraction. Yogis call this the root lock (*mūlabandha*). (76–7) When the *apāna* has turned upwards and goes together with fire to the place of *prāṇa*, then – now that fire, *prāṇa* and *apāna* have quickly come together – the coiled, sleeping Kuṇḍalinī, heated by that fire and stimulated by the breath, (78) makes her body enter the mouth of the Suṣumnā. Then, having pierced the knot of Brahmā, which is born of the quality of passion (*rajas*), (79) she quickly flashes like a streak of lightning in the mouth of the Suṣumnā. She hurries up to the knot of Viṣṇu and, after stopping at the heart, (80) with great speed she moves on, having pierced the knot of Viṣṇu, and goes to where the knot of Rudra is found, (81) between the eyebrows, having pierced which she goes to the orb of the moon, the *cakra* called Anāhata,

which has sixteen petals. (82) Once there she automatically dries up the fluid produced from the moon.

When the sun has been moved from its abode to the place of blood and bile by the force of *prāṇa*, (83) Kuṇḍalinī, having gone to where the *cakra* of the moon is found, which consists of the white fluid of phlegm, consumes there the heated phlegm which has been discharged and is by nature cold. (84) In the same way the white image of the moon is heated forcefully; agitated, Kuṇḍalinī moves upwards and thus [the fluid] flows even more. (85) As a result of tasting this, the mind is barred from the objects of the senses. Having enjoyed the best of what is inside him, one [becomes] intent on the self. (86) And Kuṇḍalinī goes to the place which takes the form of the eight constituents of nature. Having embraced it, she moves on to Śiva, after embracing whom she disappears.

5.4.4 *Yogabīja* 93–9. Kuṇḍalinī and piercing the knots:

(93) By strongly restraining the breath and using the 'stimulation of the goddess' technique (*śakticālana*)[55] in order to straighten Kuṇḍalinī, who is coiled eight times, (94) [the yogi] should contract the sun and then stimulate Kuṇḍalinī. Even for one in its jaws, there is no fear of death.

(95) What I have told you, Pārvatī, is the supreme secret. Practise it regularly for a fortnight, sitting in the thunderbolt pose (*vajrāsana*).

(96) The fire kindled by the breath continually burns Kuṇḍalinī. Heated by the fire, that goddess of the channel, who entrances the three worlds, (97) enters into the mouth of the Suṣumnā channel in the spine [and] together with the breath and the fire pierces the knot of Brahmā.

(98) Then, after piercing the knot of Viṣṇu, she resides in the knot of Rudra. Then, having inhaled again and again, when breath-retention is intense, (99) the yogi should

practise the four breath-retentions (*kumbhaka*s) called 'accompanied' (*sahita*): piercing the sun (*sūryabheda*), victorious (*ujjāyī*), cooling (*śītalī*) and bellows (*bhastrā*).

5.4.5 *Siddhasiddhāntapaddhati* 4.14–27. Kuṇḍalinī:

(14) Kuṇḍalinī is of two kinds: awakened and unawakened. The unawakened kind is in all bodies in the form of consciousness, naturally taking the form of various thoughts, actions, efforts and phenomena. She is sinuous by nature and [so] is known as Kuṇḍalinī ('she who is coiled'). It is she who is the well-known Kuṇḍalinī who goes upwards in yogis, her nature being to try to prevent the disturbances that have appeared in each of them.

(15) 'Upwards': all elements and their own forms exist on high, as a result of which she is well known as 'she who takes the form of investigation', because [thanks to her] yogis realize their true forms.

And it is said in the *Rulaka*[*tantra*]:

(16) By means of the awakening of the central goddess (*madhyaśakti*) as a result of the clenching of the lower goddess (*adhaḥśakti*) [and] by means of the descent of the upper goddess (*ūrdhvaśakti*) the supreme level is attained. (17) She is only one [but] by being classified as central, upper or lower she has three names. (18) When she consists of various thoughts produced by the activities of the external sense organs she is called the lower goddess. It is because of this that yogis are intent on contracting her. Contracting her is perfected by locking the Base support (*mūlādhārabandhana*),[56] from which this [entire] universe, moving and unmoving, conscious and unconscious, is produced. That is the Base support, which is well known as the source of consciousness.

Śivānandācārya has said:

(19) Without doubt, the creation and destruction of the universe happen because of all the emissions and

contractions of the goddess. As a result she is called the Base (*mūla*). [And] that is why almost all adepts are devoted to the Base support (*mūlādhāra*).

(20) She who is always inherently able to hold in the middle of her light the individual self, which is restless by nature and wanders in vain, is celebrated as the central goddess [manifestation of] Kuṇḍalinī. It has been ascertained that the Great Adepts know her in her gross and subtle forms.

(21) 'Gross': she who wanders through different objects in the form of consciousness even though she is by nature [both] the support of all that which is perceptible and perceptible herself is Kuṇḍalinī with form, [i.e. the] gross [Kuṇḍalinī]. Moreover that same Kuṇḍalinī, who has been determined to be the bringer of great bliss to yogis, because of her skill at extending herself, is known in the teachings of the Great Adepts as subtle, formless and awakened.

(22) Creation is called Kuṇḍalinī; she has two states. In one she has a gross form and is the individual soul in people. (23) In the other she is everywhere and subtle; she does not pervade nor is she pervaded. He who is confused by convictions does not understand her division. (24) So the supreme subtle Kuṇḍalinī, the central goddess, whose own form is consciousness, is to be awoken when she is in her own natural state by yogis who have learnt [how to do so] from the mouth of a true guru in order for them to perfect their bodies.

Now the descent of the upper goddess is taught:

(25) Because the nameless supreme place is above all the elements it is known as 'upper'. She whose nature is to reveal and point to various objects by means of self-perception is called the upper goddess. Her descent is not merely the extinction of the fallacy that one's true nature is twofold; on the contrary, it happens because of the indivisibility of one's own true nature.

And it has been said:

(26) The goddess is in Śiva; Śiva is in the goddess. One should know that there is no difference between them, in the same way [that there is no difference] between the moon and moonlight. (27) This is why it has been established that the Great Adept yogis attain the supreme level by means of the descent of the upper goddess.

5.5

Nectar, *Bindu*, Moon

5.5.1 *Amṛtasiddhi* Chapters 3, 4, 5 and 7. The moon, sun and fire, and the restraint of *bindu*:

[Chapter 3, The Inquiry into the Moon]

(1) The moon is located on the peak of [Mount] Meru and has sixteen digits. Facing downwards it rains white nectar day and night. (2) Men who are versed in the elements should know that the nectar of immortality [that comes] from it is of two sorts. The water of the [river] Maṇḍākinī goes through the Iḍā channel in order to nourish [the body]. (3) Going by way of a subtle channel it nourishes the whole body. This form of the moon is in the left path. (4) The other, its orb drawn together in rapture and looking like a cluster of jasmine flowers, goes by way of the middle of the Goddess of the Centre (Madhyamā) to bring about creation.

Thus ends the Inquiry into the Moon.

[Chapter 4, The Inquiry into the Sun]

(1) The orb of the sun is at the base of the Goddess of the Centre complete with twelve digits, shining with its own rays. (2) The lord of creatures, of intense appear-

ance, [the sun] travels upwards on the right. In the hollow pathways of the channels he pervades the entire body. (3) In every body, the sun consumes the lunar secretion, wanders in the sphere of the wind and burns up the seven bodily constituents (*dhātus*). (4) This sun is the great figure on men's right-hand pathways. It moves through the celestial intersections, causing creation and destruction. (5) When the sun, in line with Meru, stops moving on the left, know that to be the equinox, an auspicious time in the body. (6) By recognizing the equinox in their own bodies, yogis, full of the vigour [produced by] their practice, easily abandon their bodies in yogic suicide at the correct time. (7) Season, juncture, day, night, moment, instant and other measures of time, receiving and emitting: all this arises from the sun. (8) When the sun and moon meet in union (*yoga*), externally that should be known to be creation. Internally, it is yoga. (9) One should know it to be definitely an eclipse, whether external or internal. Externally it is the most meritorious time and internally it is liberation. (10) When the sun seizes the disc of the moon in the sky a mutual union (*yoga*) arises; that is why it is called yoga. (11) When the fire that is the sun happens to journey upwards in the body [and] the lunar nectar of immortality goes downwards then men die. (12) [When] all these elements move upwards in the body, then these two, the sun and the moon, are said to bestow liberation.

Thus ends the Inquiry into the Sun.

[Chapter 5, The Inquiry into Fire]

(1) In the middle of the orb of the sun in the region of the stomach, with ten digits, is the fire which digests food. (2) Fire is the sun; the sun is fire. The two look the same, [but] differ subtly. (3) While the fire of Time is in the middle of the sun in the body, then the nectarean flow of *bindu* is unbroken. (4) The fire gives strength to people,

the fire bestows longevity. When the fire is healthy, a man is free from disease.

Thus ends the Inquiry into Fire. [. . .]

[Chapter 7, The Inquiry into the Restraint of *Bindu*]

(1) A single seed is taught to be the fundamental bodily essence. Everything seen in this world arises from the seed. (2) The source of the essence of the bodily elements, the seed is Sadāśiva. In its middle are situated all the gods in subtle form. (3) This is *bindu*, this is the moon, this is the seed, this is ichor.[57] This is the element, this is the vital essence, this is the essence of everything.

(4) The [four] bodily blisses whose last is [the bliss of] cessation[58] are all taught to be born from *bindu*, just as moonlight is born from the moon. (5) *Bindu* puts one on the path, it grants heaven, it grants liberation and it grants pleasure. It provokes good and bad acts; always powerful, it grants everything.

(6) *Bindu* is mastered by the breath; there is no other method of mastering *bindu*. *Bindu* enters the state that the breath is in. (7) Stunned, it removes disease; bound, it makes one a sky-rover (*khecara*); absorbed and unmoving, it brings about all supernatural powers and bestows liberation.

(8) Know that *bindu* to be of two kinds, male and female. Seed is said to be the male (*pauruṣeya*) [*bindu*] and *rajas* [i.e. female generative fluid] is the *bindu* which is female (*strīsamudbhava*). (9) As a result of their external union people are created. When they are united internally, one is declared a yogi.

(10) *Bindu* resides in Kāmarūpa in the hollow of the multi-storeyed palace (*kūṭāgāra*) [in the head]. From contact, with delight it goes to Pūrṇagiri by way of the central channel. (11) *Rajas* resides in the great sacred field in the *yoni*. It is as red as a Javā flower and enveloped in the goddess element. (12) Know *bindu* to be

lunar and *rajas* to be solar. Their union is to be brought about in the very inaccessible multi-storeyed palace. (13) This [union] is reality (*tattva*), the ultimate teaching (*dharma*); this is considered the best yoga. This path bestows liberation. It is the ultimate secret.

(14) He who abandons *bindu* yoga and in delusion wants something else is a fool, fruitlessly keeping vigil among barren trees. (15) *Bindu* is Buddha, *bindu* is Śiva, *bindu* is Viṣṇu the lord of creatures. *Bindu* is the universal god, *bindu* is the mirror of the three worlds.

(16) *Bindu* is mastered in the same way that the breath is mastered. The mind adopts whatever condition *bindu* is in. (17) When the breath is unstable then *bindu* is taught to be unstable. The mind of he whose *bindu* is unstable is restless.

(18) The god who is lord of all the elements has the nature of existence [yet] is untainted, and he resides in all beings in the form of *bindu*. (19) As long as the breath is moving in the body, so *bindu* is said to move. As long as *bindu* is moving the mind is restless. (20) Whenever *bindu*, the mind [and] the breath are moving, people are born and die. True, true is this teaching!

(21) *Nāda* is *bindu* and that is what the mind is said to be. In practice these three are one. (22) Although these three are present as one in the body, it is when the breath is mastered that they are all certain to attain perfection. (23) When the breath stops through contact with the middle of the Goddess of the Centre, then *bindu* and the mind stop together with the breath.

(24) All these elements dwell in the body. They move when the breath moves and they stop when the breath is stopped. (25) Death comes about through the fall of *bindu*, life from its preservation. When the great jewel *bindu* is perfected, then everything is perfected. (26) [When] the lunar nectar of immortality goes down, [there is] death for all embodied beings. He whose *bindu*

is one with the indivisible is an adept in a diamond body.

Thus ends the Inquiry into the Restraint of *Bindu*.

5.5.2 *Vivekamārtaṇḍa* 126–31. Keeping the body full of *amṛta* and so immortal:

(126) Pressing the special opening at the uvula with the tip of the tongue and meditating on the goddess as made of the nectar of immortality, one becomes a sage (*kavi*) in six months. (127) When the upper opening is sealed by this process together with the nine locks, the nectar of immortality, the sixteen digits of the moon, is never released. (128) If the tongue continually touches the tip of the uvula and sour, pungent, bitter, milky, sweet and syrupy flavours flow forth [in succession], then there is the removal of disease and old age, [spontaneous] recitation of the scholarly and religious texts, immortality, the eight powers and the power to attract adept (*siddha*) women. (129) After two or three years the semen of the yogi whose body is filled with the nectar of immortality moves upwards and the powers of becoming as small as an atom and so forth arise. (130) Poison does not trouble the yogi's body if it is constantly filled with the [nectar from the] digits of the moon, even when he is bitten by a snake. (131) Just as fire does not leave fuel when a lamp has a wick in oil, so the embodied [self] does not leave a body which is full of the [nectar from the] digits of the moon.

5.5.3 *Jñāneśvarī* 6.247–70. The transformation of the body with the nectar of immortality:[59]

(247) Then the tank of moon-nectar pours from above [and], turning over, merges into the mouth of the goddess (*śakti*). (248) Through that tube the fluid fills [and] is held in the whole body, where it merges with the *prāṇa* wind. (249) Just as in a heated mould the wax disappears [and] then the filled [mould] remains with

the solidified liquid, (250) so that digit (*kalā*) [of the nectar of immortality] becomes manifest in the shape of the body, [and] is covered on top with a screen of skin. (251) As the sun has made a veil of the clouds, [but] when they disappear, cannot hold [back his] light, (252) like that is the dry crust of skin on the surface. As the husk is shed [from the grain], (253) [as] the self-existent sprouts of a crystal, or [those] arisen [from] a seed in the form of a jewel, so the lustre of the beauty of the limbs, (254) or [like] the colour of the sky at sunset, drawn out, turned [into] that body, or the *liṅga* of inner light made manifest, (255) a solid mass of red powder, mercury cast in a mould – when I see [it, it seems] embodied peace to me. (256) It [is like] the paint of a painting of bliss, or an image of supreme happiness, or like a [well-]established sapling of the tree of satisfaction. (257) It [is like] the large bud of a golden Campaka [flower] or an image of nectar, an orchard of tenderness in bloom, (258) as if the disc of the moon [had] blossomed with autumnal moisture, or solid light [were] seated on a seat: (259) like that becomes the body when Kuṇḍalinī drinks the moon. Then death fears the form of the body. (260) Then old age turns back, the knot of youth is untied, the lost state of childhood [re]appears. (261) [The yogi's] age then [is] up to this much, that he gives [to the word] 'strength' (*bala*) the meaning 'child' (*bāla*): the greatness of [his] fortitude is incomparable. (262) [As] on the foliage of a tree of gold new varieties of jewel-buds, such beautiful nails grow. (263) Also the teeth become different, but incomparably small, as if a row of diamonds [would] sit on both sides. (264) Particles of tiny rubies, by nature small like atoms, such tips of hairs rise all over the body. (265) The palms of the hands [and the soles] of the feet [are] like red lotuses, [and] the eyes become washed clean – what shall I say? (266) Just as, because of the fullness of maturity [of the pearls], the two parts of the shell do not cover the pearls, [and] then the joint of the oyster[-halves] bursts open, (267) like that, in the embrace of the eyelid, the sight [can]not [be] contained and, grasping [forward], manages to get out. [It looks] exactly as before, but [is] embracing heaven. (268) Listen, the body becomes golden, but gets the lightness of the wind, so that there is no [more] part of water and earth. (269) Then [the yogi] sees the other shore of the ocean, hears the whispering sound of heaven, [and] knows the thought of the ant. (270) He mounts the conveyance of the wind, [and when] he walks, then his foot does not touch water – on many such occasion[s] supernatural powers arise.

5.5.4 *Lallāvākyāni* 22. The moon:

The day will be extinguished, and there will be night.
The surface of the earth will spread out towards the sky.
On the new-moon day, the moon will swallow Rāhu.
This is worshipping Śiva, the illumination of the self in thought.

5.5.5 *Gorakṣa Bijaẏ* 1, 4–8. The practice of the moons:[60]

[Gorakhnāth sings:]
(1) Alas, guru Mīnanāth,
you destroyed your body.
Sinning, you have forgotten yoga.
You abandoned your guru's teaching.
Being deluded by amorous passion,
you wanted to taste death.
[. . .]
(4) Guru, there are four moons
pervading a body.
If you practise them you will be rescued.
An original moon, one's own moon,
an excited and a poisonous moon:
these four pervade the body.
(5) He who fixes the original moon,
joins the own moon
with the excited one,

restrains the three moons,
and loads [them] on himself [or: on Khemāi],
he drinks all the poisonous moon.
(6) Having restrained the four moons,
and having crossed the ocean of existence,
then he is fully protected.
But you did not do this work
and you have forgotten everything.
Tell me, guru, what is the way?
(7) You do not have the strength
to run away from here.
There is no hope for life.
I say true words of the teaching.
Think and examine them
if you have a desire to live.
(8) Do a reverse yoga,
make yourself still
and remember your own mantra.
Keep yourself reversed
and strike at Triveṇī
to fill the channels with water.

5.6

Baking and Mortification of the Body

5.6.1 *Jñāneśvarī* 6.228–40. Kuṇḍalinī's awakening:[61]

(228) Naturally hungry for many days, then awakened – that is how it starts. Then she forcefully spreads out her mouth straight upward. (229) There, Kirīṭī, she embraces all the wind that has filled [the region] below the space of the heart. (230) With the fire of her mouth she reaches up and down [and] begins to eat morsels of flesh. (231) Whatever place is endowed with flesh, there she takes a small bite. Afterwards she also fills in one or two

morsels. (232) Then she purifies the soles of the feet and the palms of the hands, pierces the upper parts [and] searches the joints of every limb. (233) Although she does not leave the [Base] support, she also draws out the essence [from] the nails, [and] after cleaning the skin unites with the skeleton. (234) [When] she scrapes the hollows of the bones [and] rubs the fibres of the head, then the outside sprout of hair-seed gets scorched. (235) Then the thirsty one takes a gulp in the ocean of the seven bodily constituents (*dhātus*) and immediately produces dry heat. (236) Holding back the neck, the wind that goes twelve fingers' breadth out of the cavity of the nose pours inside. (237) There the lower [breath] contracts above, the upper one attacks below. In that embrace the cover of the *cakra*s remains. (238) Otherwise just then the two [would] mix, but Kuṇḍalinī [would be] for a while irritated, so that she [would say] to them: 'How [come] you [are] over there?' (239) Listen, consuming the whole element belonging to the earth, she does not leave anything and then cleans away the water. (240) [When] she eats both elements in that way, then she is completely satisfied. Then, mollified, she remains near Suṣumnā.

5.6.2 *Yogabīja* 49–53. Baking the body's constituents in the fire of yoga:[62]

The Lord said:

(49) Everyone [else] is conquered by the body, [but] the body is conquered by yogis, so they are not subject to the fruits [of their actions], such as pain, pleasure and the like.

(50) When [the yogi] has conquered the senses, mind, intellect, desire, anger and so forth, he has conquered everything. Nothing can trouble him. (51) [After] the gross and [other] elements have arisen in series, the body composed of its seven constituents is slowly burnt by the fire of yoga.

(52) Even the gods cannot obtain the mighty yogic body. The great [yogi] who by severing bonds has become free possesses various supernatural powers. (53) The body is like the sky, [but] even more pure than the sky. It becomes more subtle than the subtle, more gross than the gross, more solid than the solid.

SIX
Yogic Seals

A yogic seal (*mudrā*) is a method of manipulating the breath and other vital energies. In the earliest systematic description of *haṭhayoga* named as such, found in the *c.* thirteenth-century *Dattātreyayogaśāstra*, it is the practice of yogic seals which sets *haṭha* apart from other methods of yoga; *mudrā* is one of the four stages of *haṭha* in the *Haṭhapradīpikā* (see 1.2.9) and one of its *aṅgas* ('auxiliaries') in the *Haṭharatnāvalī* (see 1.2.10). The *mudrās* taught in the *Dattātreyayogaśāstra* (6.2.2) are physical techniques whose purpose is not always explicit, but which is implicitly (and from other textual descriptions of the same techniques) to make the breath enter and rise up the central channel, and to control *bindu* (semen),[1] the preservation of which is elsewhere in the text explained to be the key to extending life and preventing death. The *Dattātreyayogaśāstra* concludes its teachings on *mudrā* by saying that their practice leads to the state of *rājayoga*, the royal yoga, in which the yogi may do whatever he wants.

Bindu is produced in the head and constantly drips downwards – to be consumed by the fire in the stomach or ejaculated – unless it is prevented from doing so by means of yogic seals. Using *khecarīmudrā* (detailed descriptions of which are found in passages from the *Khecarīvidyā* (6.2.8), the *Baḥr al-ḥayāt* (6.2.11) and the *Gherandasaṃhitā* (6.2.13)) the yogi seals *bindu* in the head by inserting his tongue into the cavity above the soft palate. Using *jālandharabandha* ('the *jālandhara* lock'), the yogi presses his chin against his chest and constricts his throat, again stopping *bindu* (equated in the *Dattātreyayogaśāstra*'s description of the practice with *amṛta*, the nectar of immortality) from dripping downwards. In *viparīta-*

karaṇī ('the inverter') the yogi turns himself upside down, adopting either a headstand or a shoulderstand, using gravity to keep *bindu* in the head. And by means of *vajrolīmudrā*[2] the yogi overcomes the ejaculatory impulse, preventing involuntary loss of semen.

Three of the *mudrā*s taught in the *Dattātreyayogaśāstra* are first taught in the *Amṛtasiddhi*, with more detail about their methods and aims (**6.2.1**). The *mahāmudrā* ('great seal'), (*mahā*)*bandha* ('(great) lock') and (*mahā*)*vedha* ('(great) piercing')[3] are physical postures which check the movement of the breath and/or make it travel upwards.

*Mudrā*s in Tantric Ritual

Prior to the *Amṛtasiddhi* and *Dattātreyayogaśāstra*, from at least the sixth century CE onwards, *mudrā*s of an altogether different sort were taught extensively in tantric texts.[4] With a small number of important exceptions,[5] tantric *mudrā*s are not methods of manipulating vital energies; they are physical attitudes and gestures adopted in ritual in order to bring about certain supernatural effects or, in fewer cases, possession by the deities with which they are associated. The deities' *mudrā*s are also said to manifest spontaneously in the practitioner when possession occurs through other means. Within the tantric tradition different levels of sophistication are evident in analyses of how such possession manifests. Thus, for example, the tantric *khecarīmudrā* (whose various methods of practice are different from those found in haṭhayogic texts) is said to bring about either possession by the sky-roving Yoginīs known as Khecarīs or direct experience of Khecarī consciousness, the highest mental state.[6]

The most common type of tantric *mudrā* is a hand gesture, and this chapter opens with the eight such *mudrā*s taught in the *Niśvāsatattvasaṃhitā* (**6.1.1**). Later tantric works taught large numbers of *mudrā*s. Some, such as the Buddhist *mahāmudrā* (which is not to be confused with the haṭhayogic *mahāmudrā*), are mental states not necessarily associated with specific practices, and this understanding of *mudrā* persisted in some later traditions (see, for example, the *Aṣṭa Mudrā* or 'Eight *Mudrā*s' attributed to

Gorakhnāth (6.2.12)). Some others do involve physical techniques other than hand gestures. The second passage in this chapter presents three of the 121 *mudrā* teachings found in the *Jayadrathayāmala* (6.1.2). The first two are hand gestures, but in the instructions for the third, the *phetkārīmudrā* ('howler seal'), the aspirant is told to assume a posture similar to the haṭhayogic *mahāmudrā*, put his clenched fists to his ears and howl like a jackal.

The Protohistory of Yogic *Mudrā*s

Notwithstanding this outward similarity with the haṭhayogic *mahāmudrā*, there is nothing in the *Jayadrathayāmala*'s description of the 'howler seal' to suggest that it was conceived of as a yogic rather than ritual technique, and in fact none of the haṭhayogic *mudrā*s is taught in any tantric text which predates the *haṭha* corpus.[7] But it seems likely that their codification in the *haṭha* corpus from about the eleventh century onwards was not because they were invented then: there are references to ascetics practising similar, perhaps even identical techniques from the time of the Buddha onwards. The Buddha himself tried forcing his tongue against his palate in the manner of *khecarīmudrā*;[8] Śramaṇa ascetics with whom the Buddha fraternized (see Introduction, p. xiii) would practise the bat penance, hanging themselves upside down in the manner of the inverter seal (*viparītakaraṇī*);[9] and Jain ascetics meditated in squatting postures which put pressure on the perineal region in the same way as the great seal, lock and piercing (see 3.1 and 3.5).[10] The *Dattātreyayogaśāstra* is a product of a tradition of non-tantric celibate ascetics whose roots are probably in these early Śramaṇa orders, and these techniques of ensuring sexual continence – which in Indian myths has always been key to the power of celibate ascetics – are likely to be of a similarly ancient pedigree.

The Purpose and Practice of Yogic *Mudrā*s

The *Gorakṣaśataka*, one of the earliest texts on physical yoga to derive from the tantric traditions, teaches four of the techniques which in later haṭhayogic works are called *mudrā*s. Three of them, the root, *uḍḍīyāna* and *jālandhara* locks (*mūlabandha*, *uḍḍīyānabandha* and *jālandharabandha*), are methods of forcing the breath upwards and into the central channel and these are also found in the *Amṛtasiddhi* and/or *Dattātreyayogaśāstra*. The fourth, *śakticālana* (the 'stimulation of the goddess'), is an innovation and introduces a new purpose to the haṭhayogic *mudrās*: the awakening of Kuṇḍalinī, which, in *śakticālana*, is performed by pulling on the tongue.

The Old Marathi *Jñāneśvarī* teaches a yogic method of raising Kuṇḍalinī by means of the three locks, which is similar to that taught in the *Gorakṣaśataka*. Its teachings (**6.2.6**) do not mention *śakticālana*, but do instruct the yogi to half-close his eyes and turn his gaze inwards in the manner of a technique taught in other haṭhayogic works as *śāmbhavīmudrā*. Unlike the more physical *mudrās* of *haṭhayoga*, *śāmbhavīmudrā* is also found in earlier Śaiva tantric texts, most commonly with the name of *bhairavamudrā*. The earliest descriptions of *śāmbhavīmudrā* by that name are those in the *Candrāvalokana* (**6.2.7**), *Amanaska* (2.10) and *Anubhavanivedanastotra* (1–2).[11]

The *Amṛtasiddhi* and *Dattātreyayogaśāstra* make no mention of Kuṇḍalinī when they teach their *mudrās*, which are for manipulating the breath and *bindu*. And when six of the *mudrās* they describe are taught in the *Vivekamārtaṇḍa* (which, like the *Gorakṣaśataka*, is attributed to Gorakṣa) some, such as *khecarīmudrā* and the inverter, are still explicitly said to be for the preservation of *bindu* (see **6.2.4**). However, their teaching is immediately preceded by a pair of verses which state, firstly, that it is by means of Kuṇḍalinī that yogis attain liberation and, secondly, that the yogi who knows the *mudrās* will be liberated.

The implication of the beginning of the *Vivekamārtaṇḍa*'s section on *mudrās* is clear: *mudrās* work on Kuṇḍalinī. This crude refashioning of the haṭhayogic *mudrās* to fit a Kaula tantric paradigm[12] is more deftly effected in two subsequent works of Kaula tantric schools, the *Khecarīvidyā* and *Śivasaṃhitā*. In the former, *khecarīmudrā*, taking on some of the characteristics of the *Gorakṣaśataka*'s 'stimulation of the goddess' technique, becomes a way of awakening Kuṇḍalinī and leading her to the store of the nectar of immortality in the head, with which she then floods the body as she returns to her home at the base of the spine. The *Khecarīvidyā*'s teachings on the practical details of the technique, together with the fruits of the tongue tasting the nectar, are included at **6.2.8**; its teachings on the ascent and descent of Kuṇḍalinī at **5.4.2**.

The *Śivasaṃhitā* includes all ten haṭhayogic *mudrā*s taught in texts which precede it, including the *Gorakṣaśataka*'s 'stimulation of the goddess'. It states at the outset of its section on *mudrā*s that their purpose is to awaken the sleeping Kuṇḍalinī and incorporates this aim into the descriptions of individual *mudrā*s in a way not found in earlier works. In this chapter we have included the *Śivasaṃhitā*'s teachings on the *vajrolī*, *sahajolī* and *amarolī mudrā*s (**6.2.10**). These descriptions are further evidence of the tantric appropriation of the haṭhayogic *mudrā*s. Whereas their aim in earlier texts, when made explicit, is to prevent the loss of the yogi's *bindu* or the yoginī's *rajas* (uterine fluid), here it is the absorption through the urethra of the mixed products of sexual intercourse (which are to be ingested orally in certain earlier Kaula tantric rites).[13]

The *Śivasaṃhitā* adds one *mudrā* not taught in earlier haṭhayogic texts, the *yonimudrā*,[14] giving it pride of place at the beginning of its chapter on *mudrā*s (**6.2.9**). The application of this *mudrā* involves a visualization conjoined with contraction of the perineal region (*yoni*) and breath-control. It is likely to be derived from the older tantric *mudrā*s of the *Śivasaṃhitā*'s tradition, in particular because of its connection with the practice of mantra-repetition.[15]

Some of the more physical haṭhayogic *mudrā*s came to be taught also as *āsana*s in later medieval texts. Thus the *Jogpradīpakā*, composed in the old Hindi dialect Braj Bhasha, includes a *mahāmudrā āsana* among its eighty-four *āsana*s. This conflation of *āsana* and *mudrā* (and other yogic methods) is already apparent in the Persian *Baḥr al-ḥayāt*, whose twenty-two *zikr*s ('remembrances' or 'meditations') use a wide range of yogic techniques. One teaches a set of methods for *khecarī* (*mudrā*) and is included in this chapter (**6.2.11**).

Like the other practices of *haṭhayoga*, there was a significant proliferation in the number of *mudrā*s taught in texts composed and compiled during the seventeenth and eighteenth centuries.

Thus the *Jogpradīpakā* teaches twenty-four *mudrās*, and the *Gheraṇḍasaṃhitā*, twenty-five. A selection of the latter, which, exceptionally, include five *dhāraṇās* or meditative fixations on the five elements (see also Chapter 8), are at **6.2.13**.

Chapter Contents

6.1

Śaiva Tantric *Mudrās*

6.1.1 *Niśvāsatattvasaṃhitā Uttarasūtra* 4.10a–23b. Hand-gesture *mudrās*:[16]

[The Seed Seal (*bījamudrā*)]

(10) Then tie up the braided hair, join and extend the little fingers of both hands and conceal the thumbs in the middle. (11) [This] is taught in this tantra under the name 'seed seal'.

[The Paying Homage Seal (*namaskāramudrā*)]

Put the hands together and extend all the pairs [of digits]. (12) This is called the paying homage [seal], [used] in venerating all gods.

[The Nectar of Immortality Seal (*amṛtāmudrā*)]

Entwine both middle fingers with the two ring fingers, (13) join together and turn back the index and middle fingers and in the same way the little fingers and ring fingers, too. (14) Point the thumbs down. This is the seal known as the nectar of immortality.

[The Point Seal (*koṭimudrā*)]

Place the hands together, back to back, with the fingers of one interlaced with those of the other, (15) and turn them round, [so] turning them into a ball: [thus] is taught the point seal.

[The Offering Seal (*dravyamudrā*)]

Next I shall teach you the definition [of] the offering seal. (16) Whenever the aspirant has in mind a particular thing [that should be offered] he should always change the arrangement of his two hands so that they are similar [to the required offering]. (17) He should raise both hands with their fingers interlaced; by moving them [to and fro] he should show them to the [ritual helper, known as the assistant aspirant] as a sign alone [without accompanying words]. (18) By this [act] alone, everything can be brought into being, and in this way one removes obstacles [that the absence of certain offerings would have produced].

[The Ananta Throne Seal (*anantāsanamudrā*)]
He should turn his two hands downwards with the fingers entwined, (19) [but] with the little fingers and thumbs hanging downwards: this is the Ananta throne seal.

[The *Sakala* Seal (*sakalamudrā*)]
Interlock the fingers of both the hands [and make] a fist. (20) This is the *sakala* seal + . . . + in the middle.

[The *Niṣkala* Seal (*niṣkalamudrā*)]
Interlock the little fingers and ring fingers (21) [and] stretch out the middle fingers joined + . . . + tips of the index fingers. Extend the thumbs between them, point them downwards and bend them. (22) This is the *niṣkala* seal, the index finger with the left thumb. On seeing this [seal, souls] are released; on forming it, one goes to the state of Śiva. (23) For all other [gods] one should show the paying homage [seal for welcoming] and the point seal for dismissal.

6.1.2 *Jayadrathayāmala* 4.2.122c–127d, 145–9, 612–22. Three *mudrā*s:

Hear about the seal called the banner (*patākā*), O Gauri, (123) which is very powerful in bestowing the ability to move through the sky and grants omniscience. Make the left hand into a fist and point the index finger upwards. (124) Spread the fingers of the right hand and hold it sideways. This is the lovely seal called the banner. (125) One should regularly make her in the cremation ground, joined with the power previously taught. After a week, O queen of all the gods, a man will obtain communion [with Yoginīs]. (126) He will become a sky-rover, bringing a wealth of great pleasures. No seal like this is taught in the three worlds. (127) Endowed with the previously taught power and imbued with emotion, she is known to be omnipotent for the aspirant of noble soul.

This is the banner observance in the *Jayadrathayāmala*.

(145) Now I shall teach the supreme great seal called the pot (*kalaśa*), which brings nourishment to all and bestows great good fortune. Completely entwine the fingers of both hands. (146) This seal, which in the middle and elsewhere is filled with the fluid from a shower of nectar, is called the pot and brings success in all matters. (147) She is said to be sure to revive mantras which are cut, lost, burnt, broken, blocked or destroyed, O goddess. (148) By means of her, O queen of the gods, one anoints one's self; it is sure to be nourished, together with the mantra. (149) When she is performed all the gods are happy. She should be known to bestow enjoyment and liberation [and] has been duly taught to you.

This is the pot seal in the *Jayadrathayāmala*.

(612) Now I shall teach the best of all the best seals, which is called the howler (*phetkārī*) and which results in the attainment of all powers. (613) In a cremation ground, full – satiated by flesh – and resolute in one's vows, go to the middle of a sacrificial altar and perform the queen of seals. (614) Or [do it] in an empty house +whose interstices have been filled in+. Do not do it in any other way: doing so brings trouble. (615) Sit down, alert, put the left foot at the anus and extend the right leg, slightly bent, my dear. (616) Bend the arms, clench the fists and put them at the earlobes. Look upwards and make the terrifying, horrific howl of a jackal. (617) With angry eyes and angry face make harsh howls [. . .] and the best middle nectar of immortality. (618) One should thus sound out a howl [. . .]; in this way one obtains communion [with Yoginīs] in two *ghaṭikā*s [i.e. forty-eight minutes]. (619) The horde of Yoginīs tremble, terrified and very distressed. They are in his power,

as if he were Lord Bhairava. (620) This that you have been taught is the queen of seals, called the howler, which accomplishes all the deeds of men and is very hard to get in this world. (621) It has been taught among the many, various seals, along with its method, O queen of the gods. When the great, best [seal] is obtained by the lords of aspirants from the mouth of a guru, (622) then the best heroes should know that there is no rebirth. When it reaches one's ears then one is sure to master yoga.

This is the howler seal observance in the *Jayadrathayāmala*.

6.2

Haṭhayogic *Mudrās*

6.2.1 *Amṛtasiddhi* Chapters 11–13. The great seal, the great lock and the piercing.

[Chapter 11 The Inquiry into the Great Seal (*mahāmudrā*)]

(1) The great seal concealed in all the tantras is being taught. Men who obtain it are worshipped by the gods. (2) Having obtained it after performing a great number of good deeds for ten billion births yogis cross the ocean of existence.

(3) Carefully press the *yoni* with the left heel, extend the right foot and hold it firmly with the hands. (4) Raise the haunches on to a seat, put the chin on the chest, close the nine [bodily] openings and fill up the abdomen with air. (5) Put the mind at the crossroads and commence breath-control. Divide the breath's movement between the moon and sun, and restrain it.

(6) This consumes impurities, holds *bindu* and *nāda*, makes all the channels flow and kindles the fire. (7) Through practice, mastery of the body, speech and mind by means of yoga of the body, speech and mind is

sure to arise for the yogi who is on the path. (8) By means of this seal yogis are sure to obtain everything, so one should zealously practise this great seal. (9) Because this self-born seal is the greatest of all seals, the best among the wise call her the great seal. (10) She stops death, so is always beneficial. Only the mind which holds her overcomes magical restraints. (11) +Her name is spelt out by the first syllables of the words+. It is taught only for the delight of those engaged in yoga.

Thus ends the Inquiry into the Great Seal.

[Chapter 12 The Inquiry into the [Great] Lock ([*mahā*]*bandha*)]

(1) That by which yogis are sure to master this great seal is called the great lock (*mahābandha*). It holds the breath in the body. (2) And the lock should be known to be of two kinds, just as *bindu*[17] was said to be, for there is the perineum lock for the goddesses and the throat lock for the gods.[18]

(3) Inhale, hold the breath, assume the [great] seal which removes danger and quickly apply the lock, which is kept secret by the gods and demons. (4) Simultaneously contract the anus and the perineum, make the *apāna* breath move upwards and join it with the *samāna* breath.[19] (5) The yogi should practise the lock at the side of the gateway of the central channel, having blocked the triple pathway, then carefully restrain the breath. (6) Put the breath in *prāṇa*, make *prāṇa* face downwards and move it so that it goes upwards by joining *prāṇa* and *apāna* together as one.

(7) This finest of yogas makes known the way of the adepts in the body. Fulfilment, conviction and growth arise through practising it, not otherwise. (8) The channels, all of which usually flow downwards, are reversed by this great lock.

(9) Like minds leaving their field of operation, the elements and essences which are excreted leave the body because of the downward flow. (10) Yogis should always

remember that this [lock] functions in the body like a dyke in the external world blocking a stream. (11) This lock is said [to work] on all the channels. By the grace of this lock, the gods become manifest. (12) This is the lock on the crossroads, which blocks the three paths.

[The yogi] should make manifest the one path by which the adepts travelled happily. (13) This downward path is said to bestow birth and death. These two [paths] which flow at [its] side cause sin and merit. (14) Put all the elements into the pot of breath-retention by means of a firm lock, and gather together the *udāna* breath through joining *prāṇa* and *apāna*. (15) This lock blocks upward movement in all the channels. By the grace of this alone is the perineum lock successful. (16) This is the casket (*saṃpuṭa*) yoga; it is also taught as the root lock (*mūlabandha*). By means of this alone the three yogas are successful for good people who practise.

Thus ends the Inquiry into the [Great] Lock.

[Chapter 13 The Inquiry into the Piercing (*vedha*)]

(1) The [great] seal should be known to be of two kinds, just as the lock is twofold: the perineum seal is for the goddesses, and the penis seal is for the gods. (2) Just as external creation arises from the female and the male, so is creation in the body destroyed by the female and the male. (3) A woman of virtue and beauty is useless without a man; the great seal and great lock are useless without the piercing.

(4) The yogi should take hold of all the breaths, perform the lock as taught and start performing the piercing with the breath, which must be joined with the mind. (5) After making the mighty *prāṇa* breath face the opening of the central channel, he should gradually pierce the crossroads with the breath. (6) Using the hands put the penis on the ground, motionless like the Pole Star. In the same way, keep the two feet facing downwards, unmoving. (7) Sitting steadily, lift the haunches and

tap the great [Mount] Meru [i.e. the central column of the body] with the heels of the upright feet using ten million diamond points of breath. (8) That makes the piercing happen. The gods in the middle of [Mount] Meru, from the underworld to the heavens, tremble because of Meru being made to move. (9) As a result of the piercing of Meru, Brahmā and the other gods are sure to die. At first this piercing happens quickly in the knot of Brahmā; (10) then, having broken the knot of Brahmā it breaks the knot of Viṣṇu. Then, having broken the knot of Viṣṇu, it breaks the knot of Rudra. (11) Then, having broken the knot of Rudra and cut the creeper of delusion, this breath opens the very secret gateway of Brahmā.[20] (12) The great seal, the great lock [and] the third, the great piercing: by means of these three elements, whose essences are secret, yoga is successful. (13) He who knows these three elements knows the three worlds. He who is lucky enough to practise them becomes omnipresent and [omni]potent. (14) The gods are in the most secret tantras. It is because of this entitlement that men have this claim [to them]. (15) A man becomes anointed with all consecrations, endowed with all entitlements and associated with the path of the adepts [by means of this] and not otherwise. (16) The pride of one who knows this seal is justified: everything is understood by him, thanks to the goddess of the channel.

Thus ends the piercing insight in the Attainment of Immortality.

6.2.2 *Dattātreyayogaśāstra* 131–64. The haṭhayogic *mudrās*:

[*Haṭhayoga*: The Way of adepts such as Kapila]

(131) 'Next I shall teach the [*haṭhayoga*] doctrine of adepts such as Kapila. The difference [from the eightfold yoga, which I have just taught] is a difference in practice, but the reward is one and the same.

[The Great Seal (*mahāmudrā*)]

(132) I shall carefully proclaim the great seal (*mahāmudrā*) as taught by Bhairava. [The yogi] should place the heel of his left foot at his perineum. (133) He should stretch out his right foot and hold it firmly with both hands. After placing his chin on his chest, he should then fill [himself] up with air. (134) Using breath-retention he should hold [his breath] for as long as he can before exhaling. After practising with the left foot, he should practise with the right.

[The Great Lock (*mahābandha*)]

(135) [The yogi] should place the outstretched foot on his thigh. This is the great lock (*mahābandha*) and he should practise it like the [great] seal.

[The Great Piercing (*mahāvedha*)]

(136) While in the great lock, [the yogi] should gently tap his buttocks on the ground. This is the great piercing (*mahāvedha*); it is practised by perfected men.

[The *Khecarī* Seal (*khecarīmudrā*)]

(137) Next [the yogi] should turn back his tongue and hold it in the hollow of the skull, while looking between the eyebrows. This is the *khecarī* seal.

[The *Jālandhara* Lock (*jālandharabandha*)]

(138) [The yogi] should constrict the throat and firmly place the chin on the chest. This is the *jālandhara* lock. It prevents loss of the nectar of immortality (*amṛta*). (139) As long as it keeps drinking the nectar of immortality that has dripped from the thousand[-petalled] lotus in the skull of embodied beings, the fire at the navel burns brightly. (140) And so that the fire might not drink that nectar of immortality, [the yogi] should drink it himself. Through constant practice in this way, it goes by the rear pathway (141) and makes the body immortal. For this reason one should practise *jālandhara*.

[The *Uḍḍiyāna* Lock (*uḍḍiyānabandha*)]

Uḍḍiyāna is easy and always taught because of its many good qualities. (142) Practising it regularly, even an old man becomes young. With special effort [the yogi] should pull his navel upwards and push it downwards. (143) Practising [like this] for six months, he is sure to conquer death.

[The Root Lock (*mūlabandha*)]

He who regularly practises the root lock is expert at yoga. (144) He should press his anus with his heel and forcefully contract his perineum over and over again, so that his breath goes upwards. (145) Becoming united by means of the root lock, the upward and downward moving breaths, and *nāda* and *bindu*, are sure to bestow complete success in yoga.

[The Inverter (*viparītakaraṇī*)]

(146) The technique called the inverter destroys all diseases. In one constantly devoted to [its] practice the digestive fire increases. (147) He must eat a lot of food, O Sāṃkṛti. If he eats little, the fire will burn [him] up. (148) Listen, Sāṃkṛti, to how the sun can be up and the moon down. On the first day the head should be down and the feet up for a short while. (149) By practising for a little while longer every day, after six months grey hair and wrinkles disappear. (150) He who regularly practises for three hours is expert at yoga.

[The *Vajrolī* Seal (*vajrolīmudrā*)]

I shall teach *vajrolī*, which is kept hidden by all yogis, (151) for it is a great secret, not to be given to all and sundry. But one should certainly teach it to one who is as dear to one as one's own life. (152) The yogi who knows *vajrolī* is worthy of success, even if he behaves self-indulgently, disregarding the rules taught in yoga. (153) I shall tell you the two things [necessary] for it which are hard for anyone to obtain, [and] which are said to bring about success for a [yogi] if he does obtain them: (154) milk and generative fluid (*āṅgirasa*). Of the two, the first is [readily] available. The second is hard for men to get; they must use some stratagem to procure it from women. (155–6) A man should strive to find a woman devoted to the practice of yoga. Either a man or a woman can obtain success if they have no regard for one another's gender and practise with only their own ends in mind. If the semen moves, then [the yogi] should draw it upwards and preserve it. (157) Semen preserved in this way truly overcomes death. Death [arises] through the fall of semen, life from its preservation. (158–60) All yogis achieve success through the preservation of semen.

The method of practice by which *amarolī* and *sahajolī* arise is taught in the tradition of the adepts.

[The yogi] should practise using these [techniques] that have been taught, each at the proper time. Then the royal yoga will arise. Without them it definitely will not happen. Success does not happen through mere superficial knowledge; it happens through practice alone. (161) After obtaining the excellent royal yoga, which subjects all beings to his will, [the yogi] can do anything or nothing, behaving as he likes. (162) When the activity of the yogi is perfect without yoga, the perfection stage [arises], which bestows the rewards of enjoyment and liberation.

(163–4) I have taught you everything, O Brahman. Practise yoga, Sāṃkṛti!'

After hearing these words of his, that Sāṃkṛti obtained complete success through the grace of Dattātreya and then attained yoga.

6.2.3 *Gorakṣaśataka* 16–28. The stimulation of the goddess:

(16) Now I shall teach in brief the stimulation of the goddess (*śakticālana*). The goddess is coiled. Making her move (17) from her home to the centre of the eyebrows is called the stimulation of the goddess. There are

two chief ways of accomplishing this: the stimulation of Sarasvatī (18) and the restraint of the breath. Through practice, Kuṇḍalinī becomes straight.

[The Stimulation of Sarasvatī]

Of the two [methods] I shall first teach you the stimulation of Sarasvatī. (19) Knowers of antiquity call Sarasvatī Arundhatī. By making her move, Kuṇḍalinī moves automatically. (20–21) With the vital breath moving in the Iḍā channel, the wise man should sit steadily in the lotus posture, spread out a cloth twelve fingers long and four fingers broad, wrap it around [Sarasvatī's] channel [i.e. the tongue] and hold it firmly with the thumbs and index fingers of both hands. (22) For two *muhūrta*s [i.e. one hour, thirty-six minutes] he should fearlessly move it left and right over and over again, as much as he can. (23) He should draw [the part of] the Suṣumnā channel which is at Kuṇḍalinī slightly upwards so that Kuṇḍalinī can enter the Suṣumnā's mouth. (24) *Prāṇa* leaves that place and automatically enters the Suṣumnā. [The yogi] should stretch his stomach and, having contracted his throat, (25) he should fill himself up with air through the solar channel; (26) the wind travels up from the chest. Therefore, one should regularly stimulate Sarasvatī, she who contains sound. (27) By stimulating her the yogi is freed from diseases such as abdominal distension, dropsy, splenitis and others which affect the stomach. (28) All those diseases are sure to be destroyed by the stimulation of the goddess.

6.2.4 *Vivekamārtaṇḍa* 47–57. On *khecarīmudrā*, *bindu* and *rajas*:

(47) The tongue turned back and into the hollow of the skull, the gaze between the brows: this is *khecarīmudrā*. (48) Neither disease, nor death, nor sleep, nor hunger, nor fainting arise for he who knows *khecarī*. (49) He who knows *khecarī* is not afflicted by disease or tainted by *karma* or troubled by death. (50) The mind moves (*carati*) in space (*khe*), because the tongue moves in

space. This is the *mudrā* called *khecarī*, honoured by the adepts.

(51) The *bindu* of he who has sealed the opening above the uvula with *khecarī* does not fall, even if he is embraced by a passionate woman. (52) When *bindu* is steady in the body then there is no fear of death. When the sky *mudrā* (*nabhomudrā*) is applied, then *bindu* does not move. (53) When *bindu* has moved and reached the fire it goes upwards on being checked by the *yoni mudrā* and struck by the goddess (*śakti*). (54) *Bindu* is [in fact] of two kinds: white and red. White is *bindu* and red is the great *rajas* (female generative fluid). (55) Looking like vermilion, *rajas* is situated in the perineal region. *Bindu* resides in the moon. Joining the two is very difficult. (56) *Bindu* is Śiva. *Rajas* is Śakti. *Bindu* is the moon. *Rajas* is the sun. Only by joining the two is the highest condition attained. (57) When *rajas* is propelled by moving the goddess by means of the breath it joins with *bindu*. He who knows this knows yoga.

6.2.5 *Vivekamārtaṇḍa* 113–15. The inverter (*viparītakaraṇī*):

(113) The sun, whose essence is fire, resides in the region of the navel. The moon, whose essence is the nectar of immortality, is always situated in the palate. (114) The moon faces downwards and rains. The sun faces upwards and takes. One must learn the technique by means of which nectar is obtained. (115) The navel up, the palate down; the sun up, the moon down. The technique called the inverter is to be obtained through the teaching of a guru.

6.2.6 *Jñāneśvarī* 6.192–210 (on *Bhagavadgītā* 6.13). The seals and the locks:[21]

Bhagavadgītā

(6.13) Holding the body and head straight, unmoving and steady, staring at the tip of the nose, not looking elsewhere [. . .]

Jñāneśvarī

(192) Hear how powerful the seal is. Join the thighs with the calves, (193) put the soles of the feet at the foot of the tree of the Base (*ādhāra*), angled, joined together and steady. (194) The right [foot] is put at the Base, thereby the perineal seam is pressed, [and] then the left foot sits on it at ease. (195) Between the anus and penis [is a space] exactly four fingers broad. There, leaving one and a half [fingers on one side] and one and a half [on the other] within [that] area, (196) one finger['s breadth] is left in between. There [the perineum] is pressed by the upper part of the heel, with the body balanced on top. (197) It is raised imperceptibly, likewise the end of the back is raised. Both ankles are held in just that measure. (198) Then the sum of the body, Pārtha, wholly in every respect, becomes balanced (?) on top of the heel.

(199) Arjuna, know that to be the characteristic of the root lock (*mūlabandha*), the thunderbolt pose (*vajrāsana*) being its secondary name. (200) Such a seal (*mudrā*) comes to be in the Base (*ādhāra*), and the path [of breath] in the lower portion [of the body] is closed. There, *apāna* begins to recede inside. (201) Then the cupped hand automatically sits on the left leg, [and] it looks [as if] the shoulders are enlarged. (202) In between, because of the raised spine, the lotus of the head becomes firm, [and] the sides of the doors of the eyes want to close. (203) The upper lids do not move, the lower ones expand on the lower part [of the eyes. Thus] for [the eyes] comes about the state of being half-open. (204) Sight, after remaining inside, fondly puts a foot outward, [and] there gets a place on the seat at the top of the nose. (205) Like that it fixes itself inside and does not step out again, therefore this half-sight remains right there. (206) Now all desire to visit the directions [of the outside world] or see forms ceases automatically. (207) Then the neck recedes, the chin presses down. Becoming firm, it presses itself to

the breast. (208) The Adam's apple disappears inside. The lock (*bandha*) which is fixed above [it] is called *jālandhara*, O son of Pāṇḍu.

(209) The navel is pushed up, the belly disappears [and], inside, the casket of the heart expands. (210) On the margin on top of the Svādhiṣṭhāna [*cakra*], at the bottom of the area of the navel: the lock (*bandha*) produced there, Arjuna, that is *uḍḍiyāna*.

6.2.7 *Candrāvalokana* 1. *Śāmbhavīmudrā*:

When [the yogi] focuses internally with his gaze, unblinking, directed outwards it is the *śāmbhavīmudrā*, which is concealed in all the tantras.

6.2.8 *Khecarīvidyā* 1.45–57, 65–72. *Khecarīmudrā*:

(45) In the manner described by his guru, [every day] for seven days the knower of the self should rub the base of his palate and clean away all impurity. (46) He should take a very sharp, well-oiled and clean blade resembling a leaf of the Snuhī plant and then cut away a hair's breadth [of the frenulum] with it. (47) After cutting, he should rub [the cut] with a powder of rock salt and Pathyā [*Terminalia chebula* Linn.]. After seven days he should again cut away a hair's breadth.

(48) [The yogi], constantly applying himself, should thus practise gradually for six months. After six months the binding tendon at the base of the tongue is destroyed. (49) Then, knowing the rules of time and limit, the yogi should gradually pull upwards the abode of the goddess of speech [i.e. the tip of the tongue] having wrapped it in cloth.

(50) Then, in six months, after regular drawing out [of the tongue], my dear, it reaches [upwards] between the eyebrows, obliquely to the ears, (51–2) and downwards it is gradually made to reach the base of the chin. Then, only after three years, upwards it easily reaches the

hairline, sideways the temples, my dear, [and] downwards the Adam's apple. (53) After three years more it covers the end of the Suṣumnā channel, O goddess; obliquely it reaches the region above the nape of the neck [and] downwards the hollow [at the base] of the throat.

(54) The practice must only be carried out gradually, not all at once. The body of him who tries to do it all at once is destroyed. (55) For this reason the practice is to be carried out very gradually, O beautiful lady.

When the tongue reaches the aperture of Brahmā (*brahmarandhra*) [i.e. the fontanelle] by the external path, (56) then [the yogi], O goddess, should rub with the tip of his finger the bolt [of the doorway] of Brahmā, [which is] hard for even the gods to pierce, [and] insert [his] tongue there. (57) Practising thus for three years the tongue enters the door of Brahmā. [. . .]

[The drinking of *amṛta* and its rewards]

(65) [The yogi] should know the great pathway in the skull in the region above the uvula between the eyebrows [to be] the Three-peaked Mountain, [which is] honoured by the perfected ones (66) [and] resembles a chickpea sprout. He should fix his mind there. Licking with his tongue the supreme nectar of immortality (*amṛta*) flowing there (67) [and progressing] gradually on the path of the practice, [the yogi] should drink [nectar] for four years, my dear. Grey hair and wrinkles are destroyed, supreme success arises (68) and, as the knower of the meaning of all scriptures, [the yogi] lives for a thousand years. Success in sciences – such as finding buried treasure, entering subterranean realms, controlling the earth and alchemy (69–71) – arise for the yogi after five years, O Pārvatī.

Duly drinking the flowing nectar with [his] tongue, the resolute yogi should curb his diet for twelve years, [living] as an ascetic. By this application of the practice, the great yogi, free of grey hair and wrinkles [and] with a body as incorruptible as diamond, lives for 100,000 years. With the strength of 10,000 elephants, my dear, (72) he has long-distance sight and hearing. Capable of punishing and rewarding [people], he becomes powerful with respect to everything.

6.2.9 *Śivasaṃhitā* 4.1–19. *Yonimudrā*:

(1) Next I shall teach the excellent yoga of *mudrā*s, by merely practising which all diseases disappear.

(2) First fix the mind in the Base (*ādhāra*) by means of inhalation. The *yoni* is between the anus and the penis. Contract it and make it active. (3) Meditate on the god of love as residing in Brahmā's *yoni* in the shape of a ball, looking like ten million suns and as cool as ten million moons. (4–5) Above it is the ultimate digit, a tiny flame whose form is consciousness. The yogi should imagine himself as having become one with it. He goes along the way of Brahmā, progressing through the three *liṅga*s, to the nectar of immortality which is in heaven, characterized by ultimate bliss, pink, abounding in vital energy and pouring forth showers of rain.

(6) After drinking the divine nectar of the Kula, the yogi should enter the Kula once more. He should go again to the Kula by means of breath-retention, not otherwise. (7) In this tantra I have called her *prāṇa*. That which begins with the fire of time and ends in Śiva is absorbed in her once more.

(8) This is the great *yonimudrā*. Its application has been taught. Merely by applying it one can do anything. (9–11) Mantras which are incomplete, pierced, paralysed, burnt out, blunt, dirty, reviled, broken, mistaken, cursed, unconscious, slow, young, old, audacious, proud of their youth, on the side of the enemy, impotent, weak, weakened or fragmented into a hundred pieces soon become powerful in conjunction with this practice. When given by a guru, they all bestow supernatural powers and liberation. (12) The yogi obtains mastery of whatever he utters

in the form of a mantra, auspicious or otherwise, by applying the *yonimudrā*.

(13) After duly initiating him and anointing him a thousand times, this *mudrā* is taught in order to grant the right to practise mantra. (14) Were he to kill a thousand Brahmans and destroy the three worlds, by applying the *yonimudrā* he would not be tainted by sin. (15) By applying the *yonimudrā*, a man who kills his guru, drinks alcohol, steals or sleeps with his guru's wife is not bound by these sins. (16) Therefore, those who desire liberation should practise regularly. Success arises through practice. Through practice one attains liberation. (17) One obtains understanding through practice. Yoga happens through practice. Mantras are mastered through practice. Mastery of the wind comes through practice.

(18) One deceives time through practice and conquers death. Through practice there arise mastery of speech and the ability to go where one wants.

(19) *Yonimudrā* is to be well guarded and not given to all and sundry. In no circumstances should it be given out, even by those at their last gasp.

6.2.10 *Śivasaṃhitā* 4.78–104. *Vajrolīmudrā* and *bindu*:

(78) I shall teach my devotees a summary of *vajrolī*, the secret of all secrets, the destroyer of the darkness of transmigration. (79) Through the practice of *vajrolī* even a householder living according to his desires and without the restrictions taught in yoga can be liberated. (80) Together with *vajrolī* this yoga grants liberation even to one who indulges his senses, so it should be regularly and zealously practised by yogis.

(81) First the wise yogi should, carefully and following prescription, draw up through his urethra the *rajas* from a woman's vagina and make it enter his body. (82) After awakening his *bindu* he should start to move his penis. If by chance his *bindu* should move it can be held up with

the *yonimudrā*. (83) He should draw his *bindu* on to the left side, remove his penis from the vagina for a moment and then start having intercourse again. (84) Following his guru's instructions, the yogi should draw up his *apāna* wind and, making the sound *huṃ huṃ*, forcibly extract the *rajas* from the vagina.

(85) In order to obtain success in yoga quickly by means of this practice, the yogi who worships his guru's lotus feet eats the products of the cow. (86) Know *bindu* to be lunar and *rajas* to be solar. One should strive to combine them both in one's own body. (87) I am *bindu*, the goddess is *rajas*. When both are combined, the body of the practising yogi becomes divine. (88) Death arises through the falling of *bindu*, life when it is retained. Therefore, one should do one's utmost to retain one's semen. (89) One is born and dies in the world through *bindu*. In this there is no doubt. Knowing this, the yogi should always retain his *bindu*. (90) When the great jewel *bindu* is mastered there is nothing on earth that cannot be mastered. Through its grace, one becomes as great as me. (91) *Bindu*, depending on its state, brings about happiness and sorrow for all the deluded inhabitants of the world who are subject to decrepitude and death.

(92) This auspicious yoga is the best of all for yogis. Through its practice a man obtains perfection even if he indulges his senses. (93) Every goal that is sought after is sure to be achieved in this world by means of this yoga, even after enjoying all pleasures. (94) Using it, yogis are sure to attain total perfection, so one should practise it while having lots of fun.

(95) *Sahajolī* and *amarolī* are variations of *vajrolī*. The yogi should use any and every means to master his *bindu*. (96) If his *bindu* should accidentally enter the vagina, then the resultant combination of the moon and the sun is called *amarolī* and he should suck it up through his urethra. (97) When his *bindu* moves the

yogi should restrain it with *yonimudrā*. This is called *sahajolī* and is kept secret in all the tantras.

(98) The difference is due to a difference in name. In practice it has the same result, so yogis continuously make every effort to master it. (99) I have taught this yoga out of great affection for my devotees. It is to be guarded well and not given to all and sundry. (100) There has never been a secret as secret as this, nor will there ever be, so the wise should always guard it very carefully.

(101–2) For the yogi who uses his wind to force back his urine when urinating and then releases it, bit by bit, while holding it up, and who practises every day according to the way taught by his guru, there arises the mastery of *bindu*, which grants great success. (103) The *bindu* of the yogi who practises daily for six months according to his guru's instructions is never lost, even if he enjoys a hundred women. (104) When the great jewel *bindu* is mastered, there is nothing on earth that cannot be mastered. By its grace, even my majesty is easily obtained.

6.2.11 *Baḥr al-ḥayāt* Chapter 4. On *khecarī*:[22]

On the Knowledge of the Heart and the Character of Discipline

The word of recollection of *khecarī*. When a seeker wants to begin the recollection of the *khecarī* one closes the door of the palate with the tongue. In the first stage, having ground the tongue for six months with rock salt and whole pepper, one spends twice the time massaging it; one squeezes it with both hands and lengthens it, [as one] soaks a garment and wrings it out. One never eats the betel leaf, and one keeps the nail of the index finger and the thumb long. Beneath the tongue there are two veins, one black and the other red; one gradually seizes them with the fingernail and holds most of the tongue open and introduces it towards the throat so that the entire tongue enters the cavity above the palate. While holding the breath, at the time when one brings the tongue to the palate, one flexes the beard on the collarbone. When one's activity reaches this point, one can remain for years in a single breath. The tongue then reaches the opening of the throat; when one brings the tongue out, the tops of the nostrils are level [with it]. At that point one realizes that one has reached the goal and one comprehends the way to practise. First one sits in the adept's pose (*siddhāsana*) in this form, holding one's seat on the ground and making the knee and shin stick to each other. One places the tip of the sole of the left foot behind the right foot, and the end of the sole of the left foot beneath the genitals, so that the exit of urine and semen is closed. One holds both hands backwards on both knees, and one also maintains the closure of the seal of the throat, as is mentioned above, and the benefits of this are also well known – until the wayfarer's activity reaches from here to there, and he realizes that the activities of sleep and waking, hunger and thirst, burning and drowning, softness and laziness, hot and cold, thoughts, death, and all diverse things, are transcended; the path of that wayfarer's travel is in the heavens. *Khecarī*, in the description of the yogis, they call 'the heavens' (*aflāk*). When this practice is perfected, one obtains a single station from the orbit of earth to the Cupola (*'arsh*), taking a single breath to go from the orbit of earth to the subterranean. Above, below and in the middle are all three a single orbit; all three worlds are under the control of the wayfarer. Other benefits of this practice will become clear.

6.2.12 The *Aṣṭa Mudrā* ('Eight *Mudrās*') of Gorakhnāth. The eight seals:

(1) Master, tell me about each of the eight seals inside the body.

O renouncer, the *mūlanī* seal is at the penis, where pleasure and desire happen. (2) When one becomes indifferent to pleasure and desire, then the *mūlanī* seal comes into being.

The *jalaśrī* seal is at the navel, [where] death and anger happen. (3) When one becomes indifferent to death and anger, then the *jalaśrī* seal comes into being.

The *ṣīraṇī* seal is at the heart, [where] the light of knowledge arises. (4) When one becomes indifferent to the light of knowledge, then the *ṣīraṇī* seal comes into being.

The *khecarī* seal is at the mouth, [where] good and bad tastes happen. (5) When one becomes indifferent to good and bad tastes, then the *khecarī* seal comes into being.

The *bhūcarī* seal is at the nose, [where] good and bad smells happen. (6) When one becomes indifferent to good and bad smells, then the *bhūcarī* seal comes into being.

The *cācarī* seal is at the eye, [where] good and bad sights happen. (7) When one becomes indifferent to good and bad sights, then the *cācarī* seal comes into being.

The *agocarī* seal is at the ear, [where] good and bad sounds happen. (8) When one becomes indifferent to good and bad sounds, then the *agocarī* seal comes into being.

The *unmanī* seal is at the skull, [where] the supreme light arises. (9) When one becomes indifferent to the supreme light, then the *unmanī* seal comes into being.

Ascetic, know the eight varieties of seal. By performing them, one becomes a god.

Thus the eight seals taught by the glorious ascetic Gorakhnāth are complete and finished. [Homage] to Śiva!

6.2.13 Selections from *Gheraṇḍasaṃhitā* Chapter 3. *Mudrās*:

(1–3) The great *mudrā* (*mahāmudrā*), the sky *mudrā* (*nabhomudrā*), *uḍḍīyāna*, *jālandhara*, the root lock (*mūlabandha*), the great lock (*mahābandha*), the great piercing (*mahāvedha*) and *khecarī*, the inverter (*viparītakaraṇī*), *yoni*, *vajrolī*, the stimulation of the goddess (*śakticālana*), the pool (*taḍāgi*), the frog *mudrā* (*maṇḍūkīmudrā*), *śāmbhavī*, the five fixations (*dhāraṇās*), *aśvinī*,[23] the trapper (*pāśinī*), the crow (*kākī*), the elephant (*mātaṅgī*) and the snake (*bhujaṅginī*): these twenty-five seals (*mudrās*) grant success in this world to yogis.

[The *Yoni* Seal (*yonimudrā*)]

(33) The yogi should sit in the adept's pose and block the ears with the thumbs, the eyes with the index fingers, the nostrils with the middle fingers and the mouth with the ring and little fingers. (34) Having drawn in *prāṇa* with repeated applications of the crow seal, he should then join it with *apāna* and meditate on the six *cakra*s in succession. Using the mantras *huṃ* and *haṃsa*, the wise yogi (35) should bring the sleeping serpent goddess to consciousness and raise her, together with the vital essence (*jīva*), to the highest lotus. (36) Having himself now become made of the goddess (*śakti*), he should visualize supreme union with Śiva, as well as various pleasures, enjoyments and ultimate bliss. (37) As a result of the union of Śiva and the goddess, he should experience the ultimate goal on earth. With blissful mind, he should realize that he is Brahman. (38) The great *yoni* seal is to be kept secret. It is hard to obtain even for the gods. As soon as he masters it the yogi is sure to enter *samādhi*.

[The Stimulation of the Goddess (*śakticālana*)]

(40) The great goddess Kuṇḍalinī, the energy (*śakti*) of the self, sleeps at the Base support (*mūlādhāra*) in the form of a snake coiled round three and a half times. (41) As long as she is asleep in the body the life essence is but a bound animal and gnosis does not arise, even if the

yogi practises innumerable yogas. (42) Just as he might open a door with a key, so should the yogi forcefully awaken Kuṇḍalinī and break open the gateway of Brahman. (43) The yogi should wrap his midriff in a cloth and, not going outside while naked, remain in a private room and practise the stimulation of the goddess (*śakticālana*). (44) The requirements of the covering cloth are that it should be nine inches long, three inches wide, soft, white and fine. The yogi should put on such a covering and tie it to the string around his waist. (45) He should smear his body with ash and sit in the adept's pose. Drawing in *prāṇa* through his nostrils, he should force it to join with *apāna*. (46) He should gently contract the anus by means of the *aśvinī* seal until breath (*vāyu*) is forced to enter the central channel (*suṣumnā*) and manifests its presence. (47) Then, because the breath has been restricted, Kuṇḍalinī holds her breath and suffocates, so she enters the upward path. (48) Without the stimulation of the goddess, the *yoni* seal does not succeed. The yogi should first practise stimulation and then practise the *yoni* seal. (49) I have thus taught you the stimulation of the goddess, O Caṇḍakapāli. The yogi should strive to keep it secret and practise it every day.

[The Pool Seal (*taḍāgimudrā*)]

(50) The yogi should draw the belly backwards and upwards so that it looks like a pool. This is the great pool seal. It destroys decrepitude and death.

[The Frog Seal (*maṇḍūkīmudrā*)]

(51) The yogi should seal the mouth and move the root of the tongue about. Then he should slowly swallow the nectar of immortality. This is called the frog seal. (52) For the man who regularly practises the frog [seal] neither wrinkles nor old age arise; he gets eternal youth and his hair does not turn grey.

[The *Śāmbhavī* Seal (*śāmbhavīmudrā*)]

(53) The yogi should look between the eyes and observe the delights of the self. This is the *śāmbhavī* seal, which is concealed in all the tantras. (54) [The sacred texts] – Vedas, Śāstras and Purāṇas – are like common courtesans; this *śāmbhavī* seal is kept hidden like a lady of good family. (55) He who knows the *śāmbhavī* seal is none other than the primal lord Ādinātha [i.e. Śiva], he is Nārāyaṇa [i.e. Viṣṇu] himself, he is Brahmā the creator. (56) Maheśvara has said, 'Truly, truly and again truly, he who knows Śāmbhavī is Brahman and no one else.'

[The Five Fixations (*pañca dhāraṇā*)]

(57) I have taught you the *śāmbhavī* seal. Now hear the five fixations. By practising the fixations, everything on earth is possible. (58) The yogi can come and go from the heavenly realms in his mortal body; he can move as fast as the mind and has the power of travelling through the ether. There is no other way of achieving this.

[Earth Fixation]

(59) The earth element shines like a piece of yellow orpiment and contains the syllable *la*. It is accompanied by Brahmā, is square and is situated at the heart. The yogi should fix his breath and his mind there for two hours. This is the earth fixation; it always brings about steadiness and conquers the earth.

[Verses 60–63 describe the Water Fixation, the Fire Fixation, the Air Fixation and the Space Fixation.][24]

[The *Āśvinī* Seal (*aśvinīmudrā*)]

(64) The yogi should contract and dilate the aperture of the anus over and over again. That is the *aśvinī* seal. It awakens the goddess.

[The Trapper Seal (*pāśinīmudrā*)]

(65) The yogi should put his feet behind his neck, making a tight restraint like a noose. That is the trapper seal. It awakens the goddess.

[The Crow Seal (*kākīmudrā*)]

(66) The yogi should make his mouth like a crow's beak and very slowly draw in air. This is the crow seal. It destroys all diseases.

[The Elephant Seal (*mātaṅginīmudrā*)]

(67) Standing in water up to his neck, the yogi should draw in water through his nostrils. Then he should expel it from his mouth before drawing it in through his mouth again. (68) Then he should expel it from his nostrils. He should do this over and over again. The great elephant seal destroys decrepitude and death.

[The Snake Seal (*bhujagīmudrā*)]

(69) The yogi should push his mouth slightly forward and draw in air through his throat. That is the snake seal. It destroys decrepitude and death. (70) The yogi who practises the snake seal quickly destroys all gastric ailments, particularly indigestion and the like.

SEVEN
Mantra

The use of verbal formulas called mantras to bring about worldly and soteriological aims has a pre-eminent place in almost all Indian religious traditions.[1] It is central to Vedic religion, whose rites involve the chanting, with great precision, of mantras from the Vedic Saṃhitās (*c.* 1500–1000 BCE), while making sacrificial fire offerings. It is equally important in the tantric traditions (*c.* 200 CE onwards), whose mantras include five from the Vedas (the *brahmamantra*s) supplemented by a vast array of additional formulas. Tantric mantras, which are repeated, either audibly or internally, and visualized, may vary from single 'seed' syllables (*bījamantra*s) to lengthy 'garland' formulas of twenty or more syllables (*mālāmantra*s). In contrast with the usually meaningful Vedic mantras,[2] tantric mantras often consist of syllables which embody tantric deities but are otherwise uninterpretable.

Mantra and Yoga

Both the Vedic and Tantric traditions greatly informed yoga. A passage in the *c.* 800–600 BCE Vedic *Jaiminīya Upaniṣad Brāhmaṇa* (7.1) instructs the primary singer of the first hymn in the Soma sacrifice to prepare himself by sitting facing north at dawn, visualizing the hymn, controlling his breath and harnessing his senses in order to yoke his mind to the hymn. This process is called *yukti*, a word cognate with the Sanskrit word *yoga*. In yoga's earliest explicit systematic formulations, however, it is not associated with mantra practice. Thus the *Mahābhārata* draws a distinction between the mantra-reciter (*jāpaka*) and the yogi, even if their aims are identical: 'Mantra-reciters and yogis get the same [ultimate] reward: in this there is no doubt' (12.193.22cd; see 11.3.2). The *Bhagavadgītā* makes no mention of mantra in its treatment of yoga,[3] and later says that mantra-repetition (*japa*) is the best of sacrificial rites (10.25).

The Vedic Syllable *Oṃ* and Yoga

The syllable *oṃ*, which became central to Brahmanical yoga systems, is first taught in the mantras of the *Sāma Veda* and *Yajur Veda* (*c.* 1000 BCE), but not in the context of yoga. *Oṃ* is mentioned (as *praṇava*, its usual name in Sanskrit texts) in Patañjali's *Yogaśāstra*, where it is said to verbalize Īśvara, the Lord, whom its repetition makes manifest (7.2).[4] The homologization of the components of *oṃ* (*a*, *u* and *m*) with the three Vedas, the three great gods and so forth – which is first found in the *Aitareya Brāhmaṇa* (5.32) and repeated in various Upaniṣads (e.g. *Māṇḍūkya Upaniṣad* 8) – is found in a wide range of later yoga texts (e.g. the *Mārkaṇḍeyapurāṇa* (7.4), *Vasiṣṭhasaṃhitā* (7.6), *Nādabindūpaniṣad* (7.8) and *Vivekamārtaṇḍa* (7.10)). Yoga texts also echo Vedic teachings found in, for example, the *Jaiminīya Upaniṣad Brāhmaṇa* (1.18.1–10) and the *Chāndogya Upaniṣad* (8.6.1–5), which say that the chanting of *oṃ* brings about transcendence of death and ascent to the sun or heaven. Thus the *Bhagavadgītā* (8.12–13) teaches that at the time of death the chanting of *oṃ* in combination with yogic methods and remembrance of Kṛṣṇa will lead one to the ultimate destination, while later texts assert that the chanting of *oṃ* can bring about dissolution in the absolute (*Mārkaṇḍeyapurāṇa* 39.9), defeat death (*Vasiṣṭhasaṃhitā* 3.29, 6.25–30 (7.7)) or, if performed at the moment of death, lead to a desirable rebirth (*Nādabindūpaniṣad* 12–16 (7.8)).

Tantric Mantras

The use of mantras is the defining practice of the non-ascetic tantric tradition, which calls itself, in both its Śaiva and Buddhist manifestations, 'the way of mantras' (*mantramārga*, *mantrayāna*, *mantranaya*, etc.).[5] Central to tantric yoga practice is *japa*, the repetition of mantras, which are understood to be phonic manifestations of deities (*Mṛgendratantra Yogapāda* 8ab (**7.3**)). Only in the *Mṛgendatantra*, however, is *japa* included among the auxiliaries of yoga (see **1.4.8**), which, Brunner suggests, is because yoga was not a part of the earliest formulations of tantric ritual.[6] As well as *japa* of a mantra, Śaiva texts also speak of its *uccāraṇa* ('raising'), in which the mantra, together with the yogi's consciousness, is joined with the breath and raised up the body's central channel.

As can be seen from instructions to hold the breath during the recitation of the Gāyatrī mantra in the *Jaiminīya Upaniṣad Brāhmaṇa* (3.3.1) and *Baudhāyanadharmasūtra* (4.1.22–30; see **4.4** and the introduction to Chapter 4), the association of breath-control and mantra predates the tantric corpus. A range of tantric and later texts make a distinction between breath-control with (*sagarbha*) and without (*agarbha*) mantra (see Chapter 4, pp. 133–4); in the *Gheraṇḍasaṃhitā*, the purification of the channels by means of breath-control must be accompanied by the repetition of *bījamantras* (**7.16**; see also **4.21**).

Many tantric works encrypt their mantras in a *mantroddhāra* ('mantra-extraction'), an example of which from the *Khecarīvidyā* is given in this chapter (**7.12**).[7] Once such a mantra has been acquired it is to be repeated, preferably internally, a certain number of times in order to attain particular benefits. Half a million repetitions of the *Khecarīvidyā*'s mantra leads to all obstacles being destroyed, as well as the more mundane benefit of the removal of wrinkles and grey hair. The *Śivasaṃhitā* (**7.14**) lists the benefits of increasing numbers of repetitions of its mantra, from 100,000 ('women tremble and become sick with love') to 10,000,000 ('the great yogi is absorbed into the absolute').

Tantric mantras can be visualized as well as repeated.[8] We have included here two of the many mantra visualizations in the eighth chapter of Hemacandra's *Yogaśāstra* (**7.5**). These involve placing individual mantras in the centre of lotuses in the body, each of whose petals has further seed-syllables on it. Combined with the breath, the mantras may be raised up the body's central axis; various benefits arise, ranging from the ability to overpower one's enemies to final liberation.

Another important tantric practice involving the visualization of mantras is fixation (*dhāraṇā*), which is covered in detail in Chapter

8. To practise *dhāraṇā*, the yogi fixes his mind on an object, usually one of the gross elements, each of which is associated with a particular seed-syllable (as well as other attributes such as colour and shape). In the *Ḥawż al-ḥayāt* we find a practice similar to the yogic elemental fixations, except that it is the mantras associated with each of the objects of meditation that are their most important feature (and the elements are not mentioned) (**7.15**).

Fixations of elements with their respective seed-syllables are found in some *haṭhayoga* texts (e.g. *Vivekamārtaṇḍa* 133–9); sometimes they are combined with visualizations of the *cakra*s (e.g. *Śivasaṃhitā* 5.77–207; cf. **5.3.8**).

Mantra's Lesser Role in *Haṭhayoga*

Haṭha texts compiled in tantric milieus teach mantra-repetition for both worldly aims and liberation (as we have seen in the cases of the *Khecarīvidyā* and *Śivasaṃhitā*), but tantric mantra-repetition is otherwise ignored or dismissed in the *haṭha* corpus. Two important early works on *haṭhayoga*, the *Amṛtasiddhi* and the *Gorakṣaśataka*, make no mention of mantra whatsoever. Mantra is mentioned twice in the *Dattātreyayogaśāstra*, the first text to teach a fourfold division of yoga methods (see **1.3.3**): it puts *mantrayoga* at the bottom of its hierarchy (it is for 'the lowest aspirant, he of little wisdom' and 'can be mastered by all and sundry' (**7.9**)), and it includes mantras among the obstacles to yoga practice (v. 52). The *Amaraughaprabodha* says that mantras which can bring about the infamous six magical acts do not in fact exist, and that constantly repeating mantras will lead to neither sovereignty nor lordship (6–7). The *Haṭhapradīpikā*, which draws on all of these *haṭha* texts, does not teach mantra practice; in the one instance that it mentions mantra (4.113cd) it says that in *samādhi* the yogi cannot be overcome by mantras or yantras.

The Kashmiri poet-mystic Lallā argues against mantras in a more poetic fashion. Despite being steeped in the tantric traditions, she declares that there is no need for tantric mantras when *oṃ* has been mastered; she then goes beyond even this rejection, saying that one should worship the Lord with the mantra of silence (**7.13**).

The contradictory attitudes to mantra may reflect the persistent tension between ascetic and non-ascetic yoga practice. Ascetic traditions are not inclined towards magical mantra practice (nor other rituals).[9] Mantra finds no place in the earliest Buddhist or Jain teachings (although it took hold in both by the beginning of the first millennium, perhaps because of the demands of non-ascetic devotees).[10] The ascetic proponents of the mantra-averse *haṭha* traditions are likely to be descendants of members of the same broad Śramaṇa milieu as the early Jains and Buddhists.[11]

Although tantric mantra-repetition is rarely a feature of *haṭha-yoga*, a yogic conception of mantra found in the early tantric corpus (see, for example, *Svacchandatantra* 7.29 and *Parākhya-tantra* 14.82)[12] is taught in some *haṭha* texts. This is the Haṃsa mantra, which is called the Ajapā ('unrecited') Gāyatrī in the *Vivekamārtaṇḍa* (7.10).[13] *Haṃsa* is constantly and involuntarily repeated – *ha* is uttered on the out-breath and *sa* on the in-breath – and when its components are reversed it becomes the Upaniṣadic dictum *so 'ham* ('I am that') (*Yogabīja* (1.3.2)).

From about 500 to 1300 CE Śaivism was India's dominant religion, but other tantric systems, namely those of Buddhists and Vaiṣṇavas, also flourished. With their demise, the popularity of tantric mantra practice waned accordingly. The use of mantra as part of yoga was subsequently reworked by the sectarian devotional traditions which came to prominence in the second half of the second millennium CE. In *Śivayogapradīpikā* 1.5, *mantrayoga* is understood to be the repetition of a one-, two-, six- or eight-syllabled mantra. These mantras are unspecified, but the first two are almost certainly the broadly popular *oṃ* and *so 'ham* (cf. Haṃsa above). The third is almost certainly the sectarian Śaiva root (*mūla*) mantra, *oṃ namaḥ śivāya*, while the fourth may refer to the Vaiṣṇava eight-syllabled mantra *oṃ namo nārāyaṇāya*. Ultimately the text privileges *so 'ham* over all other mantras (2.26–34). The *Sarvāṅgayogapradīpikā* of the seventeenth-century Dādūpanthī scholar Sundardās gives an even more simplified explanation of *mantrayoga*, reflecting the belief of north Indian devotional traditions at that time that the repetition of the name of God is the one true soteriological method. For Sundardās, the only mantra is 'Rām' (7.17).

Despite the dismissal or transcendence of tantric mantra practice evident in yoga texts over the course of the second millennium CE, it did continue to be practised in certain yogic milieus. Thus the *Jogpradīpakā* teaches an explicitly tantric breath-control in which, in order to re-enact the process of creation, the Sanskrit syllabary is internally recited in sequence while inhaling, holding the breath and exhaling; reciting it in reverse order re-enacts the process of destruction (4.23). Another old Hindi Rāmānandī work, a ritual handbook called the *Siddhānt Paṭal*, teaches a wide range of mantras with tantric features. While applying *sindūr* (the red part of his forehead marking), for example, the Rāmānandī ascetic is to recite the mantra *oṃ hrāṃ hrīṃ hrūṃ hanumantāya* [*sic*] *namaḥ* (section 16), whose second, third and fourth elements are of tantric origin.

Chapter Contents

7.11 *Vivekamārtaṇḍa* 64–70. *Oṃ*.

7.12 *Khecarīvidyā* 1.28c–40b. The Khecarī mantra.

7.13 *Lallāvākyāni* 11, 34, 39–40. Various mantras (including silence).

7.14 *Śivasaṃhitā* 5.232–51. The best mantra and its repetition.

7.15 *Ḥawż al-ḥayāt* 7.2–9. The seven great words.

7.16 *Gheraṇḍasaṃhitā* 5.35–45. Purifying the channels by breath-control with mantra-repetition.

7.17 *Sarvāṅgayogapradīpikā* 2.16–27. *Mantrayoga*.

7.1 *Jaiminīya Upaniṣad Brāhmaṇa* 3.5.4–5.[14] Breathing while chanting a Vedic mantra:

> (4) Then the [primary singer] saw the hymn spread out in the sky, shining greatly. He also saw its yoking (*yukti*). (5) He should sit down for the Bahiṣpavamāna hymn and do thus, breathing out, and also thus, breathing in, with the voice. He should wish to see with the eyes. He should wish to hear with the ears. Thus his mind becomes yoked [to the hymn] itself.

7.2 *Pātañjalayogaśāstra* 1.27–8, with selected passages from the *bhāṣya*. *Oṃ*:

> (1.27) [The Lord] is verbally signified by the syllable *oṃ*.

[...] For the yogi who understands what the signified and the signifier are,

> (1.28) repetition of [*oṃ*] makes manifest its meaning.

Repetition of *oṃ* makes manifest the Lord (*īśvara*), who is signified by *oṃ*. So the mind of the yogi who is repeating *oṃ* and making its meaning manifest becomes focused. Thus it is said:

'After repetition of the mantra (*svādhyāya*) one should undertake yoga; after yoga one should practise repetition of the mantra. Through perfection of repetition of the mantra and yoga the supreme self shines forth.'

7.3 *Mṛgendratantra Yogapāda* 8ab, with the *vṛtti* of Bhaṭṭa Nārāyaṇakaṇṭha. Mantra-repetition:[15]

He now defines the repetition of mantras (*japa*):

> (8ab) O sage, mantra-repetition (*japa*) is [the deity's] verbalization. It causes the [deity] visualized to approach.

The term *japa* refers to the repetition of the mantra [of the deity]. It is done to bring the [deity], who is the content of the meditation, into the presence [of the meditator]. The mantra may be in the mind, that is to say, verbalized internally, or it may be muttered so that it is audible only to oneself, or it may be spoken out loud, so that it is audible [to others].

7.4 *Mārkaṇḍeyapurāṇa* 39.1–14. *Oṃ*:

Dattātreya spoke:

(1) The yogi who is thus duly established in yoga cannot be recycled through hundreds of rebirths. (2) When [the yogi] has seen before him the supreme soul in its universal form, its feet, head and neck the universe, as the lord of the universe [and] the creator of the universe, (3) in order to attain it he should repeat the great blessing that is the one-syllabled [mantra] *oṃ*. That is its recitation. Now hear its form.

(4) The three syllables are *a*, and *u*, and *ma*. These three sound units consist of [the *guṇa*s] *sattva*, *rajas* and *tamas* [respectively]. (5) Free from the *guṇa*s and accessible by the yogi, another [sound unit, a] half-measure is situated above [those three]. It is known as *gāndhārī* [and] is in the *gāndhāra* musical note.

(6) When [*gāndhārī*] is chanted, it is characterized by a sensation of crawling ants in the head; in the same way, when *oṃ* is chanted it moves forth into the head.

(7) And the yogi who is filled with the syllable *oṃ* becomes imperishable in the imperishable [Viṣṇu]. *Prāṇa* is the bow [and] the self is the arrow [with which] the supreme Brahman is to be pierced.

(8) It should be pierced carefully as if with an arrow. [Then the yogi] becomes one with Brahman. This *oṃ* is the three Vedas, the three worlds, the three sacrificial fires. (9) [It is] Viṣṇu, Brahmā, and Śiva, and the *Ṛg*, *Sāma* and *Yajur* [*Veda*s]. The three-and-a-half syllables should be known as the highest reality. The yogi who practises them intently attains dissolution into Brahman.

(10) Moreover, the vowel syllable *a* is the earthly realm, the vowel syllable *u* is said to be the atmosphere and the consonantal syllable *ma* is the heavenly realm. (11) The first unit is manifest, the second is known to be unmanifest, and the third unit is the power of the mind. The half-unit is the supreme state. (12) These stages of yoga

are to be known through this sequence alone. By chanting *oṃ*, everything existent and non-existent can be grasped.

(13) The first unit is short, the second is double that and the third triple. The 'half-unit' is beyond the vocal range. (14) In this way the supreme, indestructible Brahman is known as *oṃ*.

7.5 Hemacandra's *Yogaśāstra* 8.1–5, 18–23. Two mantra visualizations:

(1) That [meditation] which is carried out with the support of sacred words is called 'on words' (*padastha*) by those who have fully understood the treatises on meditation. (2) In that [meditation], one should visualize the vowels [*a*, *ā*, *i*, *ī*, *u*, *ū*, *ṛ*, *ṝ*, *ḷ*, *ḹ*, *e*, *ai*, *o*, *au*, *aṃ* and *aḥ*] as a garland encircling a sixteen-petalled lotus at the bulb at the navel, one vowel on each petal. (3) And at the heart one should visualize a lotus with twenty-four petals and a central receptacle with the twenty-five consonants [*ka*, *kha*, *ga*, *gha*, *ṅa*, *ca*, *cha*, *ja*, *jha*, *ña*, *ṭa*, *ṭha*, *ḍa*, *ḍha*, *ṇa*, *ta*, *tha*, *da*, *dha*, *na*, *pa*, *pha*, *ba*, *bha* and *ma*] arranged on them in sequence. (4) Then one should visualize the other eight letters [*ya*, *ra*, *la*, *va*, *śa*, *ṣa*, *sa* and *ha*] on an eight-petalled lotus in the mouth. By visualizing the letters thus, one fully understands the wisdom of the sacred texts. (5) A meditator duly meditating on these letters, which have been fixed for all eternity, instantly attains knowledge of things that have been destroyed and so forth. [. . .]

(18–19) Or the wise one should visualize the king of mantras, with *ra* above and below, and a sliver of the moon and a dot next to it, together with *ha* (*anāhata*) [= *arhraṃ*], in the middle of a golden lotus as pure as the rays of the full moon, moving in space and filling the skies. (20–22) Then, holding the breath so that all parts of the body are filled, he should visualize it entering the lotus of the mouth, wandering between the brows, pulsating in the eyelashes, stopping on the forehead, emerging from the aperture of the palate, pouring forth nectar, rivalling the moon, pulsating among the stars, moving in the sky [and] causing [one] to be joined with the auspicious goddess. (23) The moment the resolute yogi meditates on this great truth (*mahātattva*), a world of bliss and beauty, with liberation as its ruling goddess, presents itself [to him].

7.6 *Vasiṣṭhasaṃhitā* 3.1–17. *Oṃ* and breath-control:

Vasiṣṭha said:

(1) Now I shall teach breath-control based on *oṃ*. Listen carefully, O devout son. (2) The union of *prāṇa* and *apāna* is called breath-control. Breath-control is said to be threefold: exhalation, inhalation and retention. (3) These, exhalation, inhalation and retention, have as their essence three letters [*a*, *u* and *ma*]. They are called Praṇava [i.e. *oṃ*] and breath-control consists of that. (4) That sound, which is taught in the Vedic texts and given a firm footing in the Upaniṣads, has as its first two sounds creation [*a*] and maintenance [*u*]; its last, the letter *ma*, is the destroyer. (5) Of these three, the syllable *a* takes the form of a virtuous girl with a red body riding on a goose, staff in hand. She is called Gāyatrī. (6) [And] of them the syllable *u* takes the form of a young woman with a white body riding on an eagle, the deity Cakradhāriṇī ('she who holds a discus'). (7) The letter *ma* takes the form of Sāvitrī, an old woman with a white body and three eyes, spear in hand, riding a bull. She is also known as Sarasvatī, Māheśvarī and Paścimā. (8) These three syllables are the three causes [creation, maintenance and destruction]. The cause of the three is the radiant Brahmā, the cause of everything. (9) Wise men call that one-syllabled supreme light Praṇava. Having learnt this correctly, one should practise breath-control with Praṇava using the three [parts], exhalation, inhalation and retention.

(10) Drawing in air from outside, the wise man should gently fill the abdomen by way of Iḍā for sixteen

measures while visualizing the syllable *a*. (11) Then he should hold the breath for sixty-four measures and repeat *oṃ* while visualizing in it the [previously taught] form of the syllable *u*. Alternatively, the breath should be held, accompanied by repetition [of *oṃ*], for as long as possible. (12) Then, my son, through Piṅgalā he should again gently exhale for thirty-two measures the held breath mixed with external air (13), while visualizing in it, with concentration, the final letter of Praṇava. This is breath-control. One should practise [it] repeatedly. (14) Then in the same way he should inhale through Piṅgalā for sixteen measures, visualizing in it, with full concentration, the form of the syllable *a*. (15) He should again hold the inhaled breath for sixty-four measures and repeat [*oṃ*], visualizing in it, with concentration, the [previously taught] form of the syllable *u*. (16) Then the wise man should exhale the breath for as long as he can, visualizing in it the form of the syllable *ma* as before. (17) And in exactly the same way as before he should practise [inhalation] through Iḍā. He should regularly practise sixteen breath-controls in this way.

7.7 *Vasiṣṭhasaṃhitā* 6.25–30. *Oṃ* as a means of defeating death:

(25) Having first restrained the breath using the method that has been taught involving either Gāyatrī or *oṃ* in order to purify the self, (26) [then], with the mind purified, having realized the supreme nectar of immortality in the body of the syllable *oṃ*, [the yogi] should insert the syllable *oṃ* in his body (27) [and], having inserted the mantra in his body, the wise one, covered in white ash, his breath mastered, having withdrawn the activities into their respective causes, enjoys himself in the supreme place of Viṣṇu which is endowed with the four [manifestations, i.e. Vāsudeva, Saṃkarṣaṇa, Pradyumna and Aniruddha]. (28) Having, by means of yoga, placed the mind in the citadel of Brahman in the body [and] kept Rudra, the embodiment of ultimate bliss, in his hideout,

+if one remains in the hideout one escapes rebirth+. (29) He who constantly repeats, by means of the salvific mantra (*tāraka*), this great-souled embodiment of ultimate bliss, the immortal inside his hideout, overcomes death, lives long and knows Brahman. (30) He who abandons his body while saying *oṃ* becomes none other than Brahman; as a result he also defeats death, my son.

7.8 *Nādabindūpaniṣad* 1–16, with section headings from the commentary of Upaniṣadbrahmayogin. The sacrificial bird that is *oṃ*:

The true form of [the great sacrificial bird that is] the Vairāja *oṃ* syllable [follows]:

(1) The syllable *a* is the right wing and the syllable *u* is the left. The syllable *ma* is said to be the tail and the [syllable] half a unit long is the head. (2) The feet and so forth are the *guṇa*s; the body is the ultimate reality; righteousness (*dharma*) is his right eye; unrighteousness (*adharma*) is the other [eye].

(3) The Bhūr realm is in his feet, the Bhuvar realm in his knee[s], the Suvar realm in the waist region, the Mahar realm in the navel region, (4) the Jana realm is in the heart region, the Tapas realm is in the throat and the Satya realm is situated at the forehead, between the brows.

(5) In it is revealed the mantra called 'She Who Has a Thousand Waves (*sahasrārṇamatī*)'. Riding upon her in this way, he who knows the yoga of Haṃsa (6) is not affected even by a billion bad deeds.

The true form of the four main parts of the syllable *oṃ* [follows]:

The first part is of fire, the next is of wind, (7) the next looks like the orb of the sun, and the last, the half-part, the wise know to be of water.

(8) That in which these parts have been fixed in the past, are now in the present and will be in the future is called the syllable *oṃ*. Know it by means of fixations.

A description, of the constituents and of the whole, of the division into twelve parts of the syllable *oṃ* [follows].

> (9) The first part is Ghoṣiṇī, then Vidyut, the third is Pataṅginī, the fourth Vāyuveginī. (10) The fifth is Nāmadheyā, the sixth is called Aindrī, the seventh is named Vaiṣṇavī and the eighth is Śāṃkarī. (11) The ninth is named Mahatī and the tenth is taught to be Dhṛti. The eleventh is Nārī and the last, the twelfth, is Brāhmī.

The results for practitioners of dying at the time of practising on each of those parts [follows].

> (12) If one is separated from one's life-breaths during the first part, one is born as the universal emperor Bharata. (13) After rising up in the second part, the great-souled one becomes a Yakṣa, in the third a sorcerer and in the fourth a celestial musician. (14) If one is separated from one's life-breaths during the fifth part, one lives with the gods, exalted in the Soma realm. (15) [If one is separated from one's life-breaths] in the sixth part [one attains] union with Indra, in the seventh [one attains] the state of Viṣṇu, and in the eighth one reaches Rudra, the lord of beasts. (16) In the ninth [one reaches] the Mahar realm, in the tenth one reaches the Jana [realm], in the eleventh the Tapas realm [and in the twelfth] the eternal Brahman.

7.9 *Dattātreyayogaśāstra* 12–14. Yoga by means of mantras (*mantrayoga*):

> (12) The wise man should recite a mantra after installing the alphabet in his limbs. That which can be mastered by all and sundry is called *mantrayoga*. (13) Lowly is the yogi entitled to practise it. After practising for twelve years he usually attains gnosis, as well as the powers starting with that of becoming as small as an atom. (14) The lowest aspirant, he of little wisdom, resorts to this yoga, for this yoga of mantras is said to be the lowest of yogas.

7.10 *Vivekamārtaṇḍa* 28–30. The Ajapā Gāyatrī:

(28) The vital principle goes out with the syllable *ha* [and] goes in and down with the syllable *sa*; it constantly repeats this mantra, *haṃsa haṃsa*. (29) [This], the Gāyatrī called Ajapā, bestows liberation upon yogis. Merely by thinking of it a man is freed from sin. (30) There never has been nor never will be a mantra like Ajapā, an austerity like Ajapā or a meritorious action like Ajapā.

7.11 *Vivekamārtaṇḍa* 64–70. *Oṃ*:

(64) Sitting in the pose of the liberated (*muktāsana*), holding the body and head straight, the gaze on the tip of the nose, alone, [the yogi] should repeat the imperishable *oṃ*. (65) That in whose letters are found the worlds – the earth, the atmosphere and the heavens – and the gods – the moon, sun and fire – that is the great light, *oṃ*. (66) That in which are found the three times, the three worlds, the three gods, the three accents [and] the three Vedas, that is the great light, *oṃ*. (67) That in which the three letters – *a*, *u* and *ma*, which is called *bindu* – are found, that is the great light, *oṃ*. (68) That in which the threefold goddess (*śakti*) – will, action and knowledge, Brāhmī, Raudrī and Vaiṣṇavī – is located, that is the great light, *oṃ*. (69) One should repeat it vocally, as a light one should exercise it using one's body (?) [and] one should constantly think of it with one's mind, the great light, *oṃ*. (70) Pure or impure, sin does not stick to he who constantly repeats the syllable *oṃ*, just as water does not stick to a lotus leaf.

7.12 *Khecarīvidyā* 1.28c–40b. The Khecarī mantra:

(28d) Now hear [the mantra and practice of] Khecarī. (29) And one should go, O goddess, to where there is a guru who has perfected the divine yoga and, after receiving the mantra (*vidyā*) called Khecarī spoken by him, (30) one should begin by scrupulously and tirelessly carrying out the practice described by him.

I shall proclaim the Khecarī mantra, which grants success in yoga, O goddess. (31) Without it a yogi cannot enjoy the Khecarī power. Practising the yoga of Khecarī by means of the Khecarī mantra preceded by the Khecarī seed-syllable, (32) [the yogi] becomes lord of the Khecaras and dwells among them for ever.

The abode of the Khecaras [and] fire, adorned with the mother and the circle, (33) is called the Khecarī seed-syllable. By means of it yoga is successful.

The great Caṇḍā, which is known as the peak, bearing the flaming, fiery thunderbolt [and] (34–5) joined with the previously described seed-syllable, is called the Vidyā [and] is extremely hard to obtain.

[Now] I shall teach the six-limbed mantra. [The yogi] should correctly perform [the mantra-repetition] with it interspersed with the six [long] vowels, O goddess, in order to obtain complete success. One should take the ninth letter back from Someśa. (36) The thirtieth letter from there, which is in the shape of the moon, is declared [to be next]. The eighth syllable back from there is next, my dear. (37) Then the fifth from there, O goddess. Then the first syllable after that is the fifth [syllable of the mantra]. Then Indra joined with an *anusvāra*. This [mantra] is called Kūṭa. (38–9) It is to be obtained from the teaching of a guru and bestows fame in all worlds.

Illusion, born of the body, with many forms [and] residing in the faculties, does not arise even in sleep for the controlled [yogi], as a result of the continuous twelvefold repetition [of this mantra]. (40) The glorious Khecarī power arises automatically for him who, totally self-controlled, recites this [mantra] 500,000 times. All obstacles are destroyed, the gods are pleased (41) and, without doubt, wrinkles and grey hair will disappear.

7.13 *Lallāvākyāni* 11, 34, 39–40. Various mantras (including silence):

(11) All the tantras dissolved and mantra remained.
Mantra dissolved and the mind remained.
The mind dissolved and there was nothing anywhere:
the empty was merged with the empty.

(34) What use are a thousand mantras
for one who has [by means of holding the breath]
regularly moved from the navel
the single mantra called *oṃ* up to the skull
and who has made the mind have *oṃ* as its only essence?

(39) Who is the flower-bearer and who is his wife?
By what flowers is the supreme deity to be worshipped?
What water pot should be used?
And tell me, what mantra is to be used?

(40) After taking the flower which is called steady
meditation
from the flower-bearers who are desire and the mind,
and having made a water offering with pots filled with
the nectar of the moon,
worship the Lord with the mantra called Silence.

7.14 *Śivasaṃhitā* 5.232–51. The best mantra and its repetition:

(232) Now I shall teach the ultimate mantra practice, by means of which the pleasures of this world and the next are sure to arise. (233) When this best of mantras is known, success in yoga, which bestows absolute dominion and pleasure, will certainly arise for the yogi who is a lord among practitioners.

(234) In the middle of the lotus with four petals in the Mūlādhāra is the Vāgbhava seed-syllable [*aiṃ*], flashing like a bolt of lightning. (235) In the heart is the Kāmarāja [*klīṃ*], which looks like a Bandhūka flower. In the Ājñā lotus is the seed-syllable called Śakti [*sauḥ*], which looks like ten million moons. (236) This triad of seed-syllables grants the rewards of both worldly enjoyment and

liberation. The yogi striving to achieve success should master these three mantras.

(237) After receiving this mantra from his guru, the yogi should repeat all of its syllables in sequence, neither quickly nor slowly, his mind free from doubt. (238) Absorbed in it, his mind focused, the wise yogi should make 100,000 oblations before the goddess in the manner described in the sacred texts and then repeat the mantra 300,000 times. (239) At the end of the repetition, the wise and clever yogi should offer an oblation of oleander blossom mixed with jaggery, milk and ghee into a fire pit in the shape of a vagina. (240) When this observance has been performed, the goddess Tripurabhairavī, created by the earlier worship, appears and grants wishes.

(241) Having duly pleased his guru and obtained this finest of mantras, even an unlucky yogi can achieve success by means of this technique.

(242) At the sight of the practitioner who repeats it 100,000 times with his senses subdued, women tremble and become sick with love. Shameless and without fear they fall before the practitioner.

(243) Repeated 200,000 times, it makes the men situated in the region come as if to a place of pilgrimage, abandoning their families and possessions. They give him all their property and are under his power.

(244) And when it is repeated 300,000 times, all the district governors are sure to be subjugated, together with their districts.

With 600,000 repetitions, the king is subjugated, together with his dependants, his troops and his vehicles.

(245) With 1,200,000 repetitions, spirits, demons and great snakes all come under his control and do his bidding for ever.

(246–7) When it is repeated 1,500,000 times, adepts and sorcerers, together with celestial musicians, heavenly nymphs and Śiva's host, are sure to come under the control of the wise master practitioner. Long-distance hearing, clairvoyance and omniscience arise.

(248) And with 1,800,000 repetitions, using this body the practitioner leaves the ground and rises up. He gets a divinc body, wanders freely about the universe and sees the earth in its perfect entirety.

(249) With 2,800,000 repetitions, the practitioner becomes the lord of the sorcerers, wise, able to assume any form he wishes and very powerful.

(250) And with three million repetitions, he becomes equal to Brahmā and Viṣṇu.

With six million, he attains the state of Rudra.

With eight million, he becomes the principle of the goddess (*śaktitattva*).

(251) With ten million repetitions, the great yogi is absorbed into the absolute. The practitioner becomes a yogi of great rarity in the three worlds.

7.15 *Ḥawż al-ḥayāt* 7.2–9. On the seven great words:[16]

(2) The philosophers agree that every charm, prayer, diagram, talisman or magical imagination that lacks these seven words, whether written, spoken or thought, will fail to be effective. Among them, these words are the greatest, as indeed the Greatest Name is among us.[17] They say that every one of these words has a station in the human being, so when imagining, one recollects the words in one's heart, not by the tongue.

(3) The first word is *hum*, and its meaning is 'O Lord' (*ya rabb*). The first diagram is as follows. Its bodily location is the seat and its basic colour is black, but in it is the colour of red gold. It is in the station of [Sanicar, which is] Saturn. If he meditates on this form in its bodily location with the colour of the form, then at the time of meditating on it, let him say *hum* continuously in his heart. As long as he remains in this 'magical

imagination' and he is gazing with the eye of the intellect at his heart in that bodily location, the affairs of the soul and its migration are suspended for him during this meditation. He attains its hidden aspect with ease, and he realizes in the heart that he sees by means of this attribute. Everyone who sees him loves him naturally, and people are in awe of him and draw hope from him. He finds in himself the following: his speech is understood, his magical imagination is correct, and his needs are satisfied.

(4) The second word is *awm* [i.e. *oṃ*], and its meaning is 'O Mighty One' (*ya qadir*). The second diagram is as follows. Its triangle should be equilateral. Its bodily location is between the seat and the genitals, and its basic colour is blood red, but in it is something like blazing fire. It is in the station of Mangal, who is Mars. If one meditates on its visual form in its bodily location as we have instructed you at the beginning, with all its preceding conditions, all of his enemies will be humbled to him, or if not humbled then destroyed; all honest men will fear him and people will naturally be fearful of him and his power.

(5) The third word is *rhin* and its meaning is 'O Creator' (*ya khaliq*). The third diagram is as follows. Its bodily location is the navel and its basic colour is like yellow gold, but it burns like a lamp. It is in the station of [Brhaspati, which is] Jupiter. If one meditates on its bodily location in its form and colour with all the previously mentioned conditions, then he is able to hear from afar and crosses distance in a moment; meanings are revealed to him that he did not comprehend through learning. Magic does not harm him, and if his gaze falls on one who is bewitched or insane, that condition goes away as soon as he looks at them.

(6) The fourth word is *brin tasrin*, which means 'O Generous, O Merciful' (*ya karim ya rahim*). The fourth diagram is as follows. Its bodily location is the heart and

its basic colour is red tinged with yellow, with flashes of lightning. It is in the station of Bhanu, which is the sun. If one meditates on its visual form, as was previously mentioned, men become as slaves, women as slave girls, kings and sultans submit to him, the people bless him and believe that no one like him is to be found in the inhabited quarter having more knowledge or greater power from God. He becomes the resort of humans and jinn, he hears the speech of angels, and things hidden are revealed to him by his inner senses.

(7) The fifth word is *ibi*, meaning 'O Controller of the Heavens and the Earth and What is in Them' (*ya musakhkhir al-samawat wal-ard wa ma fihima*). The fifth diagram is as follows. Its bodily location is the throat, its basic colour is white, but with something in it like fire, connected to a star. It is in the station of Sukr, which is Venus. If one meditates on its visual form as previously mentioned, he will attain the good things of life, and jinn and humans will love him, especially the women among them.

(8) The sixth word is *yum*, which means 'O Knowing' (*ya 'alim*). The sixth diagram is as follows. Its bodily location is the forehead near the space between the eyebrows on the bridge of the nose. Its basic colour is white, but in it is something like shining light. It is in the station of Budh, which is Mercury. If one meditates upon its visual form, as has been previously mentioned, and continually recites it, then the knowledge of the occult qualities and secrets of things appears in his soul, with a minimum of thought [on his part], without having to learn from anyone, along with obscurities and insight; whatever appears in his mind actually comes to pass. Humans and jinn serve him and visit him and are never absent from his service.

(9) The seventh word is *hansha mansha*, which means 'O Lifegiver' (*ya muhyi*). The seventh diagram is as follows. Its bodily location is the brain, and its basic colour is

white, with something like running water in it, and something like sperm in its water; it flows from its bodily location, [that is,] from his head to his feet. This is the station of Candra, which is the moon. And if one meditates on this as previously mentioned and continually recites *hansha mansha*, poisons withdraw from him, those who are stung become cured, the sick recover, and the insane regain health, as soon as his glance falls upon them. He becomes famous among the people for knowledge, excellence, asceticism, having his prayers answered and unveiling, and accounts of him become widely known.

7.16 *Gheraṇḍasaṃhitā* 5.35–45. Purifying the channels by breath-control with mantra-repetition:

(35) The wind cannot flow through channels clogged with dirt. How could breath-control succeed? How could knowledge of reality arise? Therefore, the yogi should first purify the channels and then practise breath-control.

(36) The purification of the channels is said to be of two kinds: with a mantra and without a mantra. The yogi should do it with a mantra by means of a seed mantra and without a mantra by means of the *dhauti* cleansing practice. (37) The *dhauti* cleansing practice has already been taught in the section on how to master the six cleansing practices,[18] so, Caṇḍa, hear about the technique with a mantra by which the channels can be purified.

(38) The yogi should sit on his seat and assume the lotus position. After ritually installing his teacher and the deities in his body, as taught by his guru, he should purify his channels so that he might be completely pure for breath-control. (39) The wise yogi should meditate upon the seed mantra of the wind as smoke-coloured and shiny and then inhale air through the lunar channel, repeating the seed mantra sixteen times.[19] (40) Using breath-retention (*kumbhaka*) he should hold the air for

sixty-four repetitions and exhale it through the solar channel for thirty-two repetitions.

(41) Having raised fire from the base of the navel, he should meditate on it as being joined with earth. For sixteen repetitions of the seed mantra of fire he should inhale through the solar channel. (42) Using breath-retention (*kumbhaka*) he should hold the air for sixty-four repetitions and exhale it through the lunar channel for thirty-two repetitions.

(43) Meditating on the shining orb of the moon at the tip of the nose, he should inhale through Iḍā for sixteen repetitions of the seed mantra *haṃ*. (44) He should hold his breath for sixty-four repetitions of the *vaṃ* seed mantra. Meditating on himself as being flooded with the nectar of immortality, he should imagine his channels being bathed. Keeping his visualization steady, he should exhale for thirty-two repetitions of *la*.

(45) He should purify his channels by means of this channel purification technique. Fixing himself firmly in a seated posture, he should then perform breath-control.

7.17 *Sarvāṅgayogapradīpikā* 2.16–27. *Mantrayoga*:

(16) Now hear about *mantrayoga*, brother, which cannot be understood without a good guru. It has no form or outline: how is it seen? (17) All the saints got together and meditated. They did not enjoy it without the Name (*nām*). Its home was nowhere to be found: what sort of name could it have? (18) Servants [of god] for their own happiness, after investigating that supreme brilliance they gave it the name Rām. Afterwards it was spoken of in many different ways. (19) Who will count the thousand names [of Viṣṇu]? The [one] Name has taken countless [people] across to the other side. The Rām mantra is the best of all, no other mantra is its equal. (20) The Rām mantra is the essence of all [mantras]; the others are [just] the way of the world. The Rām mantra

makes rocks float: how else could stones cross water?[20]
(21) The Rām mantra, when written on a leaf, makes it impossible to lift. Śiva told Pārvatī the Rām mantra; Nārada taught it to Dhruva. (22) Then Prahlāda learnt that mantra. He endured great tests, used his magic and without a hair out of place faced the edge of a sword. These are the benefits of the Rām mantra. (23) An easy and always effective method, he who searches for the Rām mantra, after first hearing it from a guru, should then practise saying it with his tongue. (24) After that, hold it in the heart and repeat the mantra without using the tongue. The mind focuses on it night and day, the meditation never stops for a moment. (25) Then the syllable *raṃ* manifests there, in a spontaneous unbroken stream. Body and mind are forgotten there, the sound of 'Rām' is in every pore. (26) As salt mixes with water, so the mind merges with that sound. The Rām mantra quickly works on you like this.
(27) He who yearns for Rām doing *mantrayoga* in this way, with the grace of a good guru, finds peace of mind.

EIGHT
Withdrawal, Fixation and Meditation

We now turn to three methods of cognitive and psychic refinement at the heart of traditional yoga practice. In modern, globalized settings, the primary linguistic association of the word 'yoga' is with physical practices like posture (*āsana*) and, to a lesser extent, breath-control (*prāṇāyāma*). Practices of 'meditation', on the other hand, tend to be colloquially understood as distinct from 'yoga', even though there may be an overlap in practice.[1] Notwithstanding this contemporary division, throughout most of its history the practice of yoga has in fact been primarily identified with meditative states and techniques like those presented in this chapter, as it still is today in most of South Asia. Understanding the place and function of these methods is therefore essential if one is to grasp the wider meaning and purpose of yoga.

At the risk of oversimplification, we can say that withdrawal (*pratyāhāra*), fixation (*dhāraṇā*) and meditation (*dhyāna*) are concerned, respectively, with the retraction of the mind from phenomenal objects, the concentration and placement of the mind, and the cultivation of advanced mental and ontological states. They can be considered as a continuum of practice which moves the yogi towards liberation (*mukti*, see Chapter 11), or the acquisition of special powers (*siddhi*s, see Chapter 10). Withdrawal is often an initial phase, in which the mind turns away from its habitual engagement with the sensory world and examines its cognitive functions in isolation. Then, by binding the mind to a phenomenal or imagined object, fixation sharpens perceptual clarity, as a result of which arises an effortless flow of concentrated awareness (or complete control of one's own ritually created reality), called meditation.

Commonly grouped together with fixation and meditation is

the still more advanced practice of *samādhi*. Given its importance as the most advanced meditative practice *and* its dual status in some systems as the ultimate goal – synonymous with yoga itself – we have devoted a separate chapter to it (Chapter 9).

Withdrawal (*pratyāhāra*)

Withdrawal is the pivotal phase in the turn from outer to inner practices. Insofar as its aim is to disengage the senses from their objects, withdrawal is central to, and in some instances coextensive with, yoga itself. As we saw in Chapter 1, in the earliest extant definition of yoga, in the sixth chapter of the *Kaṭha Upaniṣad*, yoga is identified as mastery of the senses (1.1.1). In the same text's third chapter (which is in fact older than the sixth chapter), we encounter the metaphor of the charioteer-as-intellect, which masters the unruly horses of the senses (3.3–8), an image which recurs at *Śvetāśvatara Upaniṣad* 2.9 (2.2.3) and *Mānavadharmaśāstra* 2.88 (8.1.1), where mastery of the senses and restraint of the mind are said to bring success without recourse to the bodily mortifications of yoga. Such mastery is closely associated with the practices of withdrawal (*pratyāhāra*), as it is by withdrawing the organs of senses from their objects that one masters them (cf. 8.1.2).

In the eight-auxiliary (*aṣṭāṅga*) schema of the *Pātañjalayogaśāstra* (see 1.4.3), withdrawal (*pratyāhāra*) is classed as the last of the 'outer' practices (which include rules, observances, posture and breath-extension), before the 'inner auxiliaries [of yoga]' (*antaraṅga*, 3.7) of fixation, meditation and *samādhi* (together termed *saṃyama*, 3.4). *Pratyāhāra* here indicates a disengagement of the senses from their objects, resulting in the senses taking on the resemblance of the mind itself (2.54).[2] Such withdrawal is said to bestow on the yogi the highest mastery of the senses (2.55). Withdrawal also tends to lie between *prāṇāyāma* and *dhāraṇā* in sixfold systems such as that of the *Vivekamārtaṇḍa* (wherein the withdrawal of the senses from objects is compared to the sun withdrawing its shadow at noon, and a tortoise withdrawing its limbs (8.1.7)).[3]

Pratyāhāra is closely related to breath-control (*prāṇāyāma*), and indeed is sometimes categorized as one of its stages rather than as a distinct auxiliary. This is hardly surprising given the close association of the control of breath with the control of mind. For instance, in Hemacandra's *Yogaśāstra* 5.8, *pratyāhāra* is named as the fourth stage of a sevenfold schema of breath-control in which the breath is drawn upwards from place to place, such as (notes the auto-commentary) from the navel to the heart.[4] In *Vimānārcanākalpa* 97 (5.1.6), the fourth and fifth stages of a fivefold withdrawal involve (respectively) circulating the breath upwards and downwards through the eighteen vital points (*marmans*) and holding the raised breath in the channels. The *Dattātreyayogaśāstra* presents withdrawal as a product of pure breath-retention (*kevala kumbhaka*) in which the yogi withdraws the sense organs from their objects (8.1.6).

Some tantras, such as the *Svacchanda* and the *Mālinīvijayottara*, present a type of *prāṇāyāma* in which the breath is moved internally along the central channel of the yogic body (known therefore as *internal* breath-control, *ābhyantaraprāṇāyāma*). In its fourth stage, 'the quiescent' (*supraśānta*), the yogi guides his vital energy from the heart to the navel and the 'mind accompanies the vital energy in its descent and is thereby withdrawn from the influence of the sense organs', with mind and breath being restrained in the navel region.[5] The commentator Kṣemarāja notes that this is 'strictly a method of withdrawal'.[6] This recalls the 'fourth [breath]' of *Pātañjalayogaśāstra* 2.51, in which there is a casting aside of external and internal objects, which in turn destroys the karmic 'covering of the light' (*prakāśāvaraṇa*, 2.52) and makes one fit for the practice of fixation (*dhāraṇā*, 2.53). This is the only time that the *Pātañjalayogaśāstra*'s expository sequence of the eight auxiliaries is broken – fixation being introduced here *before* withdrawal (2.54) – perhaps suggesting that in the *Pātañjalayogaśāstra*, as in later tantric works, advanced breath-control may function like, or be equivalent to, withdrawal.

Fixation (*dhāraṇā*)

Following on from withdrawal in many eightfold and sixfold systems is the auxiliary of fixation (*dhāraṇā*). We can draw a working distinction between fixation as described in the *Pātañjalayogaśāstra*, and as it occurs in the tantric traditions. The *Pātañjalayogaśāstra* (8.2.4) defines fixation as locking the mind (*citta*) on one point, but does not specify which. The commentary lists as suitable focuses the navel cakra (*nābhicakra*), the heart lotus (*hṛdayapuṇḍarīka*), the light in the head (*mūrdhni jyotis*), the tip of the nose (*nāsikāgra*), the tip of the tongue (*jihvāgra*) and other body parts or external objects. In his commentary on this *sūtra*, Vācaspatimiśra mentions the palate as a further locus and specifies that auspicious external focuses include Hiraṇyagarbha, Indra, Prajāpati and others, citing a lengthy visualization of Viṣṇu from the *Viṣṇu Purāṇa* (7.45).

Tantric fixation, on the other hand, typically involves a sequential visualization of the elements (*tattva*s or *bhūta*s), and does not allow for the kind of choice offered by the *Pātañjalayogaśāstra*.[7] Classical tantric *dhāraṇā* practices are almost always associated with element fixation, notwithstanding early variations in the number and names of the elements.[8] In the Śaivasiddhānta the association of fixation with element practices is so close that the term *dhāraṇā* came to indicate not just the process of fixation itself, but the actual elements.[9] In tantric contexts, the elements are visualized in divinized, ritualized form. As the *Parākhyatantra* puts it, 'The fixations have their own *maṇḍala*s, seed-syllables and locuses, and they are associated with the [characteristic] functions of the [five] elements (*bhūtakarmagāḥ*)' (14.13c–15b). In late first-millennium tantras this process was overlaid on to the yogic body, resulting in the teaching of visualizations of a series of *cakra*s along the body's central channel, each with an element (see Chapter 5). Typically, accomplishing the *dhāraṇā* of an element gives rise to a particular attainment (*siddhi*, see Chapter 10), usually mastery of that element. Thus perfection of fixation of the fire element means that the yogi cannot be burnt (*Dattātreyayogaśāstra* 116). Some haṭhayogic texts teach both *dhāraṇā*s of the elements (e.g. *Śivasaṃhitā* 3.72–5) and sequential visualizations of elemental *cakra*s (e.g. *Śivasaṃhitā* 5.77–207; cf. **5.3.8**).

It would be wrong to draw too sharp a distinction between tantric *dhāraṇā* practices and the *Pātañjalayogaśāstra* tradition, however. The *Mokṣadharma* of the *Mahābhārata* teaches both kinds of fixation (**8.2.2** and **8.2.3**); and tantric element *dhāraṇā*s, which emerge in texts like the *Niśvāsatattvasaṃhitā*'s *Nayasūtra*, may themselves derive from the third chapter of the *Pātañjala-*

yogaśāstra (on yogic powers), where *saṃyama* on the connection between the subtle and the gross is said to result in the *siddhi* of the conquest of the elements (*bhūtajaya*, 3.44).[10] Moreover, conquest of the *tattva*s in Sāṃkhya yoga (as described in the epics and Purāṇas) is correlated to a hierarchy of yogic achievements much as is the conquest of the elements in tantric texts.[11] So even though element practices are not explicitly associated with *dhāraṇā* practice in the *Pātañjalayogaśāstra*, we can discern such associations within the broader Sāṃkhya context.

Like withdrawal, fixation is closely associated with breath-control practices (*prāṇāyāma*), of which it is sometimes said to be simply a multiple (e.g. *Vivekamārtaṇḍa* 94). In the *Pātañjalayogaśāstra* breath-control is said to make the mind capable of the fixations (2.53 (**4.6**)), and the *Parākhyatantra* states that the purification of the inner spaces by breath-control is the means by which the fixations are conquered (14.13c–15b). In some texts, fixation is carried out by holding the breath in particular elements or parts of the body. The *Vasiṣṭhasaṃhitā*, for instance, instructs the yogi to lead the breath (together with the syllable and the deity) into the five elements, beginning with earth, and hold it there (**8.2.8**), and the *Dattātreyayogaśāstra* (111c–123) instructs the yogi to isolate the breath in the lower abdomen as part of the earth element *dhāraṇā*. The *Śāradātilaka* teaches a *dhāraṇā* practice in which the *prāṇa* breath is fixed in various parts of the body (**8.2.7**), and a similar practice of the placement of the mind and breath in different parts of the body is described in Hemacandra's *Yogaśāstra* (5.26–41). In *Gheraṇḍasaṃhitā* 3.57–63, the five-element fixations are included among the seals (*mudrā*s; see **6.2.13**).

Meditation (*dhyāna*)

As noted in the main introduction, around 500 BCE there emerged in northern India groups of extra-Vedic ascetics – collectively known as Śramaṇas, and including Buddhists and Jains – who sought permanent liberation (*nirvāṇa*, *mokṣa*, *mukti*, etc.) from the cycle of rebirth and *karma*-driven suffering. Although in early Buddhism the term 'yoga' refers to the emotional and psychological bond that ties one to the round of rebirth, rather than the technique of liberation from rebirth,[12] the *Mahābhārata* makes reference to Buddhist practitioners of *dhyānayoga* or the 'yoga of meditation'. While such techniques may have originated in Vedic contexts where ontological cessation was not the goal,[13] it is within Śramaṇa soteriologies of liberation that they first became widely known, before later being (re-)absorbed into the Vedic mainstream, notably through texts like the *Pātañjalayoga-śāstra*.[14] In early Jainism, austerity (*tapas*) was the only way to attain *mokṣa*. However, subsequent to Umāsvāti's *Tattvārtha-sūtra* – which is roughly contemporaneous with the *Pātañjalayoga-śāstra* and presents *dhyāna* as a tool of liberation on an equal par with austerity – the status of meditation in Jainism becomes considerably elevated.[15]

A fourfold method of *dhyānayoga*, by which sages are liberated from worldly existence (*saṃsāra*) and attain *nirvāṇa*, is announced by Bhīṣma in the twelfth book of the *Mahābhārata* (8.3.4). Puzzlingly, Bhīṣma only describes the first stage, which some scholars have taken as an indication that this is not originally a Brahmanical technique, but one borrowed from Buddhism.[16] The key Buddhist term *nirvāṇa* also suggests an originally Buddhist context. In the first stage of *dhyānayoga* the yogi pacifies the senses and the mind by withdrawing the senses from sense objects, as a result of which reflection (*vicāra*), attention (*vitarka*) and discernment (*viveka*) arise. One possible explanation for the *Mahābhārata*'s omission of the remaining stages of the Buddhist *dhyānayoga* is that while the first meditation is in keeping with the epic's broader conception of yoga (viz. withdrawal of the senses), the remaining three are not, and therefore needed to be discarded.[17]

According to Rupert Gethin there are two sorts of meditation in the early Buddhist Pali texts: one which stops the mind, probably deriving from pre-Buddhist asceticism, and a superior one which realizes the Four Noble Truths of Buddhism.[18] Bronkhorst has proposed that the Four Noble Truths were not originally part of the Buddhist doctrine of liberation, but were overlaid on to the earlier notion of *prajñā* (wisdom) 'by way of the Four Dhyānas [meditations]'.[19] Indeed, liberation by means of insight into the Four Noble Truths is clearly contradictory in early Buddhist contexts where liberation arises from states of meditation in which all mental activity ceases.[20] The fourfold *dhyāna* – an example of which, from the *Sekha Sutta*, is included in this chapter (8.3.3) – is the most basic (and perhaps the earliest) meditation scheme of Buddhism; however, commonly the list is expanded to include eight or even nine stages.[21]

In the *aṣṭāṅgayoga* scheme of the *Pātañjalayogaśāstra*, meditation is the seventh, penultimate auxiliary, following fixation and preceding *samādhi* (1.4.3). It is defined as a continuous flow of the single-pointed focus developed through fixation (8.3.8). When this shines forth 'as if it were free of its own form', it is known as *samādhi* (see 9.1.5). Thus, rather than discrete, functionally distinct practices, fixation, meditation and *samādhi* constitute the developmental stages of a single process, known as *saṃyama*. It is worth reiterating that, as we saw in Chapter 1, *samādhi* here is a preliminary or auxiliary practice which prepares one for yoga (itself defined in the *Pātañjalayogaśāstra* commentary as *samādhi*), and it is for this reason that the auxiliaries of *saṃyama* are considered internal with regard to the *aṣṭāṅga* scheme, but external with regard to the seedless (*nirbīja*) *samādhi*, identified as yoga itself (3.7, 8).[22]

Oberhammer identifies four types of meditation in the *Pātañjalayogaśāstra*. The first moves from a reduction in the contents of consciousness to the unrestricted self-awareness of the true nature of the subject (*puruṣa*).[23] The second is similar, but is theistic: the individual self becomes identified with a personal god (*īśvara*, *iṣṭadevatā*) through meditation and mantra.[24] In the third type of meditation, known as *samāpatti* (discussed in greater detail in Chapter 9), the remembered object of meditation entirely displaces the visible object, becoming refined to the point that it attains the status of primordial matter (*prakṛti*), according to the emanation hierarchy of the Sāṃkhya philosophy (see main introduction). This loosens the identification of the self with material existence and thus leads to liberation at death (see Chapter 11).[25] The fourth kind of meditation, exemplified by the third 'book' of the *Pātañjalayogaśāstra* (named *vibhūtipāda* by later redactors), aims at the cultivation of magical powers rather than liberation (see Chapter 10).[26]

Tantric texts and some Purāṇas, such as the *Bhāgavatapurāṇa*, do not allow for the contemplation of any possible object in meditation (i.e. *dhyāna* sensu stricto, as opposed to allied 'meditative' practices like *dhāraṇā*), but limit the focus to the deity, which is visualized in great and prescribed detail.[27] Rather than a method for the cessation of mental fluctuations like the *Pātañjalayogaśāstra* (see **1.1.5**), tantric meditation affords complete control over one's mentally constructed universe, and ultimately bestows liberation from the actual world, by means of a constantly maintained, creative inner vision. Tantric meditation is therefore an imaginative act, an 'intense, emotional and empathic "living out" of a dream-like goal by completely losing one-self in the image'.[28] It is thus often called *bhāvanā* (from the causative of the root √*bhū*, to 'exist' or 'come into being'). One of the earliest descriptions of such creative visualization is found in a *c.* third-century CE Buddhist Yogācāra text, the *Saddharmasmṛtyupasthānasūtra*, in which yoga is said to be the painting of pictures by the mind, using the brush of meditation (**8.3.7**).

Some tantric texts, echoing the *Pātañjalayogaśāstra*'s understanding of meditation as continuing on from fixation, present it as an extension of fixation on the elements up to the deity (e.g. the element meditation (*tattvadhyāna*) of the *Niśvāsatattvasaṃhitā*'s *Nayasūtra* 3.1–72 and *Uttarasūtra* 5:3–31 (see **8.3.9**)). However, in the majority of cases tantric fixation indicates a focus on the elements, while meditation requires visualization of the deity or deities alone, such as those of the self as Vajravārāhī in *Vajravārāhī Sādhana* (**8.3.14**) and of Śiva and Caṇḍikā at *Matsyendrasaṃhitā* (**8.3.18**). These visualizations can be very detailed and extend beyond the deity itself: the deity's throne (*āsana*), in particular, is often described in great detail in tantric texts.[29]

Tantric-style visualizations informed most subsequent formulations of yogic meditation and are found in a wide variety of texts (e.g. the visualization of Viṣṇu at *Vasiṣṭhasaṃhitā* 4.26–31; **8.3.17**). The objects of the visualizations that a text teaches are a sure indicator of its sectarian origins. When the Rāmānandī Jayatarāma wrote the *Jogpradīpakā* in 1737 he included a *dhyāna* of Sītā and Rāma at vv. 780–96 which was a simple reworking of the *Bhāgavatapurāṇa*'s *dhyāna* of Viṣṇu. Some texts on yoga, however, downplay their sectarian origins and supply a template for meditation into which the yogi may insert the deity of his choice (*iṣṭadevatā*; see, for example, *Gherаṇḍasaṃhitā* 6.2–8).

There also exist tantric 'formless' meditations in which detailed creative visualization is abandoned on the grounds that the deity is ultimately beyond such characterization. For example, in the 'unsupported' (*anālambana*) yoga described in *Mṛgendratantra* 58c–60b, one passes beyond the prescribed forms of visualization and instead meditates 'on anything in which one's consciousness becomes tranquil, mentally fashioning [any] position, form and size'. The result of this meditation *sans* icon, states the commentary, is that the yogi comes through 'the cessation of all mental activity to rest in nothing but his own identity', which is the nature of Śiva himself.[30]

Theistic context notwithstanding, the proximity of this description to the initial definition of yoga and its result in *Pātañjalayogaśāstra* 1.2 and 1.3 should make us cautious about drawing too categorical a distinction between 'tantric' and 'classical' methods of yoga. Other texts differentiate in a similar way between meditation with and without form. For example, the *Vasiṣṭhasaṃhitā* describes a fivefold meditation with attributes (*saguṇa*) involving visualization of the deity, as well as a meditation without attributes (*nirguṇa*) in which one contemplates formless space with no characteristics, while identifying oneself with Brahman (**8.3.17**). Similar twofold methods of meditation are also evident in the meditations with and without attributes of the *Vivekamārtaṇḍa* (**8.3.19**) and the *Dattātreyayogaśāstra* (**8.3.20**), as well as in the *Īśvaragītā*'s descriptions of the two types of meditation which lead to Pāśupata yoga (**8.3.13**).

Chapter Contents

8.1.5 *Śāradātilaka* 25.23. The forcible removal of the senses.

8.1.6 *Dattātreyayogaśāstra* 93–96. Causing sensory objects to exist in the self.

8.1.7 *Vivekamārtaṇḍa* 103–10. As the tortoise withdraws its limbs.

8.2 Fixation (*dhāraṇā*)

8.2.1 *Satipaṭṭhāna Sutta* 12. Meditation upon the elements.

8.2.2 *Mahābhārata* 12.228.8–15. The seven fixations.

8.2.3 *Mahābhārata* 12.289.38–41. Fixation (*yoga*) on parts of the body.

8.2.4 *Pātañjalayogaśāstra* 3.1. Fixation is fastening the mind to one place.

8.2.5 *Vairocanābhisaṃbodhi Sūtra* (from Chapter 15). Fixation on the circles of the elements.

8.2.6 *Mṛgendratantra Yogapāda* 35c–44b, with Bhaṭṭa Nārāyaṇakaṇṭha's *vṛtti*. The five elements are the appropriate fixation for beginners.

8.2.7 *Śāradātilaka* 25.24–5. Fixing the *prāṇa* breath on the parts of the body.

8.2.8 *Vasiṣṭhasaṃhitā* 4.1–16. The five fixations and their results.

8.3 Meditation (*dhyāna*)

8.3.1 *Muṇḍaka Upaniṣad* 3.1.8. The meditating man.

8.3.2 *Satipaṭṭhāna Sutta* 2–4. The four foundations of mindfulness.

8.3.3 *Sekha Sutta* 18. The four meditations (*jhānas*).

8.3.4 *Mahābhārata* 12.188.1–22. The yoga of meditation (*dhyānayoga*).

8.3.5 *Mahābhārata* 12.294.6–9. Meditation is the most powerful method of yoga.

8.3.6 *Mānavadharmaśāstra* 6.72–4. The importance of meditation.

8.3.7 *Saddharmasmṛtyupasthānasūtra* 7.12.7. The painting of images by the mind.

8.3.8 *Pātañjalayogaśāstra* 3.2. Meditation.

8.3.9 *Niśvāsatattvasaṃhitā Uttarasūtra* 5.3–31. Meditation on the elements (*tattvadhyāna*).

8.3.10 *Mṛgendra Yogapāda* 7ab, with Bhaṭṭa Nārāyaṇakaṇṭha's *vṛtti*. A definition of meditation (*dhyāna*).

8.3.11 *Mṛgendratantra Yogapāda* 32c–33b, 58c–60b, with Bhaṭṭa Nārāyaṇakaṇṭha's *vṛtti*. The choice of meditation object.

8.3.12 *Siddhayogeśvarīmata* 6.20d–24b. The visualization of the Trika goddess Parāparā.

8.3.13 *Īśvaragītā* 52–67. The two types of meditation, which lead to Pāśupata yoga.

8.3.14 *Vajravārāhī Sādhana* 19–24. Visualization of oneself as Vajravārāhī.

8.3.15 *Bhāgavatapurāṇa* 11.14.32–5, 42–6. A meditation on Kṛṣṇa.

8.3.16 *Śāradātilaka* 25.26. The definition of meditation.

8.3.17 *Vasiṣṭhasaṃhitā* 4.19–31, 45–8, 54–6. Meditation with and without attributes.

8.3.18 *Matsyendrasaṃhitā* 7.8–27. Visualization of Śiva and Caṇḍikā.

8.3.19 *Vivekamārtaṇḍa* 142a–155b. Meditation with and without attributes.

8.3.20 *Dattātreyayogaśāstra* 122c–124b. Meditation with and without attributes.

8.3.21 *Gheraṇḍasaṃhitā* 6.1–22. The three types of meditation.

8.1

Withdrawal (*pratyāhāra*)

8.1.1 *Mānavadharmaśāstra* 2.88–100. Control of the senses:

(88) The wise man should strive to restrain his sense organs as they wander among captivating objects, as a charioteer strives to restrain his horses. (89) The sages of old said that there are eleven sense organs. I shall duly teach them as they are, in the correct order.

(90) The ear, the skin, the eyes, the tongue, and the fifth, the nose; the anus, the genitals, the hands, the feet and the voice, which is said to be the tenth.

(91) The five of them beginning with the ear are the sense organs of the intellect; the five beginning with the anus are said to be the sense organs of action. (92) Know the eleventh to be the mind, which, because of its quality, belongs to both [groups]. When it is conquered, these two groups of five are [also] conquered.

(93) Through attachment to the sense organs one is sure to commit wrongdoing. By restraining them, on the other hand, one achieves success. (94) Desire is not appeased by the enjoyment of desires, just as ghee makes a fire grow bigger. (95) When one man obtains all these desires and another renounces them all, the renunciation of all desires is better than their attainment. (96) These sense organs, which are strongly attached to their objects, cannot be controlled by not indulging (in desires) as effectively as by the constant application of knowledge. (97) The Vedas, renunciation, sacrifices, observances and austerities do not bring success for a dissolute man.

(98) Know the man who, on hearing, touching, seeing, eating or smelling, is neither happy nor sad, to have conquered his senses. (99) If one of all the senses falls [from

control] then a man's wisdom falls away from him like water falls from the foot of an animal skin used as a water-carrier. (100) After bringing all the senses under control and restraining the mind, one can attain all ends without mortifying the body through yoga.

8.1.2 *Mṛgendratantra Yogapāda* 5–6, with Bhaṭṭa Nārāyaṇakaṇṭha's *vṛtti*. Withdrawing the mind from sense objects:[31]

Now the definition of withdrawal:

(5) Then he should practise withdrawal, the complete retraction of the mind engaged in savouring the paltry joys of those [faculties].

Then, that is to say, when he has finished practising breath-control, he should practise withdrawal. This means that the mind intent on savouring the petty sensual pleasures associated with those [faculties] should be withdrawn from contact with any sense object.

He goes on to say what happens to a person who does this:

(6) By this means consciousness loses all contact with the objects of the senses, and therefore the mind becomes fit for fixation (*dhāraṇā*) on any focus he chooses.

By this process of retraction his awareness ceases to have any contact with sense objects. Being withdrawn from this contact it loses its natural function, and as a result the mind is prepared for fixation on any focus he may choose.

8.1.3 *Parākhyatantra* 14.11a–12b. Drawing the mind into the heart:

(11) [There is] repeated withdrawal of the mind, which goes to external objects; it is drawn into the space in the heart. Because one establishes [the mind there, this process] is called drawing (*āhṛti*). (12) Because of being drawn into that [place], the mind becomes firm and a suitable locus for yoga.

8.1.4 *Vimānārcanākalpa* 97. Withdrawal by raising breath through the eighteen *marmans*:[32]

The particular nature of withdrawal [and] its divisions.

Now, withdrawal is fivefold.[33] Forcefully retracting the senses from all [their] objects; seeing everything in the soul as like the soul; performing enjoined actions externally without the mind; raising the breath through the eighteen vital points (*marmans*) from the big toes to the head, holding it [in them] and drawing it up and down from one place to another; raising the breath into the channels and holding [it in them].[34]

8.1.5 *Śāradātilaka* 25.23. The forcible removal of the senses:

When the senses are moving about freely among sense objects, their forcible removal from those [sense objects] is called withdrawal.

8.1.6 *Dattātreyayogaśāstra* 93–96. Causing sensory objects to exist in the self:

(93) He should practise unaccompanied breath-retention (*kevala kumbhaka*) once a day for three hours, either by day or by night. Withdrawal will thus arise for the yogi practising in this way. (94) When the yogi, while holding his breath, completely withdraws his sense organs from their objects, that is called withdrawal.

(95) Whatever he sees with his eyes he should cause to exist in his self. Whatever he smells with his nostrils he should cause to exist in his self. (96) Whatever he tastes with his tongue he should cause to exist in his self. Whatever he touches with his skin he should cause to exist in his self.

8.1.7 *Vivekamārtaṇḍa* 103–10. As the tortoise withdraws its limbs:

(103) Withdrawing in succession the sight and other [senses] as they move among their objects is called withdrawal. (104) As the sun at noon withdraws the shadow,

so the yogi practising the third auxiliary gets rid of mental disturbance. (105) Just as a tortoise draws its limbs into itself, so does the yogi withdraw his senses into himself.

(106) Whatever he hears with his ears, good or bad, the knower of yoga draws it in, recognizing it as the self. (107) Whatever he sees with his eyes, beautiful or not, the knower of yoga draws it in, recognizing it as the self. (108) Whatever he touches with his skin, hot or not, the knower of yoga draws it in, recognizing it as the self. (109) Whatever he touches with his tongue, sweet or not, the knower of yoga draws it in, recognizing it as the self. (110) Whatever he smells with his nose, fragrant or not, the knower of yoga draws it in, recognizing it as the self.

8.2

Fixation (*dhāraṇā*)

8.2.1 *Satipaṭṭhāna Sutta* 12. Meditation upon the elements:

And next, O monks, a monk contemplates how this same body is established and arranged with reference to the elements, thinking, 'In this body there is the earth element, the water element, the fire element [and] the wind element.' In the same way, O monks, that a skilled butcher or a butcher's apprentice, having killed a cow and cut it into pieces might sit at a crossroads, so indeed, monks, does a monk contemplate how this body is established and arranged with reference to the elements, thinking, 'In this body there is the earth element, the water element, the fire element [and] the wind element.'

8.2.2 *Mahābhārata* 12.228.8–15. The seven fixations:

Vyāsa said:

(8) *Dharma* its box, modesty its bumper, coming and going its yoke poles, the *apāna* breath its axle, the *prāṇa* breath its yoke, wisdom, health and the vital principle its reins, (9) consciousness its seat, beautiful, good conduct its wheel-rims, sight and touch its yoke shoulders, smell and hearing its horses, (10) wisdom its wheel-hub, all the scriptures its whip, wisdom its driver, overseen by the self (*kṣetrajña*), determined, faith and restraint its vanguard, (11) the road of renunciation its route, peaceful, pure, meditation its domain [and] yoked to the vital principle, the divine chariot shines forth in the world of Brahman.

(12) Now I shall teach a rapid method for someone who wants quickly to yoke [himself] to this chariot, intent on reaching the imperishable. (13–15) He is performing yoga by means of yoga who silently performs all seven fixations (other [fixation]s [operate] to the rear [or] side, these are forward), attains in sequence sovereignty over earth, air, space, water, light, egoism [and] the intellect, gradually acquires sovereignty over the unmanifest, and possesses powers.

8.2.3 *Mahābhārata* 12.289.38–41. Fixation (*yoga*) on parts of the body:

(38) The yogi who remains unmoving, having inserted his self in his self, [destroys] sin like a hunter kills fish [and] obtains the undecaying state. (39–40) On the navel, the throat, the head, the chest, the sides [and] the [organs] of sight, touch and [smell], O you of boundless valour: the yogi who, by means of the special observance of focusing on these locations, duly joins the subtle self with the self, O king, (41) quickly attains spotless wisdom, burns up good and bad *karma*, attains the highest yoga and, if he wants, is [completely] liberated.

8.2.4 *Pātañjalayogaśāstra* 3.1. Fixation is fastening the mind to one place:

The five external auxiliary methods have been described. Fixation (*dhāraṇā*) should [now] be spoken of:

(3.1) Fixation is fastening the mind to [one] place.

Fixation is fastening the mind by means of only [a modification of its] state to places such as the circle of the navel (*nābhicakra*), the heart lotus (*hṛdayapuṇḍarīka*), the light in the head, the tip of the nose and the tip of the tongue or to an external object.

8.2.5 *Vairocanābhisaṃbodhi Sūtra* (from Chapter 15). Fixation on the circles of the elements:[35]

> First, with the meditation on the golden [i.e. earth] circle, and dwelling in the great Indra [circle], one should bind the *vajra* seal and drink milk so as to nourish the body, and when one month has passed, the practitioner will be able to control his breath going out and coming in. Next, in the second month, carefully arranging himself in the water circle, he should use the lotus-flower seal and imbibe pure water. Next, in the third month, with the meditation on the most wondrous fire circle, he eats food which he has not sought out, and for the seal he uses the great wisdom sword; he will burn up all sins produced by body, speech and mind. In the fourth month, with [the meditation on] the wind circle, the practitioner constantly ingests wind, and, binding the seal for turning the Dharma wheel, he recites with his mind concentrated. With the meditation on the adamantine [i.e. earth] and water circles, he abides in yoga: this is in the fifth month and, far removed from gain and non-gain, the practitioner, without attachment, becomes like a perfected Buddha.

8.2.6 *Mṛgendratantra Yogapāda* 35c–44b, with Bhaṭṭa Nārāyaṇakaṇṭha's *vṛtti*. The five elements are the appropriate fixation for beginners:[36]

> (35c–36b) The word *dhāraṇā* ('fixation') means stasis; [but] it also refers by extension to the focus [of this

> stasis]. For the beginner the only appropriate focus is one of these [elements] beginning with earth.

[. . .] The beginner, the aspirant who has just begun to practise, should take the five elements (*tattvas*), beginning with earth as the focus of his practice. [He should] not [attempt stasis on] other elements, such as the intellect (*mahān* [= *buddhi*]) and the 'I'-factor (*ahaṅkāra*), [since] these are not directly perceptible. Rather, through practice on these elements which he can perceive, [the five] beginning with earth, practice on the others becomes much easier. This is why the fixations are taught in that order in all [our] texts on yoga. Now he states the colour, shape, function and symbol of each of these [basic] focuses:

> (36c–38b) In colour they are [like] gold, [like] snow, [like] fire, black and transparent. In shape they are a square, [the bottom] half of a circle, a triangle, a circle and a lotus. Their function is to stabilize, to revitalize, to burn, to impel and to empty. They are [marked] with a 'thunderbolt', a lotus, a flame, a dot and a zero.
>
> (38c–39b) When he has understood which of them are hostile, which indifferent and which favourable, singly and in sets, the yogi should hold them to achieve the perfections he desires.

Next, the sage [Bharadvāja] puts a request [to Indra], desiring to understand [these] fixations and their effects:

> (39c–40b) In which sites should the expert contemplate the forms of these focuses? Also explain, O king of the gods, their individual and collective effect.
>
> (40c–44b) A [yogi] who knows [their] functions should focus on earth in his heart if his mind is distracted; on water in his throat if he is thirsty; on fire in his belly, if his digestion is sluggish; on wind in his heart, throat and other [centres] if he wishes to master the functions of the outgoing and other breaths; and on ether to overcome poison and the like at these [points or] wherever it is required. Ether is in all the [other] elements. Water and wind, fire and earth, water and fire, earth and wind, water and earth, fire and wind. Recognizing the indifferent, foes and friends

in the pairs within these [three] sets of four, the intelligent man should employ them to accomplish his goals.

8.2.7 *Śāradātilaka* 25.24–5. Fixing the *prāṇa* breath on the parts of the body:

(24) Fixing the *prāṇa* breath, according to the rules, on the big toe, ankle, knee, thigh, perineal seam, penis, navel, the regions of the heart, neck and throat, the uvula, nose, (25) centre of the eyebrows, skull, top of the head and twelve finger-widths above the head (*dvādaśānta*) is called fixation.

8.2.8 *Vasiṣṭhasaṃhitā* 4.1–16. The five fixations and their results:

Vasiṣṭha said:

(1) Now I shall teach the five fixations as they truly are. Listen carefully, O devout son.

(2) Good men who know the meaning of the texts on yoga say that fixation is steadiness of the mind in a self endowed with the qualities of restraint (*yama*) and so forth.

(3) Now, fixation is also said to be [fixing the mind] on the internal space in the heart and fixing [the mind] on external space. [By practising] thus, one can move through space.

(4) Fixation is [also] said to be fixing [the mind] on the five letters found in [the elements] earth, water, fire, air and space.

(5) Fixation is also fixing [the mind] on the five gods found in those [elements]. (6) From the feet to the knees is said to be the place of earth. From the knees to the anus is taught as the place of water. From the anus to the heart is said to be the place of fire. (7) From the centre of the heart to the centre of the eyebrows is considered to be the place of the air. From the centre of the eyebrows to the top of the head is said to be [the place of] space.

(8) From among these the wise [yogi] should fix the syllable *la* in the place of earth; he should fix the syllable *va*

in water and he should fix *ra* in fire; he should fix *ya* in the air [and] he should fix *ha* in space. (9) The wise [yogi] should fix the great god Brahmā in earth, Viṣṇu in water, Rudra in fire, the intellect (*mahat-tattva*) in air [and], in space, the unmanifest god who is the lord of the universe (*jagadīśvara*).

(10) [If the yogi] leads the breath together with the letter and deity [i.e. *la* and Brahmā] into earth and holds it there for two hours, he will attain mastery over the earth [element]. (11) And [if one] holds the breath, together with the letter and god as taught [i.e. *va* and Viṣṇu], in water for two hours, one is freed from all diseases. (12) By fixing on fire as before, the [yogi] is not burnt by fire. (13) [If the yogi] fixes the breath, together with the letter and god [i.e. *ya* and the intellect], in the air for two hours, he moves through the air like the wind. (14) [If the yogi] puts the breath, together with the letter and deity [i.e. *ha* and Jagadīśvara], in space for two hours, he will become liberated while living. Within a year his urine and faeces will diminish. (15) This fifth fixation gets rid of all sorrows. (16) When this fixing of the breath [is performed] in these five locations, the yogi cannot be extracted from his seat or vehicle.

8.3

Meditation (*dhyāna*)

8.3.1 *Muṇḍaka Upaniṣad* 3.1.8. The meditating man:

Not by the eye is it perceived, nor by the voice, nor by the other senses, nor by asceticism, nor by action; it is by the grace of knowledge that a man whose being has been purified sees that which is undivided while he is meditating.

8.3.2 *Satipaṭṭhāna Sutta* 2–4. The four foundations of mindfulness:

The Lord said the following: (2) Monks, this is the direct path for the purification of good people, for the overcoming of grief and lamentation, for the annihilation of suffering and sorrow, for the attainment of the way [and] for the experiencing of *nirvāṇa*: the four foundations of mindfulness. (3) What are the four? In those [four foundations of mindfulness], O monks, a monk, continuously perceives the body as the body, while ardent, attentive [and] mindful, having dispelled worldly desire and sorrow; he continuously perceives sensations as sensations, while ardent, attentive [and] mindful, having dispelled worldly desire and sorrow; he continuously perceives the mind as the mind, while ardent, attentive [and] mindful, having dispelled worldly desire and sorrow; [and] he continuously perceives the constituents of experience as the constituents of experience, while ardent, attentive [and] mindful, having dispelled worldly desire and sorrow.

(4) And how, O monks, does a monk continuously perceive the body as the body? When this happens, O monks, a monk goes to the forest or the foot of a tree or an empty house, sits down cross-legged, holds his body erect, concentrates on mindfulness and, mindful, exhales and, mindful, inhales. Exhaling at length, he has the awareness 'I am exhaling at length'; inhaling at length, he has the awareness 'I am inhaling at length'. Exhaling shallowly, he has the awareness 'I am exhaling shallowly'; inhaling shallowly, he has the awareness 'I am inhaling shallowly'. He learns by being aware of the whole body while exhaling. He learns by being aware of the whole body while inhaling. He learns by pacifying the aggregate of the body while exhaling. He learns by pacifying the aggregate of the body while inhaling. In just the same way, O monks, that a skilful lathe-worker or lathe-worker's apprentice is aware that he is making a long pull when he makes a long pull and is aware that he

is making a short pull when he makes a short pull, O monks, the monk is aware that he is exhaling at length when he exhales at length [. . .] he learns by exhaling, while pacifying the aggregate of the body.

8.3.3 *Sekha Sutta* 18. The four meditations (*jhāna*s):

And how, Mahānāma, does a noble disciple freely obtain, without difficulty or hardship, the four meditations (*jhāna*s) of higher consciousness, in which one abides taking pleasure in the elements of experience? Here, Mahānāma, a noble disciple free from desires, free from unwholesome experiences, enters and remains in the first meditation, which is accompanied by attention and reflection, produced by discrimination [and] pleasurable. Through the cessation of attention and reflection one enters and remains in the second meditation which is inner calming of the mind, focused, without attention or reflection, produced by *samādhi* [and] pleasurable. Through detachment from joy, one remains disinterested and mindful and alert and one experiences pleasure with the body, [and] one enters and abides in the third meditation, about which the noble ones say, 'One is disinterested, mindful and abiding in pleasure.' Through abandoning pleasure and suffering, and the cessation of happiness and sorrow, one enters and remains in the fourth meditation which is without suffering and pleasure [and] purified by disinterestedness and mindfulness. That is how, Mahānāma, a noble disciple freely obtains, without difficulty or hardship, the four meditations (*jhāna*s) of higher consciousness, in which one abides taking pleasure in the elements of experience.

8.3.4 *Mahābhārata* 12.188.1–22. The yoga of meditation (*dhyānayoga*):

Bhīṣma said: (1) So now, Pārtha, I will explain to you the fourfold yoga of meditation, knowing which the great sages reach eternal perfection. (2) Yogis practise so that [their] meditation is well established. [By practising thus] great sages satiated by knowledge (*jñāna*), whose minds have attained *nirvāṇa*, (3) are not reborn, Pārtha, and are liberated from the ills of worldly existence (*saṃsāra*). Freed from the faults of birth (*janmadoṣa*s), they are established in their own nature, (4) indifferent to pairs of opposites [such as pleasure and pain], established for ever in purity (*sattva*), liberated, [and] always seeking refuge in [things which are] without attachment or quarrel and bring peace to the mind. (5) The sage, sitting as still as a piece of wood, should, after joining it with his sense faculties, fix his studious and focused mind on those things. (6) He should not hear a sound with his ear, nor feel touch with his skin, nor perceive form with his eye, nor tastes with his tongue. (7) And through meditation, the knower of yoga should abandon all smells; the powerful [yogi] should have no desire for these things which excite the five [senses].

(8) Then the wise [yogi] should join the five senses with the mind, and keep the wandering mind, together with the five sense organs, focused. (9) The mind, with its five doorways [i.e. senses], is unanchored and strays, unsteady. [Therefore] in the first stage of meditation the wise man should focus the mind within. (10) When [the yogi] joins the senses and the mind, it is the first stage of meditation, as I have explained. (11) When he first confines the mind and senses within, they will burst out, agitated, like lightning in a cloud. (12) His mind on the path of meditation becomes just like a drop of water rolling around on a leaf, moving in every direction.

(13) The mind on the path of meditation stays focused for a moment or so, then once again it strays into the path of the wind, becoming like the wind [itself]. (14) Free from despondency, cares, fatigue and envy, the knower of the yoga of meditation (*dhyānayoga*) should once again focus his mind using meditation.

(15) In the beginning, when the sage is absorbed in the first meditation, reflection (*vicāra*), attention (*vitarka*) and discernment (*viveka*) arise in him. (16) When he is being tormented by the mind, he should practise *samādhi*. The silent sage should not despair, but should do what is advantageous for himself.

(17) Just as piled-up heaps of earth, ash or cow dung do not come together in a ball when suddenly drenched with water, (18) but dry powder that is slightly moistened slowly and gradually sticks together, (19) so should one gently bring together the sense faculties and gradually withdraw them [from their objects]. [Thus] one becomes completely peaceful.

(20) Once the mind and the five senses automatically attain the first stage of meditation, O Bharata, they become peaceful by constant [practice of] yoga. (21) One will not attain the bliss of the yogi who has controlled himself thus through human action, nor through any kind of divine will. (22) Conjoined with this bliss, he will delight in the practice of meditation. It is in this way that yogis reach *nirvāṇa*, the state of well-being.

8.3.5 *Mahābhārata* 12.294.6–9. Meditation is the most powerful method of yoga:

Vasiṣṭha said: (6) Now I shall tell you what you are asking about. Hear from me in secret how yoga should be performed, O great king. (7) Of the different ways in which yoga should be performed, meditation is the most powerful. And people who know the Vedas say that meditation is of two kinds: (8) focus of the mind and breath-control. Breath-control has attributes (*saguṇa*) and [focus] of the mind is without attributes (*nirguṇa*). (9) At three times, urination, defecation and eating, O king, one should not practise yoga. One should practise it intently the rest of the time.

8.3.6 *Mānavadharmaśāstra* 6.72–4. The importance of meditation:

> (72) One should burn up faults by restraints of the breath, sin by fixations, attachment by withdrawal, and unlordly qualities by means of meditation. (73) By means of the yoga of meditation one should observe the journey of the internal self through various kinds of beings, which is hard to know for those who have not realized their selves [through meditation]. (74) He who has the correct insight is not bound by actions, but the man devoid of insight remains on the wheel of rebirth.

8.3.7 *Saddharmasmṛtyupasthānasūtra* 7.12.7.[37] The painting of images by the mind:

> Further, that monk is [thus] established in the practice of yoga: "This very painting of the flow [of existence] has three realms, five destinations in five pigments, and states of existence on three levels: [1.] the level of the sphere of sensuality, [2. the level of] the sphere of subtle materiality, and [3. the level of] the sphere of immateriality. On that [painting], the actions of the mind, like a painter, by engaging in sensuality, paint various images [based on] objects [of consciousness] of the sphere of sensuality. With the brush of the four meditations in the sphere of subtle materiality, [it] paints twenty types of [images], which are based on objects [of consciousness] of the subtle material sphere, and which are separate from sensuality. [These images appear in] sixteen states of existence that have these [meditations] as a support. The action of the mind, like a painter, [also] paints [images] in the sphere of immateriality. They are separated from the objects of the sphere of subtle materiality, and have as their basis the four [immaterial] attainments. [In this way,] this painting of the three realms is extensive."

8.3.8 *Pātañjalayogaśāstra* 3.2. Meditation:

(3.2) Meditation (*dhyāna*) is continuity of cognition on that [object of fixation].

Meditation is continuity of a cognition whose support is that which is the object of meditation on that place [of fixation], an even flow untouched by any other cognition.

8.3.9 *Niśvāsatattvasaṃhitā Uttarasūtra* 5.3–31. Meditation on the elements (*tattvadhyāna*):[38]

(3) Matter (*prakṛti*), soul (*puruṣa*), binding fate (*niyati*), time (*kāla*), illusion (*māyā*), knowledge (*vidyā*) and the Lord (*īśa*) – these [elements] are to be meditated upon one by one. (4) And eightfold Sadāśiva, and day, night and the half-years, and celestial transits, and the equinox,[39] and [the state in which everything has] the same flavour as the goddess (*śaktisamarasa*). (5) By knowing all these one attains union with Śiva. Through meditation one attains success (*siddhi*) [and] omniscience arises.

(6) The first is meditation on the element; the second is meditation on its form; the third is meditation on its sound; the fourth is meditation upon the target.

[Meditation on Matter (*prakṛti*)]

(7) After meditating upon the twenty-four [lower] elements, he should reflect on them by means of the seed-syllable mantra. This meditation using the seed-syllable mantra of matter is held to be elemental. (8) First entering into an awareness of the form [of matter], the wise man should meditate upon it until it becomes white, at which he attains success. (9) Meditation upon the sound is third. It bestows the supernatural power associated with matter. [He who knows it] becomes omniscient and free. (10) For one who stares into space, a letter *ū*, with its crooked shape, [appears]. After seeing the meditation-focus of matter, one is freed from bondage. (11) He who practises yoga and meditates [thus] will

achieve success in yoga. This yoga of matter which has been taught to you is the best means of achieving liberation.

[Meditation on the Soul (*puruṣa*)]

(12) [The first of the four meditations on the soul] is the awareness that one is conscious but not an agent. The second is a buzzing sound. The third has smoke as its object; the fourth has the form as its object. (13) 'I am not an agent and I am without the characteristics of material creation (*nirguṇa*); action is caused by matter' – such is the meditation of awareness [of the nature of the soul]: one is freed from latent impressions. (14) A buzz is the sound of the soul element. One should meditate upon it with one's mind engaged in yoga. Through meditation one obtains success and union with Viṣṇu. (15) Smoke that has emerged from the door to the fourth mental state is the meditation-focus of the soul element. By meditating upon it, that smoke catches fire. Seeing its brilliance one attains success. (16) Focusing on one's awareness of [the soul's] form, a man sees it in the sky. Practising thus one attains success and becomes Śiva.

[Meditation on Binding Fate (*niyati*)]

(17) In the case of great gains and losses, one should concentrate on water or other liquids, or a mirror, in order to have successes in conquering binding fate. (18) [Then] one is neither happy nor sad when great gains or losses occur. Having understood the true nature of binding fate, it will be defeated. (19) One should practise concentration on binding fate in water or in ghee, for it has the nature of water. On seeing binding fate, one attains success. (20) [Or] he should meditate on binding fate in a mirror. It arises in fiery form. And then, seeing binding fate, he is sure to attain success by means of it.

[Meditation on Time (*kāla*)]

(21) Moments, junctures and lunar days, and in fortnights, months and seasons: time is worshipped thus at

all auspicious times. (22) At all times he should [strive to] see time as dwindling. One who meditates thus on time will soon see time. (23) He becomes one whose form is that of time; he attains success, [being] a yogi of time. Omniscient and able to assume any form at will, he becomes pure like Śiva.

[Meditation on Illusion (*māyā*)]

(24) One who has no desire for love and is intent on seeking knowledge, who shudders at transmigration (*saṃsāra*) and wants liberation, has gone beyond illusion (*māyā*). (25) He should make an effigy of illusion from wood or clay and meditate on it. When it catches fire he attains success. (26) One should perform meditation on illusion [while staring] into sapphires, [other] jewels, or lamps. When there are [spontaneous] flames, the aspirant succeeds with his meditation on illusion.

[Meditation on Knowledge (*vidyā*)]

(27) He should meditate on Śiva as the alphabet, focusing on each phoneme in turn. He will obtain the supernatural power associated with the element knowledge and he will become equal to Śiva. (28) One should visualize each dissolution (*laya*). Alternatively one should visualize + . . . + as having the form of fire, of wind, of earth, of water, of ether. (29) By means of that form he will attain success and union with Śiva. The yoga connected with the knowledge element has been taught. Now hear the meditation related to the element that is the Lord element.

[Meditation on the Lord (*īśvara*)]

(30) He who desires the attainments associated with the element that is the Lord should meditate constantly on the sound of a bell. Then he will see the Lord, attain success [and] become Śiva. (31) Alternatively he may practise a visual meditation on two *liṅga*s in the sky. He will then see a subtle *liṅga* [above them]. When that catches fire he attains success.

8.3.10 *Mṛgendratantra Yogapāda* 7ab, with Bhaṭṭa Nārāyaṇakaṇṭha's *vṛtti*. A definition of meditation (*dhyāna*):[40]

> Meditation is the [continued] contemplation of that [focus]; and it has been taught already many times.

Meditation occurs when the mind focused by fixation contemplates a [divine] form with its various attributes, [visualizing it,] for example, as three-eyed, five-faced and so on. Such [visualizations] have been taught several times on other occasions, as in the following passage:

'[Let him visualize the form of Lord Śiva] with four lotus-like faces coloured yellow, black, white and red.'

8.3.11 *Mṛgendratantra Yogapāda* 32c–33b, 58c–60b, with Bhaṭṭa Nārāyaṇakaṇṭha's *vṛtti*. The choice of meditation object: [41]

> (32c–33b) One should meditate upon [such elements (*tattvas*)] as the body of Śiva, because no [meditation on an] inert element [in itself] could be of value even if perfected. Provided one does this [one may meditate on] anything one chooses.

One may master inherently inert entities such as [the element] earth by repeatedly practising meditation on them. But even so they cannot benefit one, except [if they are seen] as substrates of Śiva's nature. Thus it is that one is to meditate on all of this as the body of Parameśvara. By this means one may take anything as the object of meditation, even if it is something whose nature is inert.

> (58c–60b) Or rather what is this limitation on the form of the being who empowers the universe, who benefits all creatures at all times in all [kinds of] aspects? So one may meditate again and again on anything in which one's consciousness becomes tranquil, mentally fashioning [any] position, form and size.

Or rather what is this rule that one may visualize the Supreme Lord (*parameśvara*) who empowers the whole universe only as white and so forth in colour, and ten-armed, five-faced and so on in form? There is no such rule, implies the text. As the Lord is manifest everywhere in his vast pervasive power it is certainly false to meditate upon him as having one specific colour, form and location. Therefore, fashioning location, colour, dimensions, form and the rest with one's mind fixed motionless within or without, one should meditate constantly with all one's strength, and with the method one has learnt from one's master, on any focus in which one's consciousness becomes tranquil, whether it be mental (*bhāvaśarīre*) or physical (*bhūtaśarīre*).

8.3.12 *Siddhayogeśvarīmata* 6.20d–24b. The visualization of the Trika goddess Parāparā:[42]

> [Red] as blazing fire, (21) wearing a garland of skulls, with three glowing eyes, she sits with trident and skull-staff in her hands on [the shoulders of Sadāśiva,] the 'Great Transcended'. (22) Her tongue flickers in and out like lightning. She is gross-bodied and adorned with great serpents. Her mouth yawns wide and at its corners are terrible fangs. Ferocious, with her brows knitted in rage, (23) wearing a sacred thread in the form of a huge snake, adorned with a string of human corpses around her neck, with the [severed] hands of a human corpse for lotuses to deck her ears, (24) her voice like the thunder of clouds at the world's end, she seems to swallow space itself.

8.3.13 *Īśvaragītā* 52–67. The two types of meditation, which lead to Pāśupata yoga:

> (52) After paying homage to the lords of yoga and their disciples, to Gaṇeśa and to [his] guru, the yogi should practise my yoga with full concentration. (53–4) Sitting in either the auspicious (*svastika*), lotus (*padma*) or half[-moon] (*ardha*) pose, he should keep his gaze fixed on the tip of his nose [and] his eyes slightly open, fearlessly and calmly turn away from the world, which is made of delusion, and visualize the deity, the Supreme Lord, situated in his self.
>
> (55–6) Then on the tip of a flame which measures twelve fingers he should visualize a beautiful pure white lotus arising from the bulb of righteousness, knowledge its

stem, the supernatural powers its eight petals, detachment its central receptacle [and] in that a great golden seed pod, (57) which is said to be made of all the potentialities, a direct manifestation of the divine imperishable, that which is designated by the syllable *oṃ*, unmanifest, abounding in rays of light.

(58) In that the yogi should visualize a completely pure, steady light. In that light he should insert his self, with no differentiation from the light (59) and meditate on [it] in the middle of a void as the Lord, the supreme cause. Then, when his self has become all-pervasive, he should think of nothing. (60) This is a most secret meditation. Now another meditation is taught.

[The yogi] should visualize in the heart the excellent lotus that was described earlier (61) and then, in that, the self as the agent, shining like fire, [and] in [its] middle the twenty-fifth [element, namely] the person (*puruṣa*), in the form of a flame, (62) and in the middle of that he should visualize the supreme self as the great sky, the element communicated by the syllable *oṃ*, the eternal, imperishable Śiva, (63) unmanifest, dissolved in the material element (*prakṛti*), a great light, unsurpassed, [and] in that the supreme element, the substrate of the self, without attributes.

(64) Alternatively, [having become] one with it, [the yogi] should meditate upon the eternal Śiva, who has a single form, after purifying all the elements by means of *oṃ*. (65) After fixing the self in me, the pure highest level, [the yogi] should flood his body with that same water of knowledge (66) [and], his self having become me, consisting of me, he should take some ash from a sacrificial fire, rub his whole body with it while repeating the mantra that begins with 'fire' (*agni*), and visualize in his self the lord as a great light having his own form. (67) This is the Pāśupata yoga, which leads to bound souls being liberated from bondage. It is the essence of all the Vedānta and is said in the revealed texts (*śruti*) to transcend the stages of life.

8.3.14 *Vajravārāhī Sādhana* 19–24. Visualization of oneself as Vajravārāhī:

(19) Born from the seed-syllables of the moon and sun, three-eyed, saffron-coloured, with two arms and one face, treading, in the archer's stance, on the heads and chests of the supine Bhairava and Kālarātri, (20) drinking blood streaming down from the lotus bowl in her raised left [hand], a *vajra* in her right hand + . . . + her scolding [i.e. index] finger pointing to the ground scolding the wicked, (21) [her] left side adorned with a skull staff, a garland of blood-smeared human skulls hanging [around her neck], naked, her feet embellished by tinkling anklets, bearing a face terrific with fangs, (22) her head crowned by a *vajra* together with a sound [resonating] through the world, her top-knot loose, five skulls in her headband resplendent in the middle of a row of *vajra*s, (23) head, ears, throat, both wrists, [and] hips sparkling with [respectively] a chaplet, swinging earrings, a lovely necklace, glittering bracelets, [and] a girdle, (24) her flashing rays covering the three worlds, her body completely in the bloom of youth, [and] filled with nothing but the taste that is the great bliss: one should visualize oneself thus, as [Vajra]vārāhī.

8.3.15 *Bhāgavatapurāṇa* 11.14.32–5, 42–6. A meditation on Kṛṣṇa:

The Lord said: (32) Sitting comfortably on a level seat with the body straight, put the hands in the lap, look at the tip of the nose, (33) purify the path of the breath (*prāṇa*) with inhalation, breath-retention and exhalation, [then] practise slowly in reverse, too, with the sense organs subdued. (34) Using the breath, raise the uninterrupted *oṃ* syllable in the heart, which has the sound of a bell and resembles a fibre of a lotus stalk, and then reinsert the sound there. (35) Practise in this way on the breath joined with the syllable *oṃ* ten times at dawn, noon and dusk [every day]; after a month the breath is mastered.

[Verses 36–42 give a detailed visualization of Kṛṣṇa within the heart lotus.]

(42) [. . .] Meditate on [me] thus, placing the mind (*manas*) in all the parts of [my] body. The wise man, having used the mind (*manas*) to draw the sense organs away from their objects, should use the intellect (*buddhi*) as a charioteer to drive that mind completely into me. (43) Draw back the all-pervading mind (*citta*) and hold it in one place. Do not think of other things again. Visualize [my] smiling face. (44) When the mind has reached that state draw it back and fix it in space. Having abandoned that too and risen to me think of nothing. (45) With the mind thus in the state of *samādhi*, [the yogi] sees me as the self in the self, O universal soul, a light united with a light. (46) The mistaken understanding of substances, knowledge and actions had by a yogi practising yoga of his mind by means of this very powerful meditation is quickly extinguished.

8.3.16 *Śāradātilaka* 25.26. The definition of meditation:

Meditation (*dhyāna*) on one's own chosen deities with an absorbed mind moving [only] in the consciousness is what is called meditation in this system.

8.3.17 *Vasiṣṭhasaṃhitā* 4.19–31, 45–8, 54–6. Meditation with and without attributes:

(19) Meditation is perception of the self's own form by means of the mind. It is said to be of two kinds: with attributes (*saguṇa*) and without attributes (*nirguṇa*). (20) [Meditation] with attributes is said to be fivefold; there is only one [meditation] without attributes.

(21) One, luminous, pure, omnipresent like space, firm, very clear, free from impurity, eternal, devoid of beginning, middle or end, (22) +gross, subtle, not space, untouched [by the wind], invisible, without taste or smell+, unmeasurable, incomparable, (23) bliss, unageing, eternal,

the cause of everything both existent and non-existent, the base of everything, having the form of the universe, formless, unborn, undying, (24) invisible, residing in the visible, residing outside [of the visible], facing all directions, all-seeing, having feet in all directions, touching everything and having its head in all directions: (25) the thought 'May I be Brahman and made of Brahman' [which arises on meditating thus] is the meditation without attributes.

And [now] I shall teach you [meditation] with attributes.

(26) In the eight-petalled heart lotus which grows from the middle of the bulb, has a stem twelve fingers long and a face four fingers wide, has been made to blossom through repeated breath-control [and] whose central receptacle has filaments, (27–31) one should visualize Vāsudeva,[43] the lord of the universe, Nārāyaṇa, perfectly healthy, with four arms and a magnificent body, holding a conch, a discus and a club, wearing a crown and armlets, with eyes like lotus petals, the Śrīvatsa curl on his chest, Viṣṇu, his face like the full moon, his lips like the petals at the centre of a lotus, very content, smiling brightly, looking like pure crystal, wearing a yellow robe, Acyuta, his two feet the colour of a lotus, the supreme self, the Lord, his form shining rays all around, the ultimate person, the lord of gods who resides in the heart of all beings; the realization in the self that 'I am that' (*so 'ham*) [which arises on visualizing thus] is said to be meditation with attributes.

(45) The perception 'It is I who am the great Brahman; I am the imperishable supreme self' which thus [arises] is said to be meditation with attributes. (46) After six months of cultivating the nectar of meditation in this way [the yogi] conquers death. After a year he is sure to become liberated while living. (47) He who is liberated while alive (*jīvanmukta*) never experiences suffering, to say nothing of he who is eternally liberated (*nityamukta*).

That is why liberation is so precious. (48) Therefore, O lord of Brahmans, in order to attain liberation do what I say [and] always perform your duties, which have no rewards, with knowledge.

(54) Meditation alone is the high road to liberation, O great ascetic. (55) By means of this solar meditation wise men attain liberation in this world, so you too, O lord of Brahmans, must practise nothing but meditation. (56) Many other meditations are taught, O best of sages; these are the chief ones among them and the others are not important.

8.3.18 *Matsyendrasaṃhitā* 7.8–27. Visualization of Śiva and Caṇḍikā:[44]

(8) Having thus steadied the mind [the yogi] should start meditation. He should visualize in his heart a great lotus consisting of Śiva and Śakti, (9) its bulb the mantra *oṃ*, its stalk Śakti, its receptacle the Prāsāda mantra [*hauṃ*], all its petals the *maṇḍala* of fire, its fibres the *maṇḍala* of the sun, (10) its filaments the *maṇḍala* of the moon. It shines like ten thousand rising suns [and] contains the nine Śaktis. The knower of the self should for a long time visualize it thus. (11) In order to purify himself [the yogi] should visualize Parameśāna in its middle, looking like a black cloud, great serpents tied into his matted locks, (12) his crest the young moon, fearsome, filling the directions with the syllable *huṃ*, holding a sword and a spike, making the gesture of freedom from danger, carrying a noose for snakes, mighty, (13) holding a skull and a bell, + . . . +, [showing] the gesture of generosity, wearing a red robe [and] adorned with red garlands and scents.

(14) He has a huge necklace made from the eight snakes. He is roaring to dispel fear. He is wearing a tiger-skin with a lion-skin covering it. (15) He is decorated with ornaments such as ankle-bells and a double sacred thread. His [three] eyes are the moon, sun and fire. His huge mouth +has crooked tusks+. (16) He is laughing,

gets rid of all faults and the ten million obstructions, annihilates all enemies, [and] is the great destroyer of death. (17) He destroys wrinkles, grey hair, bad luck, old age and disease. Lord Bhairava, he produces all powers [and] protects his devotees. (18) All three of his eyes are rolling with intoxication from mead. His mind is blissful from alcohol. He is Hara, the guru of all the worlds. (19) [The yogi] should visualize him thus with focused mind in order to pacify all obstructive forces and so forth.

On his left thigh is Caṇḍikā, who destroys sorrow. (20) She is as black as a storm cloud, her wild hair sticks up, she is adorned with a garland of severed heads and earrings of black snakes. (21) She is decorated with red [paint], scents and flowers, as well as jewels. She has six faces, each with three eyes, and twelve arms. (22) She is wearing a tiger-skin covered with a lion-skin. She is holding a thunderbolt, a goad, a discus, a conch, a shield, a trident, (23) a knife, a staff and a pestle and is showing the gestures of generosity and freedom from danger. She is benevolent, has three eyes, removes the suffering of her devotees, has the moon as her crest, (24) dispels the three torments [which are caused by the self, the gods and the elements] from her devotees, has the form of the devourer of time, carries a skull filled with mead, is in the first flush of youth, (25) is the leader of the troop of Yoginīs, Bhairavī, the remover of fear. She causes the attainment of all desired rewards. She is the three causes (?). (26) The yogi should visualize the goddess in this way for a long time in order to obtain the rewards of yoga, to appease all calamities [and] to fulfil all desires. (27) By means of this yoga of meditation [the yogi] is freed even from time and death, O Parameśāni. What I say cannot be false.

8.3.19 *Vivekamārtaṇḍa* 142a–155b. Meditation with and without attributes:

> (142) Meditation is of two kinds, with attributes (*saguṇa*) and without attributes (*nirguṇa*). [Meditation] with attributes takes different forms, [meditation] without attributes is not connected with anything else. (143) With the mind within [and] the gaze outward, sit up straight in a comfortable pose: this is the Meditation *mudrā* (*dhyānamudrā*), which bestows success. (144) If, with the gaze on the tip of the nose, the yogi meditates on the self in the Base *cakra*, which looks like molten gold, he is freed from faults. (145) If, with the gaze on the tip of the nose, the yogi meditates on the self in the beautiful Svādhiṣṭhāna *cakra*, which looks like a flawless ruby, he is happy. (146) If, with the gaze on the tip of the nose, the yogi meditates on the self in the Maṇipūra *cakra*, which looks like the morning sun, he can shake the world. (147) If, with the gaze on the tip of the nose, the yogi meditates on the self in the heart lotus, using varieties of breath-control, he becomes Brahman. (148) If, with the gaze on the tip of the nose, the yogi continuously meditates on the self in the Viśuddha [*cakra*] in the throat, which looks like a lamp, he is freed from sadness. (149) If, with the gaze on the tip of the nose, the yogi meditates on the self in the orb of the moon at the uvula, full of flowing nectar, he attains bliss. (150) ____________[45] (151) If, with the gaze between the eyebrows, the yogi meditates on the self as the unconditioned, quiescent, resplendent Śiva in the skull, he becomes Brahman. (152) If the yogi meditates on his self as Śiva in the space which is called the Ājñā *cakra*, then he becomes made of knowledge (*jñānamaya*). (153) If the yogi mediates on his self as omnipresent, pure, with the appearance of space, like a mass of rays of light, he attains liberation (*mukti*). (154) The penis, the anus, the navel, the heart and above that the place of the uvula, the space between the brows and the aperture

into space: (155ab) these are said to be the locations of the yogi's meditation.

8.3.20 *Dattātreyayogaśāstra* 122c–124b. Meditation with and without attributes:

Then [the yogi] should practise meditation. (123) He should hold his breath for twenty-four hours and meditate on the deity who will grant what he wants. Thus the meditation with attributes arises, which bestows the powers of becoming infinitesimal and so forth. (124) By meditating on something without attributes, such as space, he enters on the path to liberation.

8.3.21 *Gheraṇḍasaṃhitā* 6.1–22. The three types of meditation:

(1) There are said to be three types of meditation: gross, luminous and subtle. Gross is of an image and luminous is of light. Subtle meditation is of the point (*bindu*). It is Brahman and Kuṇḍalinī is the ultimate deity.

(2) The yogi should visualize a sublime ocean of nectar in his heart, with an island of jewels in its middle whose sand is made of gemstones. (3) In every direction there are Kadamba trees with abundant flowers and it is ringed with a thick Kadamba forest like a stockade, (4) where the scent of Mālatī, Mallikā, Jātī, Kesara, Campaka, Pārijāta and Sthalapadma flowers perfumes every quarter. (5) In its middle the yogi should imagine an enchanting wish-fulfilling tree whose four branches are the four Vedas and which permanently bears flowers and fruit. (6) Bees and koels buzz and call there. He should steady himself and visualize a great jewelled pavilion there. (7) In its middle he should imagine a delightful throne on which he should visualize his tutelary deity in the meditation taught by his guru. (8) That deity should regularly be meditated upon with its associated form, ornaments and vehicle. This is called gross meditation.

(9) The yogi should visualize a lotus attached to the pericarp of the great thousand-petalled lotus. (10) It is white, luminous and has twelve seed-syllables, *ha*, *sa*, *kṣa*, *ma*, *la*, *va*, *ra*, *yuṃ*, *ha*, *sa*, *kha* and *phreṃ*, in that order. (11) In the middle of its pericarp is a triangle made of the syllables *a*, *ka*, *tha* and so forth, at whose corners are *ha*, *la* and *kṣa*. Inside it is *oṃ*. (12) The yogi should imagine a beautiful seat there consisting of *nāda* and *bindu*. On it are a pair of swans and a pair of wooden sandals. (13) He should visualize his guru there as a god with two arms and three eyes, dressed in white, bedaubed with white, scented paste, (14) wearing a garland of white flowers and together with his crimson consort. By meditation on the guru like this, the gross meditation is perfected.

(15) I have described the gross meditation; hear from me the luminous meditation, by which yoga is perfected and the soul is directly perceived. (16) Kuṇḍalinī is in the Base (*mūlādhāra*) in the form of a snake. The individual self (*jīvātman*) dwells there in the form of the flame of a lamp. The yogi should meditate on Brahman as made of light. This is the supreme luminous meditation. (17) Between the eyebrows and above the mind is a light consisting of *oṃ*. The yogi should meditate on it as joined with a ring of fire. That is the luminous meditation.

(18) You have heard the luminous meditation, Caṇḍa; I shall describe the subtle meditation. When through abundant good fortune the yogi's Kuṇḍalinī awakens, (19) she joins with the self, exits through the sockets of the eyes and roams about the royal road. Because she flits about, she cannot be seen. (20) The yogi attains success through the Śāmbhavī *mudrā* and the yoga of meditation. This subtle meditation is to be kept secret: it is hard for even the gods to attain. (21) The luminous meditation is considered to be a hundred times better than the gross meditation, and the supreme subtle

meditation is a hundred thousand times better than the luminous meditation.

(22) Thus have I taught you the very precious yoga of meditation. By means of it, the self becomes directly perceptible: that is why meditation is special.

NINE
Samādhi

In the Pātañjalayoga tradition and the systems which draw inspiration from it, *samādhi* is the highest state of cognitive refinement, synonymous with yoga itself. Patañjali's descriptions of the levels of *samādhi* provide a rare exposition of the most elevated states of consciousness, which carry the yogi even beyond individual existence. In theistic, tantric systems, *samādhi* is the mastery of meditative visualizations – such as those described in the previous chapter – to the point when the aspirant's elemental make-up is dissolved and he becomes completely merged with the deity. Thereafter, he ascends the levels of consciousness within the godhead itself. In other systems, especially *haṭhayoga*, *samādhi* is a death-like trance in which the yogi is insensible to stimuli and even unaware of himself, a variant that fascinated ethnographic writers on India and later became a common theme in (Western) popular culture.

This chapter offers a wide range of descriptions and interpretations of *samādhi*. The first section presents definitions and descriptions of *samādhi* from different yoga-practising traditions. The second considers the techniques of *samādhi* under the rubric of 'dissolution' (*laya*), while the third presents the specialized technique of dissolution known as 'listening to the inner sound' (*nādānusaṃdhāna*).

There is no consensus across traditions regarding the nature of *samādhi* and here, as elsewhere, our groupings are not hard and fast.[1] Nevertheless – indeed because of this – the category of *samādhi* provides an invaluable prism through which to consider the farthest reaches of the yogic endeavour.

Samādhi in the *Pātañjalayogaśāstra*

Samādhi is the last of the *Pātañjalayogaśāstra*'s triad of 'inner auxiliaries' (*antaraṅga*) collectively known as *saṃyama*, which also includes fixation (*dhāraṇā*) and meditation (*dhyāna*), examined in the previous chapter. In this context, *samādhi* is a further development of the meditation stage, in which the object of meditation appears 'as if free of its own form' (**9.1.5**). As we saw in Chapter 1, *samādhi* is also synonymous in the *Pātañjalayogaśāstra* with the state of yoga, in which all activities of the mind are suppressed (**1.1.5**).

The *Pātañjalayogaśāstra*'s taxonomy of *samādhi* is twofold. The first, *samādhi* with cognition (*saṃprajñāta samādhi*), is accompanied by some or all of four mental states (attention (*vitarka*), reflection (*vicāra*), bliss (*ānanda*) and egoism (*asmitā*)),[2] and is said to be 'with seed' (*sabīja*, 1.46) on account of the karmic traces which arise from it (**9.1.3**). *Samādhi* without cognition (*asaṃprajñāta samādhi*, simply called 'the other [*samādhi*]' in *sūtra* 1.18) is characterized by the contemplation of cessation itself, which is declared to be the highest practice of dispassion (*vairāgya*). This stage is free of meditative support or focus, in that cessation (as the absence of materiality and activity) lacks a referent. It is called '*samādhi* without seed' (*nirbīja samādhi*) because it produces no further karmic traces.

Samādhi in Vedānta-influenced Texts

In texts influenced by the various Vedāntic philosophical traditions, *samādhi* is commonly defined as identification or merger of the individual self (*jīvātman*) with the supreme self (*paramātman*) (see **9.1.11**, **13**, **16**, **17** and **18** in this chapter), a metaphysical vision at odds with the *Pātañjalayogaśāstra*'s Sāṃkhya orientation, where the final goal is a *separation* of the material and spiritual principles of existence (*prakṛti* and *puruṣa*).[3]

Jogpradīpakā 942 (**9.1.18**) offers a slightly different account of the types of *samādhi*, where *samādhi* without cognition is a permanent, post-mortem state, while *saṃādhi* with cognition is continued existence in the body (see Chapter 11 on living liberation).

Samādhi in Tantric Texts

In tantric texts, *samādhi* is not synonymous with yoga, as in the *Pātañjalayogaśāstra*, nor even necessarily the final or most elevated auxiliary of yoga.[4] Tantric texts present the goal of yoga as union with (or, in dualist systems, proximity to) the deity, rather than the ontological cessation presented by the *Pātañjalayogaśāstra*. This partly explains why texts like the *Mṛgendratantra* (1.1.17) must reject the etymologically derived definition of the word 'yoga' as meaning 'to be absorbed [in contemplation]' (from the root √*yuj*), in favour of the meaning 'to unite' (from a different root √*yuj*: see Chapter 1). This is also why the Pāśupata commentator Kauṇḍinya can consider practitioners of Pātañjalayoga to be 'beasts', as they remain in the inferior state of *samādhi* and therefore separated from the deity (see 1.5.4).[5] Unlike in the *Pātañjalayogaśāstra*, then, in tantric texts *samādhi* does not do the double work of *aṅga* and goal, but remains an auxiliary, and therefore preliminary to yoga as such. Tantric texts tend instead to use terms like *mukti*, *mokṣa*, *siddhi* and, in the case of Śaiva works, *śivatva* ('Śiva-ness') to indicate the ultimate state and goal of yoga (see Chapter 11).[6]

While not the final goal, this *aṅga* nevertheless plays a vital role in tantric yoga systems. In the *Parākhyatantra* (9.1.7) *samādhi* is defined as an absorption of the self into the supreme reality. In the *Matsyendrasaṃhitā*, *samādhi* is the means for the yogi to become Śiva through complete mastery of the empathically imagined universe created in meditation (*dhyāna*) (9.1.8). This work of empathic imagination puts the *Matsyendrasaṃhitā*'s *samādhi* very far from that of the *Pātañjalayogaśāstra*, in which all ideation and cognition cease.[7]

Kṣemarāja's commentary on the *Spandakārikā* presents two varieties of *samādhi*: eyes closed (*nimīlana samādhi*), representing the introspective state of the godhead, and eyes open (*unmīlana samādhi*), representing the power of phenomenal manifestation (*visargaśakti*). When the yogi realizes that the outer and the inner are essentially the same, he reaches a stage of mystical awareness known as the seal of Bhairavī (*bhairavīmudrā*) (9.1.9).[8]

Samādhi as a Temporal Extension of Prior Practices

In the same way that withdrawal and fixation may be presented as temporal extensions of breath-control or of each other, in *haṭha* texts *samādhi* may be characterized as a multiple of the preceding *aṅgas*, usually beginning with *prāṇāyāma*. For example, the *Gorakṣaśataka* (9.1.12) declares incrementally increased breath-retentions to be the best method of *samādhi*, and *Vivekamārtaṇḍa* 94–5 quantifies withdrawal, fixation, meditation and *samādhi* as multiples of twelve of the practice which precedes them, with breath-control preceding withdrawal. The *Matsyendrasaṃhitā* declares that *samādhi* has a duration seven times that of meditation (9.1.8) and, in similar fashion, the *Haṭhatattvakaumudī* states that *samādhi* without cognition (*asaṃprajñāta*) is a multiple of twelve meditations (51.17). The *Jogpradīpakā* offers a more organic metaphor for the relationship between the *aṅgas*, describing fixation, meditation and *samādhi* as the fruit of which the rules (*yama*) and observances (*niyama*) are the seed, posture (*āsana*) and breath-control (*prāṇāyāma*) the leaves, and withdrawal (*pratyāhāra*) the flowers (see 9.1.18). *Haṭhatattvakaumudī*, echoing *Vivekamārtaṇḍa* 160, offers the rule of thumb that while sounds are still heard in the ears (51.11) and sense objects perceived (51.12), it is meditation; thereafter it is *samādhi*.

Samādhi as Death-like Trance

After having been an auxiliary practice in tantric works, *samādhi* again comes to prominence in *haṭhayoga*, but as a death-like state in which the yogi is insensible to stimuli, rather than as the graded cognitive *samādhi* of the *Pātañjalayogaśāstra*.[9] *Vivekamārtaṇḍa* 166–9 notes that the yogi in *samādhi* perceives nothing (not even himself), is immune from sorrow and pleasure, and even invulnerable to weapons (9.1.13). In similar fashion, the *Haṭhatattvakaumudī* remarks that the yogi in the final state of *samādhi* has no perception and is like a block of wood (51.15, 18, 54, 73; see also *Amanaska* 1.26–7 (9.2.3)). We might note in this context that the term *yoganidrā* (yogic sleep) is used as a synonym of the 'fourth state' of *samādhi* (*turīya*) in some twelfth-century yogic texts.[10] It does not appear to refer to a specific technique of yoga until the twentieth-century Satyananda Yoga Nidra, as taught by modern yoga guru Satyananda Saraswati (1923–2009).[11]

The yogi's trance-like state of *samādhi* became something of a trope in ethnographic writing on India, in particular when it was used to survive long periods of burial underground. We include here an account by Sir Claude Wade on the *samādhi* of the renowned yogi Hari Dās, who in 1837 was interred in a locked chest in a garden in Lahore for forty days before being revived in front of many witnesses.[12] Also included is an extract from the *Tashrīh al-Aqvāṃ*'s chapter on Saṃnyāsīs, which equates the burial of the yogi (dead or alive) with *samādhi*, noting that living interments are carried out either with the aid of cannabis (*bhāṅg*) or by the power of ritual and ascetic practice (**9.1.22**);[13] and a comparable account from 1342 by the Moroccan explorer Ibn Baṭṭūṭa of year-long *samādhi* burials (**9.1.20**). Public *samādhi* burials still occur today, such as the case of the yogi known as Pilot Baba, who, along with his female Japanese disciple, has remained in an open pit for up to a week at every Kumbh Melā since 1992.[14]

It is worth noting that the figure of the *jīvanmukta* ('one who is liberated while living'; see Chapter 11) offers a version of *samādhi* quite different from both the death-like trance of the *haṭha* yogi and the graded *samādhi*s of the *Pātañjalayogaśāstra*. The pre-tenth-century *Mokṣopāya* (better known in its *Yogavāsiṣṭha* recension) presents the *samādhi* of the *jīvanmukta* as simply the calm state of mind arising from certainty of one's real nature and the constant awareness of being already liberated (see **11.2.2**).[15] Such composure-in-action, which accompanies all the yogi's activities, distinguishes it both from the inert haṭhayogic *samādhi* and the *Pātañjalayogaśāstra*'s 'cessative' states.[16]

Dissolution (*laya*) and Inner Sound (*nāda*)

This chapter also contains passages on techniques of dissolution (*laya*), including the practice of listening to internal sounds (*nāda*). We have placed them here by virtue of dissolution's common identification in haṭhayoga texts with *samādhi* and with royal yoga (*rājayoga*), itself often understood as equivalent to *samādhi*. For example, the haṭhayogic *Gheraṇḍasaṃhitā* (9.1.17) lists six types of *samādhi*, which it calls the 'sixfold *rājayoga*': meditation (*dhyāna*), sound (*nāda*), bliss in taste (*rasānanda*), success in dissolution (*layasiddhi*), devotion (*bhakti*) and stupefaction of the mind (*manomūrcchā*).[17] *Haṭhapradīpikā* 4.3–4 gives a list of synonyms of *samādhi* which includes both royal yoga and dissolution (see 1.3.8), and categorizes the practice of listening to the inner sound (*nāda*) as both *samādhi* and dissolution (e.g. 1.43 and 4.80; see 9.3.1 and 9.2.6). Echoing the *Haṭhapradīpikā*, the *Haṭhatattvakaumudī* unequivocally identifies the technique of dissolution through sound (*nāda*) as a form of *samādhi* (9.3.6).

The *Dattātreyayogaśāstra* claims that Śiva taught 80 million esoteric techniques (*saṃketas*) of dissolution (9.2.2), while the *Haṭhapradīpikā* (9.3.1) puts the number at 12.5 million and the *Yogatārāvalī* at 125,000 (9.3.5). The *Haṭhapradīpikā*'s definition of dissolution (9.3.1) begins with a question: 'They say "dissolution, dissolution" [but] what are the characteristic features of dissolution (*layalakṣaṇa*)?', a rhetorical structure which perhaps indicates the popularity of dissolution methods at the time of the text's composition, as well as the lack of consensus as to their essential features.

As we saw in Chapter 1, *layayoga* is categorized as a distinct *type* of yoga in the fourfold typologies of yoga which appear from the thirteenth century, and which also include *mantrayoga*, *haṭhayoga* and *rājayoga*. However, the distinction between *layayoga* and *rājayoga* is slight in practice because 'as meditative states of mind, the term *laya* is synonymous with *rājayoga*', itself conceived as the practice of *samādhi*.[18]

In the context of four yogas, the *Amaraughaprabodha* specifies that dissolution means the dissolution of the mind's flow, in contradistinction to *haṭha*, which is said to be the stopping of the breath (1.3.1). The *Yogabīja* similarly describes *layayoga* as the dissolution of the mind, as a result of which the breath becomes steady, and the highest state of happiness – characterized as 'bliss in one's own self' (*svātmānanda*) – is obtained (9.2.1). In the *Vivekamārtaṇḍa*, dissolution is characterized by the destruction of *prāṇa* and the dissolution of the mind (163),[19] as it is in the *Haṭhapradīpikā*, in which the air in the central channel dissolves: i.e. the breath is extinguished, and the mind becomes steady, and then itself dissolves (9.2.6).[20] *Haṭhapradīpikā* 4.34, answering its own rhetorical question about the features of dissolution, defines dissolution as 'the non-remembrance of the objects of the senses as a result of karmic traces (*vāsanā*s) not recurring' (9.3.1). In keeping with its anti-*haṭha* sensibilities, *Amanaska* 2.27–8 also prescribes the destruction of breath and mind – but (as is made clear earlier in the text) in this case it is the breath which dissolves as a consequence of the dissolution of the mind, and not vice versa, with the result that external knowledge does not arise (see 9.1.15 and 9.2.3).

As mentioned in Chapter 1 (pp. 6–7), *layayoga* is also associated with tantric visualizations of the dissolution of the elements, which may include the rising of the breath (and, in later works, Kuṇḍalinī) up the central channel.[21] This orientation is apparent in the *Śārṅgadharapaddhati*'s description of a power- and liberation-bestowing dissolution carried out via the nine *cakra*s (v. 4350).[22] However, not all texts understand dissolution in these terms: for example, the *Dattātreyayogaśāstra* lists seven 'esoteric techniques' (*saṃketa*) of dissolution, which include staring at the tip of the nose or between the eyebrows, meditating on the rear of the head and lying supine like a corpse, but does not mention tantric element visualization in this context. These practices are also described in the *Śivasaṃhitā* (9.2.5), although they are not explicitly named there as practices of dissolution. The *saṃketa*s are similar to the simple techniques for *samādhi*/dissolution taught in the *Vijñānabhairava*[23] (9.2.4) and the *Amanaska*, and are suggestive of the subitist *rājayoga* model of *samādhi* in which there are no sequential steps towards *samādhi* (such as ascending through the *cakra*s).

Finally, we include some passages pertaining to the practice of listening to the inner sound (*nāda*), also sometimes referred to as the unstruck (*anāhata*) sound. The inner sound is declared in the *Haṭhapradīpikā* (9.3.1), *Śivasaṃhitā* 5.47, *Yogamārgaprakāśikā* (9.3.3), *Yogatārāvalī* (9.3.5) and *Haṭhatattvakaumudī* (9.3.6) to be the best of the dissolutions, while the *Rājayogāmṛta* identifies unity of the mind with the inner sound as *layayoga* itself (9.3.4). Most of the *Haṭhapradīpikā*'s verses on concentration on the inner sound (*nādānusandhāna*) have yet to be traced to earlier texts, although it appears to have precedents in practices of the Śaiva tantras.[24] Our textual sources subsequent to the *Haṭhapradīpikā* suggest that the practice of the inner sound was commonly taught,[25] as perhaps also indicated by its appearance in the Tamil *Tirumandiram* and the Persian *Baḥr al-ḥayāt* (9.3.8).

Chapter Contents

9.1.16 *Śāradātilaka* 25.27abc. Absorption as the identity of the individual and supreme selves.

9.1.17 *Gheraṇḍasaṃhitā* 7.1–6, 17. The six *samādhis* of royal yoga.

9.1.18 *Jogpradīpakā* 942–50. The best *samādhi* is thinking only of Sītā and Rāma.

9.1.20 Ibn Baṭṭūṭa's *Reḥla*. The *samādhi* of the yogis.

9.1.21 *Tashrīh al-Aqvāṃ*. The *samādhi* of the Saṃnyāsīs.

9.1.22 Sir Claude Wade. The 1837 CE *samādhi* of Hari Dās.

9.1.23 *Bṛhatkhecarīprakāśa* commentary on *Khecarīvidyā* 3.27–9. Placing Kuṇḍalinī in the skull as the means to long-term *samādhi*.

9.2 Dissolution (*laya*)

9.2.1 *Yogabīja* 150c–151d. Yoga by means of dissolution.

9.2.2 *Dattātreyayogaśāstra* 15–26. Dissolution by means of esoteric techniques.

9.2.3 *Amanaska* 1.17–30. Dissolution through focusing the mind on nothing.

9.2.4 *Vijñānabhairava* 34, 36, 56, 58, 69–74, 78, 113–16, with the *Uddyota* commentary of Śivopādhyāya. Simple means to attain *samādhi*.

9.2.5 *Śivasaṃhitā* 5.60–71. Techniques of dissolution.

9.2.6 *Haṭhapradīpikā* 4.50–54, 78–80. Dissolution of the mind and the royal yoga (*rājayoga*).

9.3 The Inner Sound (*nāda*)

9.3.1 *Haṭhapradīpikā* 1.43, 4.29–31, 34, 65–8, 81–107. *Nāda*, listening to the internal sounds.

9.3.2 *Śivayogapradīpikā* 1.6. The true *laya* yogi.

9.3.3 *Yogamārgaprakāśikā* 4.20ab. The inner sound is the best dissolution.

9.3.4 *Rājayogāmṛta* 2.5c–6b. The single inner sound.

9.3.5 *Yogatārāvalī* 2–4, 14, 28. Concentration on the inner sound is the most important dissolution.

9.3.6 *Haṭhatattvakaumudī* 54.1. Sound as the best method of dissolution.

9.3.7 *Tirumandiram* 607–8. The unstruck sound.

9.3.8 *Baḥr al-ḥayāt* 4.12–13. The unstruck sound.

9.3.9 *Jogpradīpakā* 932–4. Sītā, Rāma and the unstruck sound.

9.1

Samādhi

9.1.1 *Cūḷavedalla Sutta* 12. *Samādhi* as focus:

> 'And what, noble lady, is *samādhi*? What are the causes of *samādhi*? What are the requisites for *samādhi*? What is the cultivation of *samādhi*?'
>
> 'Dear Visākha, *samādhi* is focus of the mind. The causes of *samādhi* are the four foundations of mindfulness [the body, the sense-experiences, the mind and phenomena], the requisites for concentration are the four exertions [restraint of the senses, giving up sinful thoughts, meditation and safeguarding one's character],[26] [and] the cultivation of *samādhi* is the repetition, cultivation and regular practice of these same states.'

9.1.2 *Mahābhārata* 12.245.13cd. Yoga in *samādhi*:

> Śāṇḍilya said that this tranquillity is yoga in *samādhi*.

9.1.3 *Pātañjalayogaśāstra* 1.17–18. *Samādhi* with and without cognition:

Now, what is the description of *samādhi* with cognition (*saṃprajñāta samādhi*) of someone whose mental fluctuations have been stopped by means of the two methods [i.e. practice and dispassion]?

> (1.17) Because it takes on the form of attention (*vitarka*), reflection (*vicāra*), bliss (*ānanda*) and egoism (*asmitā*) it is '[*samādhi*] with cognition'.

Attention is the gross expansion of the mind on to its support. Reflection is [the same, but] subtle. Bliss is delight. Egoism is unitary consciousness.

Of these the first *samādhi*, accompanied by those four [i.e. attention, etc.], is [*samādhi*] with attention (*savitarka*). The second, shorn of attention, is [*samādhi*] with reflection (*savicāra*). The third, shorn of reflection, is [*samādhi*] with bliss (*sānanda*). The fourth, shorn of that, is pure egoism. All these *samādhi*s are with a support.

Now, what are the methods, and what is the nature, of *samādhi* without cognition (*asaṃprajñāta samādhi*)?

> (1.18) The other [*samādhi*] is preceded by the practice of contemplation of cessation and is the residue of karmic traces.

When all fluctuations [of the mind] are cast off and there is cessation of the mind [which is] the residue of karmic traces, that is '*samādhi* without cognition' (*asaṃprajñāta samādhi*). Its method is supreme dispassion. Because a practice with a [meditative] support is not suitable for accomplishing it, contemplation of cessation, which has no substance, is made the support. And that is without object.

Because the mind becomes supportless, as if it has attained non-existence, after the practice of that [contemplation of cessation], this seedless *samādhi* is [called] 'without cognition'.

9.1.4 *Pātañjalayogaśāstra* 1.41. The state of identity (*samāpatti*):

Now the true nature and sphere of operation of the state of identity (*samāpatti*) of a mind that has attained steadiness is taught:

> (1.41) The state of identity (*samāpatti*) of [a mind] whose fluctuations have been attenuated with regard to the perceiver, the organ of perception and the perceived is like that of a precious gem: the condition of being coloured by that which is near it.

The meaning of 'of one whose fluctuations have been attenuated' is 'of one whose cognition has stopped'. 'Like a precious gem' is the use of an example. Just as a crystal is tinged by the colour of – and takes on the appearance of – whatever it is resting on, so the mind is coloured by the object which is its support [and], having become the same as the object, takes on its appearance. Coloured by a subtle element [and] having become one with a subtle element, the mind resembles the subtle element's true form. Likewise, coloured by a gross mental support [and] having become one with the appearance of the gross [object, the mind] assumes the form of the gross [object]. Likewise, coloured by the various [phenomena] of the world [and] having become one with those phenomena, [the mind] assumes their form.

This is to be understood with regard to the means of perception, the sense organs, too. Coloured by the support of a means of perception [and] having become one with a means of perception, [the mind] takes on the appearance of the true form of [that] means of perception. Likewise, coloured by the support of the perceiver, i.e. the self, [and] having become one with the perceiver, i.e. the self, [the mind] assumes the appearance of the perceiver, i.e. the self. Likewise, coloured by the support of a liberated self [and] having become one with that liberated self, [the mind] assumes the appearance of that liberated self. So the state of identity (*samāpatti*) is thus said to be the assumption of the form of the things in which the mind is situated with regard to the perceiver, the organ of perception and the perceived (i.e. the self, the sense organs and the object), i.e. the condition of being coloured by that which is near it, like a precious gem, of the mind.

9.1.5 *Pātañjalayogaśāstra* 3.3. A definition of *samādhi*:

> (3.3) [When] that same [meditation (*dhyāna*)] has the appearance of only [its] object, as if it were free of its own form, that is *samādhi*.

When, as a result of immersion in the true being of the object of meditation, meditation has the appearance of the form of its object, as if free of its own form, which consists of cognition, that is said to be *samādhi*.

9.1.6 *Mṛgendratantra Yogapāda* 7cd, with Bhaṭṭa Nārāyaṇakaṇṭha's *vṛtti*. When meditation becomes coextensive with its object:[27]

Next the character of *samādhi*:

> 7cd. That [meditation] is termed *samādhi* [when] it becomes coextensive (*ekatāna*).

When that meditation becomes coextensive [with its object], when, that is, it reaches a state in which it appears to be nothing but its content, then the texts term it *samādhi*. Patañjali defines it in the same way:

'*Samādhi* is that same [meditation] when it appears as the object alone, as though empty of any identity of its own.'

9.1.7 *Parākhyatantra* 14.16c–17b. Absorption as dissolution into the supreme reality:[28]

> *Samādhi*, in which there is dissolution (*laya*) into the supreme reality level (*paratattva*), is what accomplishes union (*yoga*). (17) [The soul is] placed (*samāhita*) in the supreme reality level, and that is why it is called *samādhi*.

9.1.8 *Matsyendrasaṃhitā* 7.75–81, 88–9. *Samādhi* and its results:

The Lord spoke:

> (75) I shall teach [you] *samādhi*, by means of which the yogi may become Śiva, on whose image, perfected by visualization, [the yogi] should gaze by means of yogic sight (76) over and over again with a pure heart and all his attention. Whenever that image melts away together with the attention (77) he should focus on it with yogic sight and make it firm.
>
> A duration seven times that of meditation is called *samādhi*. (78) Empathetic imagination (*bhāva*)[29] on this and that will be shaky, because of its nature. He who perceives with a focused attention is said to be in *samādhi*. (79) With his thoughts focused, undistracted, steady, his senses unwavering, he who is in *samādhi* constantly sees Śiva by means of a lack of differentiation from [his] self. (80) In *samādhi*, O goddess, the light of fire, a great splendour, is seen. When this is seen, liberation arises for the yogi in *samādhi*. (81) When *samādhi* is completely mastered, the yogi is sure to see by means of yogic sight whatever image he brings to mind.
>
> [Verses 82–7 describe further special powers attained through *samādhi*, including strength, good health, sky-walking and omniscience (see Chapter 10 on *siddhis* (special powers)).]
>
> (88) If obstacles have arisen for the yogi in *samādhi*, he should completely remove them using the previously taught method, O Pārvatī, (89) and having thus mastered *samādhi*, he should +slowly move upwards+.

9.1.9 Kṣemarāja's *Spandasaṃdoha* commentary on the *Spandakārikā* 1.11. *Samādhi* with open and closed eyes:

> By means of the *samādhi*s in which the eyes are closed and open (*nimīlana* and *unmīlana samādhi*) the yogi resorts to the middle ground that simultaneously pervades both, as a result of which all thought is dried up by [the fire produced by] the coming together of the churning sticks into which these two have transformed, a state in which all the sense organs expand at once. This is the Bhairavī *mudrā*[30] concealed in all the tantras, in which the gaze, unblinking, is turned outwards, but focuses inwards.

9.1.10 *Lallāvākyāni* 1–2, 9, 25. The supreme teaching:

(1) Through practice, the expanse of the sky meets
that which has form, becoming one – WHACK!
The empty melts, and the pure remains
This, O scholar, is the teaching.

(2) Speech, thought, Kula and Akula are not there.
The silent seal (*mudrā*), there, is no way in.
There, Śiva and Śakti do not dwell
If there's anything left (?), that is the teaching.

(9) When the sun disappears, the moon's orb shines.
When that disappears only the mind shines.
When the mind disappears, the earth, sky and heavens –
all these visible phenomena – instantly go elsewhere.

(25) Having cut [down] these six forests of desire and so forth,
I obtained the nectar of immortality, which is made of
awakening.
After burning up matter by restraining the breath and
parching the mind with the fire of devotion, I reached Śiva.

9.1.11 *Vasiṣṭhasaṃhitā* 4.57–66. Focuses for *samādhi*:

> (57) Now I shall teach *samādhi*, which destroys the bonds of existence. You are bound by the bonds of

existence: you should listen carefully. (58) Equipped with restraint (*yama*) and the other virtues, your breath and senses conquered [and] endowed with fixation and meditation, practise *samādhi*, my son. (59) *Samādhi* is the state of identity of the individual and supreme selves (*jīvātman* and *paramātman*). *Samādhi* is taught to be the abiding of the individual self in the supreme self.

(60) *Samādhi* arises in whichever way [the yogi] is meditating on the self. By means of meditation he should establish [his self] in the self in such a way that it does not become otherwise. (61) Meditating on the self as bliss, knowledge of truth, unending [and] Brahman, free from attributes, [the yogi] attains *samādhi* in it alone. (62) Meditating on the self in the heart lotus as the supreme self in the form of Vāsudeva, [the yogi] attains *samādhi* in it alone. (63) Meditating on the god of fire as the Lord in the middle of the heart lotus, abiding in its flames, [the yogi] attains *samādhi* in him.

(64) Meditating on one's self in the heart lotus as the embodied [supreme] person (*puruṣa*) flooded with the nectar of immortality, [the yogi] attains *samādhi* in that alone. (65) Meditating on the self in between the brows as the sovereign Lord, golden-brown, [the yogi] attains *samādhi* in that alone. (66) Meditating on the self as the god Viṣṇu (*hari*) with a golden body [in the form of] the orb of the sun, [the yogi] attains *samādhi* in that alone.

9.1.12 *Gorakṣaśataka* 63d–67b. Breath-retention is the best method of *samādhi*:

Now I shall teach the best way to *samādhi*, (64) an enjoyable method which conquers death and always brings about the bliss of [*samādhi* in] Brahman. Correctly assuming a posture in exactly the same way as was taught earlier, (65) [the yogi] should stimulate Sarasvatī and control his breath. On the first day he should perform the four breath-retentions,[31] (66) [holding] each of them ten times. On the second day [he should increase] that by five. Adding five each day, on the third day he should do twenty, which is enough. (67ab) Breath-retention should always be performed in conjunction with the three locks (*bandhas*).

9.1.13 *Vivekamārtaṇḍa* 160–69. The difference between meditation and *samādhi*:

(160) As long as the subtle elements of sound and so forth are situated in the ears and other sense organs it is called meditation. *Samādhi* follows meditation. (161) Fixation is for five *nāḍīs* [i.e. two hours] [and] meditation is for six *nāḍīs* [i.e. two hours and twenty-four minutes]. *Samādhi* arises in twelve days as a result of restraining the breath. (162) When the mind and the self of the yogi unite like salt mixes with water it is called *samādhi*.

(163) When *prāṇa* is completely destroyed and the mind dissolves, then all experience is the same (*samarasatva*). That is called *samādhi*. (164) When the individual self and the supreme self are joined and all conceptions are destroyed, that is *samādhi*.

(165) The activity of the mind in the sense organs is a different process. When the breath and the vital principle have gone upwards, there is no mind, there are no sense organs.

(166) The yogi in *samādhi* perceives neither smell, nor taste, nor form, nor touch, nor sound, nor self, nor other. (167) The yogi in *samādhi* knows neither cold nor heat, neither sorrow nor pleasure, respect nor disrespect.

(168) The yogi in *samādhi* is not troubled by death, nor bound by *karma*, nor troubled by disease. (169) The yogi in *samādhi* is invulnerable to weapons, invincible to all people, and unassailable by mantras and yantras.

9.1.14 *Haṭhapradīpikā* 4.1–5, 10–12. Synonyms of *samādhi* and dissolving *prāṇa* and mind:

(1) Homage to Śiva, the guru Śiva, who consists of *nāda*, *bindu* and *kalā*, devoted to whom one always attains the immaculate state. (2) Now I will explain the highest process of *samādhi*, which destroys death, is a means to happiness [and] the best producer of the bliss of Brahman. (3) Royal yoga (*rājayoga*), *samādhi*, beyond the mind (*unmanī*), beyond and in the mind (*manonmanī*), non-dying (*amaratva*), dissolution (*laya*), empty and not empty (*śūnyāśūnya*), supreme state (*paraṃ padam*), (4) no mind (*amanaska*), non-dual (*advaita*), supportless (*nirālamba*), immaculate (*nirañjana*), liberation in life (*jīvanmukti*), natural [state] (*sahajā*) and the fourth state (*turyā*) are synonyms. (5) Oneness of the self and mind in the same way that salt dissolves in water as a result of [their] union (*yoga*) is called *samādhi*. [. . .]

(10) When the great goddess (*mahāśaktī*) is awakened by various postures and techniques (*karaṇa*s) of breath-control, and by the many *mudrā*s, then *prāṇa* dissolves into emptiness. (11) For the yogi in whom the goddess has awakened [and] who has abandoned all actions, the natural state (*sahajāvasthā*) arises automatically. (12) When *prāṇa* is flowing in the Suṣumnā channel and the mind is entering emptiness, then the knower of yoga eradicates all actions.

9.1.15 *Amanaska* 2.27–8. The relationship between breath and mind:

(27) Like mixed milk and water, mind and breath have the same action. Wherever there is breath, mind will appear, and wherever there is mind, breath will appear. (28) When one is destroyed, the other is destroyed. When one manifests, the other manifests. If they are not destroyed, the group of senses continues to function. If they are destroyed, the state of liberation is attained.

9.1.16 *Śāradātilaka* 25.27abc. Absorption as the identity of the individual and supreme selves:

> Constant mental cultivation (*bhāvanā*) of the identity of the individual self (*jīvātman*) and the supreme self (*paramātman*) is called *samādhi* by the sages (*munis*).

9.1.17 *Gheraṇḍasaṃhitā* 7.1–6, 17. The six *samādhi*s of royal yoga:

> (1) *Samādhi*, the highest level of reality, is attained by he who is very fortunate. It is received through the compassion and grace of the guru, and by devotion to the guru. (2) The yogi who day by day develops conviction in his learning, conviction in his guru, conviction in his self [and] awakening of his mind quickly attains the most beautiful practice. (3) The yogi, his consciousness free from its [various] states and so forth, should separate the mind from the body and unite it with the supreme self and know that to be *samādhi*.
>
> (4) I am Brahman and nothing else. I am Brahman alone and do not suffer. My form is truth, consciousness and bliss. I am eternally free. I abide in my own nature.
>
> (5) By means of the *śāmbhavī*, *bhrāmarī*, *khecarī* and *yoni mudrā*s four types of *samādhi* arise: meditation (*dhyāna*), resonance (*nāda*), bliss in aesthetic experience (*rasānanda*) and success in dissolution (*layasiddhi*). (6) The fifth is by means of devotion and the sixth is stupefaction of the mind. The royal yoga (*rājayoga*) has six varieties. One should learn each of them. [. . .]
>
> (17) I have thus taught you, O Caṇḍa, *samādhi*, which is a characteristic of liberation. *Samādhi* is the royal yoga, the means to oneness. Together with the beyond-mind state (*unmanī*) and the natural state (*sahajāvasthā*) they are synonyms of oneness.

9.1.18 *Jogpradīpakā* 942–50. The best *samādhi* is thinking only of Sītā and Rāma:

(942) It is called [*samādhi*] without cognition when one holds meditation [and] enters into [final] *samādhi*.[32] The [*samādhi* experienced] when one continues in the body is called [*samādhi*] with cognition. (943) Lord Rāma, who is in the entire universe, is in the water and the earth. +This is the observer of vows (*vrata dhārā*)+; he is the complete Brahman.

(944) Know there to be [the three states of] wakefulness, dreaming and deep sleep; *samādhi* is unconsciousness, but its scope is knowledge and ignorance, while only Sītā and Rāma are all-pervasive. (945) Know that the greedy person thinks only of money, the lustful only of lust [and] the thirsty only of water, but the yogi thinks only of Sītā and Rāma.

(946) Standing, sitting, waking [and] sleeping are mundane physical activities; mundane activities call out the slogan 'know that suffering is certain'. (947) The vow of the devotee is, having made a firm decision, that he will see nothing but Sītā and Rāma everywhere. (948) This is the best *samādhi*; there is no other way. Jayatarāma remains fixed in this *samādhi*. (949) Know rules and regulations to be the seed, posture and breath-control to be the leaves, withdrawal to be the flowers and fixation, meditation and *samādhi* to be the fruit. (950) Yoga is the wish-fulfilling tree; it removes exhaustion. Coming near it, Jayatarāma [obtains] the reward of easy liberation.

9.1.20 Ibn Baṭṭūṭa's *Reḥla*. The *samādhi* of the yogis:[33]

These people work wonders. For instance, one of them remains for months without food and drink; many of them dig a pit under the earth which is closed over them, leaving therein no opening except one through which the air might enter. There one remains for months and I have heard that some jogis hold out in this manner for a year.

9.1.21 *Tashrīh al-Aqvāṃ*. The *samādhi* of the Saṃnyāsīs:[34]

In this sect the dead body is buried in the ground or thrown in the river. Whenever someone is buried in the ground that is called *samādh*. When they throw someone in the river, that is called 'casting into water' (*jala-pravāha*). Some take *samādh* when they are still alive and of these there are two types. One takes *samādh* in a state of intoxication with cannabis (*bhāṅg*) and other intoxicants, imagining that they are leaving the world, and this is entirely devoid of spiritual benefits. Those who take *samādh* by the power of their ritual worship and ascetic practices, whatever they say to anybody will come to pass. And these people can appear in another city 500 or even 1,000 leagues (*kos*) distant in their own shape and form, appearing from under the ground.

9.1.22 Sir Claude Wade. The 1837 CE *samādhi* of Hari Dās:[35]

[The author accompanies Runjeet [sic] Singh to a garden adjoining the Lahore palace where the fakir Hari Dās has been buried in an apparently sealed, air-tight and guarded building.]

After our examination [of the building], we seated ourselves in the verandah opposite the door, while some of Runjeet Singh's people dug away the mud wall, and one of his officers broke the seal and opened the padlock. When the door was thrown open, nothing but a dark room was to be seen. Runjeet Singh and myself then entered it, in company with the servant of the Fakeer; and a light being brought, we descended about three feet below the floor of the room, into a sort of cell, where a wooden box, about four feet long by three broad, with a sloping roof, containing the Fakeer, was placed upright, the door of which had also a padlock and seal similar to that on the outside. On opening it, we saw a figure enclosed in a bag of white linen, fastened by a string over the head – on the exposure of which a grand salute was fired and the surrounding multitude came crowding to the door to see the spectacle. After they had gratified their curiosity, the Fakeer's servant, putting his arms into the box, took the figure out, and closing the door, placed it with its back against it, exactly as the Fakeer had been squatted (like a Hindoo idol) in the box itself.

Runjeet Singh and myself then descended into the cell, which was so small, that we were only able to sit on the ground in front of the body, and so close to it as to touch it with our hands and knees.

The servant then began pouring warm water over the figure; but, as my object was to see if any fraudulent practices could be detected, I proposed to Runjeet Singh to tear open the bag, and have a perfect view of the body before any means of resuscitation were employed. I accordingly did so; and may here remark, that the bag, when first seen by us, looked mildewed, as if it had been buried some time. The legs and arms of the body were shrivelled and stiff, the face full, the head reclining on the shoulder like that of a corpse. I then called to the medical gentleman who was attending me to come down and inspect the body, which he did, but could discover no pulsation in the heart, the temples or the arm. There was, however, a heat about the region of the brain, which no other part of the body exhibited.

The servant then recommenced bathing him with hot water, and gradually relaxing his arms and legs from the rigid state in which they were contracted, Runjeet Singh taking his right and I his left leg, to aid by friction in restoring them to their proper action, during which time the servant placed a hot wheaten cake, about an inch thick, on the top of the head, – a process which he twice or thrice renewed. He then pulled out of his nostrils and ears the wax and cotton with which they were stopped; and after great exertion opened his mouth by inserting the point of a knife between his teeth, and, while holding his jaws open with his left hand, drew the tongue forward with his right, – in the course of which the tongue flew back several times to its curved position upwards, in which it had originally been, so as to close the gullet.

He then rubbed his eyelids with ghee (or clarified butter) for some seconds, until he succeeded in opening them, when the eyes appeared quite motionless and glazed. After the cake had been applied for the third time to the top of his head, the body was violently convulsed, the nostrils became inflated, when respiration ensued, and the limbs began to assume a natural fullness; but the pulsation was still faintly perceptible. The servant then put some of the ghee on his tongue and made him swallow it. A few minutes afterwards, the eyeballs became dilated, and recovered their natural colour, when the Fakeer, recognizing Runjeet Singh sitting close to him, articulated, in a low sepulchral tone, scarcely audible: 'Do you believe me now?'

Runjeet Singh replied in the affirmative, and invested the Fakeer with a pearl necklace, and a superb pair of gold bracelets and pieces of silk and muslin, and shawls, forming what is termed a *khelat*; such as is usually conferred by the princes of India on persons of distinction.

From the time of the box being opened to the recovery of the voice, not more than half an hour could have elapsed; and in another half an hour, the Fakeer talked with myself and those about him freely, though feebly, like a sick person; and we then left him, convinced that there had been no fraud or collusion in the exhibition we had witnessed.

9.1.23 *Bṛhatkhecarīprakāśa* commentary on *Khecarīvidyā* 3.27–9. Placing Kuṇḍalinī in the skull as the means to long-term *samādhi*:

(27–9) Holding his breath by stopping Iḍā and Piṅgalā, [the yogi] should awaken Kuṇḍalinī and pierce the six lotuses. Inserting [Kuṇḍalinī], who has the appearance of a thousand lightning bolts, into the very middle of the skull in the place that is an ocean of cool *amṛta*, he

> should remain there for a long time. When the yogi resides at will in the abode of Brahmā, then [with him] at that place the body appears (*bhāti*) lifeless.

This is the means to long-term *samādhi*. This *samādhi* is to be done by one who is free from all worry, has mastered all methods and is capable, on a mountain or such like, in a cave or in the ground in a cell +dug out of rocks+ with features such as a small, covered opening and a group of pupils to protect him, because the body [of the yogi] must be taken care of. 'When the yogi resides' [. . .] At the time of such *samādhi*, when the adept yogi goes at will, i.e. without effort, like a bee going from one flower to another, into the abode of Brahmā, which has the previously mentioned characteristics, then the body, even though it is alive, appears lifeless, like a piece of wood. If the objection is raised from this that in a lifeless body bad smells and features of a corpse arise, it is refuted by the word 'appears' (*bhāti*) [. . .]

Some practise *samādhi* until the end of the world (? *maṇḍalaparyanta*). Others, after lots of practice, use a special massage of an internal channel that they have discovered to enter [*samādhi*] and cause others to enter it. Some enter it by assuming the corpse pose and focusing their minds on both their big toes. Others dissolve their mind and breath by the royal yoga, dissolution. The touch of fresh air [or] massaging the head with butter, ghee, etc., are the means of bringing [the yogi] round from *samādhi*. When bringing him round one should hold an image of a deity or such like in front of his eyes. Pupils, etc., should not stand [in front of him].

9.2

Dissolution (*laya*)

9.2.1 *Yogabīja* 150c–151d. Yoga by means of dissolution:

> (150c) Then, when union has been attained, O goddess, the mind is dissolved. (151) The breath becomes steady when dissolution arises. From dissolution, happiness, the highest state of bliss in one's own self, is obtained.

9.2.2 *Dattātreyayogaśāstra* 15–26. Dissolution by means of esoteric techniques:

> (15) 'Yoga by means of dissolution (*layayoga*) happens as a result of the dissolution of the mind by means of esoteric techniques (*saṃketas*). Ādinātha has taught 80 million esoteric techniques.'
>
> Sāṃkṛti said: (16) 'Please tell me, what form does Lord Ādinātha take? Who is he?'
>
> Dattātreya said: (17) 'The names of Mahādeva, the great god, are Ādinātha, Bhairava and Lord of the Śabaras. While that mighty god was sporting playfully (18–19) with Pārvatī in the company of the leaders of his troop in [various places such as] Mount Śrīkaṇṭha, Śrīparvata, the top of a mountain in the region of the Banana Forest, [and] the mountain at Citrakūṭa covered with beautiful trees, he, Śaṅkara, out of compassion secretly told an esoteric technique to each of them in those places. (20) I, however, cannot teach all of them in detail. [But] I shall gladly proclaim some of them, [such as this one] which consists of a simple practice and is easy: (21) while staying still [or] moving, sleeping [or] eating, day and night one should meditate on emptiness. This is one esoteric technique taught by Śiva. (22) Another is said to be merely staring at the tip of the nose. And meditation on the rear part of the head conquers death. (23) The next esoteric technique is said to be merely staring between the eyebrows. And that which is [staring] at the flat part of the forehead between the brows is said to be excellent. (24) [Another] excellent dissolution (*laya*) is [staring] at the big toes of the left and right feet. Lying supine on the ground like a corpse is also said to be an excellent [dissolution]. (25) If one practises in a place free from people while relaxed, one will achieve success.
>
> (26) 'Thus Śaṅkara has taught many esoteric techniques. That dissolution of the mind which occurs by means of [these] and several other esoteric techniques is yoga by

means of dissolution (*layayoga*). Next hear about yoga by means of force (*haṭhayoga*).'

9.2.3 *Amanaska* 1.17–30. Dissolution through focusing the mind on nothing:

(17) In a solitary place, sitting comfortably on a level seat, slightly hunched, the gaze fixed at arm's length, limbs relaxed, and free from worries, engage in practice. (18) Sitting in a comfortable posture, [the yogi] should undertake the practice of the elements (*tattva*s). By regular practice, he causes the ultimate element to be revealed. (19) 'The universe is produced from the five gross elements; the body is made from the five elements; everything is made from the elements.' Abandoning [such thoughts] one should cultivate the thought that nothing exists. (20) The yogi should focus the mind on nothing, free from all worries about internal and external [matters]. He [becomes] oriented towards the [ultimate] element. (21) When he has become oriented towards the [ultimate] element, the no-mind state manifests. When the no-mind state arises, the dissolution of the mind and other [faculties] ensues. (22) When the dissolution of the mind and other [faculties] has ensued, the breath dissolves. As a result of the disappearance of the breath and the mind, he relinquishes the objects of the senses. (23) When the sense objects have been relinquished, external knowledge does not arise. When external knowledge is destroyed, then he becomes equanimous towards everything. (24) When he has become equanimous towards everything, he is free from action. Joined with the great Brahman, the yogi has then attained dissolution.

(25) I will describe the features of that great dissolution, free from the mind, which arises for those devoted to regular practice. (26) When [the yogi] is in dissolution, he knows neither happiness nor suffering, recognizes neither cold nor heat and is not conscious of the

activities of the sense objects. (27) Neither dead nor alive, he neither sees nor blinks. He remains lifeless like a piece of wood and is said to be in dissolution. (28) In the same way that a lamp placed in a sheltered spot shines unwaveringly, the yogi in dissolution is free from worldly activity. (29) Just as a windless lake appears still and clear, so [the yogi] in dissolution appears to have abandoned sound and the other objects of the senses. (30) Just as salt thrown in water gradually dissolves, so by means of practice the mind dissolves into Brahman.

9.2.4 *Vijñānabhairava* 34, 36, 56, 58, 69–74, 78, 113–16, with the *Uddyota* commentary of Śivopādhyāya. Simple means to attain *samādhi*:

(34) Insert the mind into the [hollow in the] skull [and], remaining with the eyes shut, use the steadiness of the mind to focus gradually on the ultimate focus.

(36) When, through piercing [the knot] of the brows [and] blocking the doors by means of the weapon that is the eyes being blocked by the hands, the point (*bindu*) is seen and one gradually becomes dissolved in it, the ultimate state [arises].

(56) Meditate upon the absolute in the form of the paths beginning with earth moving from gross to subtle to beyond until finally the mind dissolves.

(58) Meditate upon all this, O great goddess, as empty, and the mind becomes dissolved in it; then one becomes worthy of dissolution in the ultimate.

(69) The pleasure at the culmination of possession by the partner/goddess (*śakti*) stirred up by sexual intercourse with a partner, is [the pleasure] of the reality level of Brahman; that pleasure is said to be within oneself. (70) The weight of the memory of the pleasure of kissing, embracing and scratching a woman, even in the absence of a partner, O great goddess, results in a flood of bliss. (71) When great bliss is attained or when a

friend is seen after a long time, meditate on the bliss that has arisen. Dissolved in that one's mind becomes [fixed] on the ultimate. (72) When one meditates upon the feeling of being full after the arising of the sweet bliss of the happiness produced by eating and drinking, then the great bliss arises. (73) The ascent of the mind produced by the identification with the absolute of the yogi who is united with the peerless happiness that arises from the enjoyment of song and other objects of the senses leads to his becoming the absolute. (74) Fix the mind in whatever place the mind is content. In that place the true nature of supreme bliss [arises].

(78) On a soft seat [sit] on one buttock and hold a hand and foot [out] without a support; by concentrating on this the mind becomes pure and complete.

(113) Listen, O goddess, to this tradition. I shall tell it to you in full. Isolation (*kaivalya*) arises immediately merely by holding the eyes steady. (114) By clenching the ears and the lower openings, and meditating upon that which has no vowels or consonants, one enters the eternal Brahman. (115) When one's mind is free from thought as a result of standing in a deep hole such as a well and looking upwards, complete dissolution of the mind manifests immediately. (116) Wherever the mind goes, internally or externally, is the state of Śiva. It is all-pervasive: where can it go?

This state is the permanent *samādhi*, attained after the six *samādhi*s [taught] in treatises on yoga have been perfected. Its form is as a revealer [of the absolute], it is effortless [and] it is said to be the seventh *samādhi*.

9.2.5 *Śivasaṃhitā* 5.60–71. Techniques of dissolution:

(60) When the yogi sits in the lotus position, concentrates on his Adam's apple and puts his tongue at the base of his palate, he feels neither hunger nor thirst. (61) In the place below the Adam's apple is the lovely Kūrma channel. When the yogi concentrates on it, his mind

becomes completely still. (62) When the yogi visualizes the eye of Śiva as an aperture in his skull, then there arises a shining light as brilliant as a ball of lightning. (63) Merely by visualizing it sins are destroyed. Even a wicked man attains the ultimate state. (64) Then, when the wise man continually performs the visualization, he is sure to see and speak with the adepts.

(65) If the yogi meditates on emptiness day and night, while standing still, moving, sleeping and eating, he becomes made of space and is absorbed in the space of consciousness. (66) This meditation should be done regularly by the yogi desirous of success. Through constant practice, he is sure to become my equal. (67) By the power of this meditation the yogi becomes dear to everyone. After conquering all the elements, he is free from desire and acquisitiveness.

(68) When the yogi sits in the lotus position and looks at the tip of his nose, his mind dies and he successfully becomes a sky-rover. (69) The lord of yogis sees a bright light like a white mountain. Through the power of practising on it, he himself becomes its guardian. (70) To remove his fatigue quickly, the wise yogi should lie on his back on the ground and meditate without pause on that light. (71) When the rear part of the head is meditated upon, death is conquered. The unrivalled reward produced merely by looking between the eyebrows has been taught.

9.2.6 *Haṭhapradīpikā* 4.50–54, 78–80. Dissolution of the mind and the royal yoga (*rājayoga*):

(50) One should make the mind supportless and think of nothing: [thereby] one is sure to be situated in internal and external space, like a pot. (51) In the same way that the external air (*vāyu*) comes to rest, so the breath in the centre, along with the mind, is sure to attain steadiness in its own place. (52) The breath of one who practises on

the path of the breath night and day in this way is extinguished through practice [and] the mind dissolves in the very same place. (53) One should flood the body, from the soles of the feet to the head, with the nectar of immortality. [The yogi] is thus perfected, with a mighty body, great strength and great courage. (54) One should place the mind in the midst of the goddess (*śakti*), and the goddess in the midst of the mind. Observing the mind with the mind, one should focus on the supreme state.

(78) Whether there is liberation or not, in this very state there is unbroken happiness. This happiness which springs from dissolution is attained through the royal yoga. (79) I consider those practitioners who, ignorant of the royal yoga, practise only *haṭha* to be toiling without results. (80) To quickly attain the beyond-mind state (*unmanī*), I recommend meditation on the eyebrows. [This is] an easy way for those of little intelligence to attain the state of royal yoga. Dissolution produced by sound instantly bestows results.

9.3

The Inner Sound (*nāda*)

9.3.1 *Haṭhapradīpikā* 1.43; 4.29–31, 34, 65–8, 81–107. *Nāda*, listening to the internal sounds:

(1.43) There is no posture like the adept's pose, no breath-retention like the pure retention, no seal like *khecarī* and no dissolution like [listening to] the inner sound (*nāda*).

(4.29) The mind is the lord of the senses, but the breath is the lord of the mind. Dissolution is the lord of the breath, and that dissolution is dependent on the inner sound (*nāda*). (30) This is called liberation [by some], but others are of the opinion that it is not [liberation].

When mind and *prāṇa* dissolve, a certain bliss arises. (31) Dissolution in which inhalation and exhalation disappear and grasping of the objects of the senses ceases, and which is inactive and unchanging, is the best for yogis.

(34) They say 'dissolution, dissolution' [but] what are the characteristic features of dissolution? Dissolution is the non-remembrance of the objects of the senses as a result of karmic traces (*vāsanā*s) not recurring.

Now concentration on internal sound (*nādānusandhāna*). (65) The [internal] sound practice, which is approved even for those fools who are incapable of realizing the truth, and was taught by Gorakṣanātha, is [now] explained. (66) The 12,500,000 kinds of dissolution (*laya*) taught by the glorious Ādinātha [i.e Śiva] are the best. We consider one of [those] dissolutions, concentration on the [internal] sound, to be pre-eminent.

(67) Seated in the posture of the liberated (*muktāsana*), the yogi should adopt the Śāmbhavī *mudrā* and listen single-mindedly to the sound situated in the right ear. (68) Block the ear holes, both eyes, the nose and the mouth. An unsullied sound is clearly heard in the purified Suṣumnā channel. [. . .]

(81) The one glorious lord of gurus knows the unique, indescribable bliss growing in the hearts of the lords of yoga, who enjoy *samādhi* in concentration on the [internal] sound. Only the blessed lord guru knows this. (82) The sage who presses his ears with his hands hears the resonance (*dhvani*). He should steady his mind there until he attains the steady state. (83) On being practised, this inner sound (*nāda*) blocks out external sound. After a fortnight, with distractions completely conquered, the yogi is happy.

(84) In the initial stage of practice, various kinds of loud noises are heard. As the practice develops, increasingly subtle sounds are heard. (85) In the beginning [the

sounds] of the ocean, thunder, a kettledrum and a *jharjhara* drum occur. In the intermediate [stage], [the sounds] of *mardala* drum and conch arise, then of a bell and a *kāhala* drum. (86) In the last [stage there arise] the sounds of a small bell, a flute, a veena and a bee. These are the various sounds that are heard within the body.

(87) When he hears loud sounds like thunder, kettledrums and so on, he should focus only on the very subtlest sound. (88) Whether it has put a loud sound in a quiet one or a quiet one in a loud one, one should not move one's distracted mind elsewhere, even if it is taking pleasure. (89) The mind becomes steady exactly where it first cleaves to a sound, and dissolves together with it.

(90) Just as a bee drinking nectar pays no attention to the perfume, so a mind attached to sound does not desire the objects of the senses. (91) The mind, a rutting elephant wandering about in the garden of sense objects, can be brought under control by this sharp goad of sound.[36] (92) The mind which is bound by the fetter of sound is entirely free of unsteadiness. It becomes completely still, like a bird with clipped wings.

(93) He who desires the kingdom of yoga should abandon all anxiety and, with an attentive mind, concentrate on the inner sound. (94) The inner sound is the snare that captures the deer of the mind. And it is the hunter who slays the antelope of the mind. (95) For the horse that is the mind of the ascetic, the technique of the inner sound is the bolt [to lock it in], so the yogi should practise it regularly.

(96) By being oxidized in the sulphur of sound, the mercury of the mind is bound and its unsteadiness eradicated, [and] it wanders in the space called 'supportless'. (97) By hearing the inner sound the snake of the mind forgets everything and, single-pointed, does not rush off anywhere. (98) [Just as] fire kindled with wood burns out along with the wood, [so] the mind started with sound dissolves along with the sound. (99) If one is a

good shot with an arrow, it is easy to hit the deer of the mind when it is motionless and fixed on the sounds of the bell and so forth. (100) That which is to be known is inside the noise of the unstruck sound which is heard and inside that which is to be known is the mind. The mind gets dissolved there. That is the supreme state of Viṣṇu. (101) As long as sound continues, there is the conception of space. The soundless great Brahman is praised as the supreme self. (102) Whatsoever is heard in the form of inner sound is nothing but the goddess (*śakti*). Only the formless (*nirākāra*) ultimate reality is the supreme Lord.

(103) All the methods of *haṭha* and dissolution (*laya*) are for the sake of attaining *rājayoga*. The man who has surmounted *rājayoga* cheats death. (104) Truth (*tattva*) is the seed, *haṭha* is the field, indifference is the water. By means of these three, the wish-fulfilling vine of the beyond mind [state] (*unmanī*) spontaneously grows. (105) By constantly concentrating on the inner sound, accumulations of sins are destroyed, and mind and breath are without a doubt dissolved into the immaculate (*nirañjana*). (106) By means of the beyond-mind state, one never hears the sound of the conch or the kettledrum, and one's body is sure to become like wood. (107) The yogi who is freed from all states and devoid of all thought remains as if dead. He is liberated. In this there is no doubt.

9.3.2 *Śivayogapradīpikā* 1.6. The true *laya* yogi:

He whose own thoughts, having been meditated upon,[37] become, together with the mind and breath, dissolved in the inner sound (*nāda*), is truly a dissolution (*laya*) yogi.

9.3.3 *Yogamārgaprakāśikā* 4.20ab. The inner sound is the best dissolution:

There is no science like yoga, no dissolution like the inner sound; 'beyond and in the mind' (*manonmanī*) is [the best] among states like Śāmbhavī is [the best] among seals.

9.3.4 *Rājayogāmṛta* 2.5c–6b. The single inner sound:

One should insert the breath into the Suṣumnā and [then] a single inner sound is heard. (6) Unity of the mind with that inner sound is said to be the yoga of dissolution.

9.3.5 *Yogatārāvalī* 2–4, 14, 28. Concentration on the inner sound is the most important dissolution:

(2) In the world there are 125,000 focuses of dissolution (*laya*) taught by Sadāśiva. We consider *samādhi* by means of concentrating on the inner sound to be the single most important of the dissolutions. (3) When all the channels have been purified by means of retention of the breath, together with exhalation and inhalation, then internally the sound called 'unstruck' (*anāhata*) constantly arises in several forms. (4) O concentration on the [unstruck] sound, homage to you! I consider you the means of reaching the state of [the highest] reality. Through your grace my mind dissolves in the abode of Viṣṇu together with my breath.

(14) When the state of *rājayoga* is attained and flourishing, there are no focuses for the gaze, there is no locking of the mind, no place or time [for practice], no holding of the breath [and] no exertion of oneself with fixation or meditation. [. . .]

(28) When will I, on the peaks and in the caves of Śrīśailam, obtain the perfection which is this dissolution of the mind in *samādhi*? When creepers entwine my body and birds make nests in my ears!

9.3.6 *Haṭhatattvakaumudī* 54.1. Sound as the best method of dissolution:

Among the dissolutions (*laya*s), the most eminent one is *samādhi* by means of concentration on the inner sound.

9.3.7 *Tirumandiram* 607–8. The unstruck sound:[38]

(607) Bell, sea, elephant, flute, cloud, bee, dragonfly, conch, drum and lute: the subtle sounds of these ten are heard only by those who have stilled their minds in God. (608) The roar of the sea, the thundering of a cloud, the trumpeting of an elephant, the euphony of a lute, the music of the orbs, the melody of the flute, the resonance of the conch: by the grace of the glow of the vastness of space only the true yogi hears all these.

9.3.8 *Baḥr al-ḥayāt* 4.12–13. The unstruck sound:[39]

(12) The recollection of *anāhad*. When the wayfarer wants to be continually occupied with a single presence, but essentially has no time at his disposal, he should perform the *anāhad* practice. They call *anāhad* that which is of the eternal. One sits on both knees, holding the buttocks on the soles of the feet. One places the hands even with the ears, inserting both index fingers into the ears, with the thumb behind the ears, and the other three fingers spread out evenly, to the point that a sound arises. In this sound is the sign without a sign, perpetually. When one can no longer hold the hands up, one takes round pepper grain and performs the posture, throwing it into fresh cotton and placing the cotton into each ear, so that the voice arises from the finger. By holding the cotton it will arise even so; the mystical adepts act so that, expecting that time, the fruits of this are more plentiful. This will become clear in practice.

(13) The word of recollection of *nād*. When someone wants to practise the *nād*, first one should sit cross-legged, holding the head, stomach and back straight. Keeping both hands upright, joining the two thumbs together, one holds the elbows below and places both elbows on the stomach over the navel. One takes one's thought to the base of the brain. Now the base of the brain is a window that the Jogis call *brahmarandhra*

('the aperture of Brahman'). In that enters the window of the place of life, death, sleep, the settled abode of manifestation, the determination of the source of the essence, and the heaven of life, so that it is the testimony of the state of this word.

9.3.9 *Jogpradīpakā* 932–4. Sītā, Rāma and the unstruck sound:

Now the description of *samādhi*.

(932) The yogi should enter *samādhi* in the bee cave on the thousand-petalled lotus described earlier. (933) It shines with the splendour of countless suns and is completely and supremely blissful. The unstruck sound continues unceasingly and one obtains [union of] the individual and supreme selves. (934) Sītā and Rāma are there in that which has countless petals in the form of truth, consciousness and bliss, the bliss of consciousness with the form of special knowledge.

TEN
Yogic Powers

The Importance of Supernatural Powers in Yoga's History

Yoga's ability to bestow supernatural powers[1] upon its practitioners has always been central to its textual descriptions. Yogic powers run the gamut of human fantasies. They include flight, long-distance hearing and sight, omniscience, the ability to become infinitely small, large, light, heavy or invisible, the ability to locate buried treasure, mastery of alchemy, and control over other people. One frequently mentioned power is simply the ability to do whatever one wants. In this chapter we have included descriptions of such powers and the methods of attaining them from a wide variety of manuals of yoga practice.[2] The extraordinary capabilities of accomplished yogis are a widespread motif in other literary genres, including yogis' own legends, narrative tales and travellers' reports, and we have also included examples of these.

Despite their fantastical nature, belief in such powers was not restricted to the credulous. Though sceptical voices are sometimes heard – such as that of the Kashmiri poetess-*yoginī* Lallā (10.21) – of the many distinct Indian intellectual traditions only the Mīmāṃsakas, the strictest proponents of Vedic ritualism, denied their existence outright.[3] Other scholastic traditions taught *yogipratyakṣa* ('the perception of the yogi') to be one of the means of acquiring authoritative knowledge, and they discussed its characteristics at length.[4] We have included in this chapter a brief description of yogic perception from a sixth-century CE text of the Vaiśeṣika philosophical tradition (10.6) and a simple method of attaining it through yogic meditation taught in the sixth- to seventh-century CE *Skandapurāṇa* (10.10).

Nor was belief in the powers of India's yogis found only in their devotees. Visitors to India have often remarked approvingly of Indian yogis' marvellous attainments. At the end of the eighteenth century the head teacher of Hindustani at Fort William in Calcutta was commissioned by the East India Company to write an Urdu translation of an account of the yogis from a Mughal imperial gazetteer completed in 1695–6. The translation's section on the myriad supernatural powers of the yogis is included in this chapter (10.25).[5]

Ambivalence towards Yogic Powers

Belief in yogic powers may have been almost universal, but the attitude towards them in texts on yoga is ambivalent as far as their usefulness for reaching yoga's final goal is concerned. Some powers are said to arise automatically as the yogi advances in his or her yoga practice and are thus helpful indicators of progress (some such signs are in fact not powers at all, but unpleasant symptoms, such as trembling). However, as shown by several of the passages in this chapter, in many schools of yoga such powers must then be ignored or rejected in order for the yogi to go on and achieve the final goal, liberation. The *Dattātreyayogaśāstra* explains that the yogi should not take pleasure in his powers and must conceal them because otherwise he will acquire too many devotees and, busy attending to them, will be unable to carry out his yoga practice (10.17). Allowances are made in some texts for displaying powers in order to draw people on to the right path. Thus the *Pañcārthabhāṣya* (1.20.26) says that yogic powers are like a flag for attracting a student, but later warns against taking pleasure in them, and the Buddha uses his ability to be in two places at once to refute the doctrines of others,[6] but elsewhere rejects the display of such powers because it could lead to the gullible being tricked into believing that they may be bought for money (10.1).

In contrast with this widespread understanding of yogic powers as ultimately a hindrance to yoga practice, some texts teach them to be a necessary prerequisite of the attainment of the ultimate goal. Thus in the *Mahābhārata*, Śuka, in order to become finally liberated, needs to use the powers that he has previously kept concealed,[7] and in many later tantric and yogic texts in order to attain final liberation the yogi must use the power of *utkrānti* ('yogic suicide') to project the life force out of the top of the skull.[8] Furthermore, as can be seen in many of the passages in this book, the final state of yoga is itself accompanied by great powers. In early formulations of yoga, such as those found in the *Mahābhārata*, yoga, like asceticism (*tapas*), is seen as a glorious power in itself, through which the yogi becomes mightier than the gods and can even burn up the entire universe (**10.2**).

Although *sūtra* 3.37 ('Those powers are hindrances when [the yogi is] in *samādhi*; when the mind is active they are perfections') of the *Pātañjalayogaśāstra* is often cited by Indian commentators and modern scholars in order to demonstrate that Patañjali considered powers to be an obstacle to the goal of yoga, his position is not in fact clear-cut. If we read his auto-commentary to 3.37 we see that it is only the powers mentioned in *sūtra* 3.36 ('luminous cognition and [divine] hearing, sensation, sight, taste and smell') that are said in *sūtra* 3.37 to be hindrances to *samādhi* (see **10.4**). Meanwhile, Patañjali devotes the rest of the third of the four chapters of his *Yogaśāstra* to descriptions of other powers, and these are not said to be obstacles; indeed, included among them at *sūtra* 3.50 is isolation (*kaivalya*), the ultimate aim of Pātañjala yoga. Furthermore, although elsewhere in the *Pātañjalayogaśāstra* (in the *bhāṣya* preceding *sūtra* 2.35) yogic powers are said to signal success in yoga, nowhere are they said to arise automatically; on the contrary, to attain each power a specific object must be concentrated upon.

Intentional and Unintentional Powers

A distinction between powers which arise automatically and those which are sought deliberately is formalized in the *c.* fourteenth-century CE *Yogabīja*, which classifies them into two types: unintentional (*akalpita*) and intentional (*kalpita*) (**10.20**). Intentional powers, which are inferior to unintentional ones, are acquired deliberately by means of directed practices, including alchemy, ritual and mantra. These methods are typical of the tantric traditions and it is only in tantric works that we find an unambiguously positive attitude towards the acquisition of supernatural powers; when theorized, their enjoyment is seen as an emulation of divine cosmic play.[9] Tantric systems distinguish two types of practitioner: the seeker of liberation (the *mumukṣu*, who is usually an ascetic) and the seeker of powers (the *bubhukṣu*, who is usually a householder); the majority of tantric texts are aimed at the latter and contain extensive descriptions of directed methods of obtaining specific supernatural powers. Mantra-based ritual is the central means of doing so, with yoga as an additional method.[10] In some tantric teachings, yoga is specifically for the *sādhaka*, i.e. the aspirant who has taken the initiation which allows him to pursue supernatural powers, and is 'a precious help (according to some texts, a necessity) in his effort to obtain *siddhi*s'.[11]

The *c.* 325–425 CE *Pātañjalayogaśāstra*, which predates the texts of mainstream tantra (i.e. those of the Mantramārga, the 'way of mantras'), gives a list of things other than yoga which may produce supernatural powers: birth (*janma*), medicinal herbs (*oṣadhi*), mantra and asceticism (*tapas*). Examples of these may be found in various texts which predate the *Pātañjalayogaśāstra*. In the twelfth book of the *Mahābhārata* the sage Śuka is born with the ability to fly, thanks to a boon won from Śiva by Śuka's father Vyāsa as a result of his performance of *tapas* (12.312). Elsewhere in the *Mahābhārata* – as well as in the *Rāmāyaṇa* and the later Purāṇic corpus – we find numerous stories of sages undertaking fearsome austerities in order to gain powers from the gods. Perhaps the most famous Indian story involving magical medicinal herbs occurs in the *Rāmāyaṇa*, when Rāma's unconscious brother Lakṣmaṇa is revived by divine herbs brought by Hanumān from the Himālaya (*Yuddhakāṇḍa* 40). Detailed descriptions of medicinal herbs that produce powers are rare in yoga texts, but the many tantra-inflected works that teach *rasāyana*, elixir medicine, give extensive descriptions of herbal preparations which can bring about a variety of powers, in particular perfection of the body. Often this is to be effected by a process called *kāyakalpa*, in which the practitioner consumes nothing but a single preparation for a lunar month, while confined in a dark room or cave. Unusually for a yoga text, the short final chapter of the *c.* fourteenth-century CE *Khecarīvidyā* (10.19) details various such preparations. The *Mahābhārata* does not give detailed teachings on magical herbs, but it does contain a short passage on diets that produce yogic power (*bala*) (10.3). The practice of repeating mantras or sacred formulas in order to bring about supernatural effects dates back to the Vedic period and, as noted above, this is the central rite of the tantric traditions (on mantra, see Chapter 7).

All of the powers available through these methods may also be acquired through yoga. This is stated explicitly in the *c.* ninth-century *Bhāgavatapurāṇa* (10.13), which, clearly invoking the *Pātañjalayogaśāstra*, says that yoga can bring about all the powers that birth, elixirs, mantra and austerities may produce.

Several texts explain the mechanisms by which the powers arise. In the *Pātañjalayogaśāstra*, as we have seen, they result from intense concentration on a particular object. Thus concentration on the Adam's apple gets rid of hunger and thirst (3.30). The *Pātañjalayogaśāstra*'s metaphysical underpinning is that of Sāṃkhya and later commentators understand the powers to result from the ability to manipulate *prakṛti*, the material aspect of Sāṃkhya's dualism of spirit and matter. In Sāṃkhya *prakṛti* is divided into twenty-four elemental constituents (*tattva*s). Other metaphysical traditions have different systems of *tattva*s, but there is a broad consensus that yoga may be achieved by a sequential meditation on the *tattva*s, however they may be conceived, leading from the gross to the subtle in a reversal of the process of creation. The powers that arise along the way match the *tattva* that is the focus of meditation. This notion is first found in the *Mahābhārata* (12.228.13–26), wherein fixation on select Sāṃkhyan *tattva*s – the five gross elements, egoism, intellect and 'the unmanifest' (*avyakta*, i.e. *prakṛti* ('matter') before the onset of creation) – leads to the yogi being able to manipulate the *tattva* that has been the object of fixation. Thus fixation on the earth element makes the yogi as immobile as a mountain and able to shake the earth with his thumb or big toe. A similar system is found in the *Bhāgavatapurāṇa* (see 10.13), where the eight classical powers first detailed in the *Pātañjalayogaśāstra* are said to be innate, but there are ten more, which arise through fixation on the *tattva*s. In more straightforward schemata, the *Amanaska* teaches that greater and greater powers arise simply as the result of longer and longer durations of dissolution (*laya*) (10.23), the *Śivasaṃhitā* promises more powerful *siddhi*s for greater numbers of mantra-repetitions (7.14) and the *Siddhasiddhāntapaddhati* correlates the arising of powers with the length of time that the yogi has been practising yoga (10.24).

Classifications and Hierarchies of Yogic Powers

Many texts, from those of the Buddhist Pali canon through the *Pātañjalayogaśāstra* to haṭhayogic works such as the *Śivasaṃhitā*, list, and in some cases describe, the powers that a yogi may attain. These lists are often unsystematic, but ordered classifications are also found. Several texts of the Buddhist Pali canon give a stock list of ten, an example of which from the *Dīghanikāya* we have included at 10.1. In the *Mahābhārata*[12] there are passing mentions of an unspecified group of eight powers, which may be a precursor of the group of eight first described in detail in the *Pātañjalayogaśāstra* (10.4) and which subsequently became a widespread trope in yoga texts of all traditions. This group is very rarely listed in full, being usually invoked by reference only to its first member, *aṇimā*, the power to become as small as an atom.[13] Included in this chapter is a passage from Hemacandra's *Yogaśāstra* in which the eight powers are individually described (10.15).

Not surprisingly in the light of powers being the main aim of the practices taught therein, Śaiva tantric texts contain extensive lists and a variety of systematizations of yogic powers. Thus the earliest work of initiatory Śaivism, the *c.* second-century CE *Pāśupatasūtra* of the ascetic Atimārga tradition, gives a list which includes many powers similar to those of the *Pātañjalayogaśāstra*. Kauṇḍinya's commentary on *Pāśupatasūtra* 2.12 (*c.* 400–550 CE) mentions the group of eight powers taught in the *Pātañjalayogaśāstra* and adds that they are further subdivided into sixty-four. A group of sixty-four powers is mentioned in other Śaiva texts;[14] a description of all of them is found in the *Vāyavīyasaṃhitā* of the *Śivapurāṇa* (10.11).[15]

The *c.* sixth-century CE *Brahmayāmala* describes a group of eight magical powers quite different from those of the *Pātañjalayogaśāstra* (10.9). These esoteric powers, and the means of attaining them, reflect the *Brahmayāmala*'s status as a text of the

Śaiva Vidyāpīṭha, in which worship of the goddess and transgressive rites predominate. An early Buddhist tantra, the seventh-century or earlier *Subāhuparipṛcchā*, gives another eightfold list of powers,[16] some of which it shares with the *Brahmayāmala* (Śaiva, Vaiṣṇava and Buddhist tantric systems have much in common). The *Subāhuparipṛcchā*'s eight powers are divided into a threefold hierarchy of inferior, middling and superior, which is taught in several other tantric works, both Buddhist and Śaiva.[17] Its earliest occurrences are in the *Guhyasūtra* of the Śaiva *Niśvāsatattvasaṃhitā* and in the *Mañjuśriyamūlakalpa*, one of the earliest Buddhist tantras. Descriptions from the latter and the *Brahmayāmala* of similar rituals for mastering a ghoul and attaining a lesser, middling or superior power according to its success are given in this chapter at **10.7** and **10.9**.

The threefold classification of powers is applied in various ways in tantric texts. The simplest scheme is that found in the *Siddhayogeśvarīmata* (translated here at **10.12**), in which the highest powers are the eight of the *Pātañjalayogaśāstra* and liberation, the middling are magical abilities such as becoming invisible, and the inferior are various means of subjugating people. Here, as in other texts, the hierarchy of powers reflects the methods of attaining them and the division into intentional and unintentional mentioned above. Thus in the *Niśvāsatattvasaṃhitā* (*Mūlasūtra* 7.19a–20b) the practice of yoga leads to the spontaneous arising of the highest powers (which match closely the powers detailed in the *Pātañjalayogaśāstra*), while the other powers are achieved through directed rituals.

Many of the middling powers are also taught in texts which are devoted solely to yoga, although only those such as the *Śivasaṃhitā* and *Khecarīvidyā*, which retain a strong link with tantric traditions, teach that yoga may produce more specifically tantric powers such as alchemy and the ability to find buried treasure. These texts appear, however, to be somewhat mischievously trumping tantric practices with yoga: the *Śivasaṃhitā* and the *Dattātreyayogaśāstra* (**10.17**) say that the yogi may turn iron into gold by smearing it with his urine or faeces, while, in a passage full of terms borrowed from alchemical texts, *Khecarīvidyā* 2.72–9 says that the yogi may perfect his body by rubbing it with his excreta. This is a development of a notion found in Hemacandra's *Yogaśāstra*, in which the perfected yogi's excreta and even his touch are said to have supernatural powers (10.15).

The malefic, inferior tantric powers, which give the practitioner control over others, are absent in yoga texts.[18] The compound *ṣaṭkarma* ('the six techniques') is commonly used in later tantric traditions to denote a group of six such magical acts. Its use in haṭhayogic texts as a collective name for the physical cleansing techniques specific to *haṭhayoga* (on which, see Chapter 2, pp. 49–50) seems to be an implicit rejection of these tantric powers.

It is the middling powers that occur most commonly in narrative tales and legends. Included in this chapter are a story of a wicked Buddhist ascetic being thwarted in his attempt to use a cremation-ground ritual to gain the power of flight (10.14) and an early (*c.* 1320 CE) Indian Sufi tale in which the famous master Nizām al-Dīn outdoes a yogi at levitation (10.18). In the second millennium CE, tales of magical contests like this become very common, and often allegorize a historical reality in which one tradition wins from another religious dominion over a territory.[19]

Chapter Contents

10.9 *Brahmayāmala* 15.13–15, 58–64. Eight varieties of supernatural power.

10.10 *Skandapurāṇa* 179.28–31. The attainment of yogic perception.

10.11 *Vāyavīyasaṃhitā* 2.29.84c–114d. The sixty-four powers.

10.12 *Siddhayogeśvarīmata* 29.8–11. The three grades of supernatural power.

10.13 *Bhāgavatapurāṇa* 11.15.3–9, 31–6. The eighteen supernatural powers.

10.14 *Kathāsaritsāgara* 7.4.45–72. A deceitful Buddhist monk seeking supernatural power.

10.15 Hemacandra's *Yogaśāstra* 1.8–9, with selected passages from his *Svopajñavṛtti* auto-commentary. Lesser powers arising in the body and the great powers.

10.16 *Dattātreyayogaśāstra* 75–88. The powers resulting from pure breath-retention.

10.17 *Dattātreyayogaśāstra* 99–107. The powers resulting from withdrawal of the senses (*pratyāhāra*).

10.18 The *Fawā'id al-fu'ād* of Amīr Hasan Dehlavī. A battle of powers between a Sufi and a yogi.

10.19 *Khecarīvidyā* 4.1–4. Elixirs that bring about perfection of the body.

10.20 *Yogabīja* 164–82. Intentional and unintentional powers.

10.21 *Lallāvākyāni* 38. Fraudulent powers.

10.22 *Śārṅgadharapaddhati* 4505–7. The greatness of the yogi.

10.23 *Amanaska* 1.36–40, 82–6. The powers attained through increasing durations of dissolution.

10.24 *Siddhasiddhāntapaddhati* 5.32–41. The powers produced in each year of yogic mastery.

10.25 *Arayish-i maḥfil* ('The Adornment of the Assembly'), pp. 39–40. The powers of the yogis.

10.1 *Kevaddha Sutta* 11.1, 3–5, 8. Superhuman powers:

(1) [The householder Kevaddha said to the Buddha:] 'Please, venerable sir, the Blessed One should instruct a monk to perform superhuman acts and miracles. As a result [the people of] this [place] Nālandā will be devoted to the Blessed One in greater measure.' The Blessed One replied to the householder Kevaddha, 'But, Kevaddha, I do not instruct monks to go and perform superhuman acts and miracles for laypeople in white clothes.'

[In verses 2–3 Kevaddha repeats his request twice more, and the Buddha replies in the same way.]

(3) [. . .] [The Blessed One said,] 'I have declared there to be three miraculous powers, having experienced them myself. What three? The miraculous power of superhuman capability, the miraculous power of telepathy and the miraculous power of instruction. (4) And what, Kevaddha, is the miraculous power of superhuman capability? When it has arisen, Kevaddha, a monk experiences various kinds of attainments. Though one, he becomes many; though many he becomes one. He can appear and disappear [at will], pass through walls, ramparts and mountains unimpeded, as if through air, enter and emerge from the earth as if it were water, walk without sinking on water as if it were earth, fly in the sky cross-legged like a bird, even touch and stroke with his hand the moon and the sun, greatly powerful and majestic as they are, [and] travel in his body as far as the world of Brahmā.

'Then someone who is a pious believer sees that monk possessing these various powers [. . .] (5) [. . .] and he tells someone who is not a pious believer about him: "How amazing, how wonderful is the great superhuman capability and majesty of [this] ascetic! Yes, I have seen a monk who possesses these various powers! [. . .]"[20]

'Then the one who is not a pious believer might say to

the pious believer, "Yes, there is a spell called Gandhārī by means of which that monk possesses these various powers [. . .]"

'What do you think of that, Kevaddha? Surely the one who is not a pious believer might say that to the pious believer?'

'He might say it, venerable sir.'

'Indeed, Kevaddha, seeing the wretchedness of the miraculous power of superhuman capability, it worries me, I am shamed by it, I despise it.'

[In verses 6–7 the Buddha describes in similar terms the problems that can arise from the power of telepathy, and once again dismisses it as wretched.]

(8) 'And what, Kevaddha, is the miraculous power of instruction? When that occurs, a monk teaches thus: "Think this, not that; make your mind like this, not like that; abandon this, adopt that; remain [a monk]." This, Kevaddha, is said to be the miraculous power of instruction.'

[In verses 9–66 the Buddha evokes the enlightened teacher who arises in the world and preaches the *dharma* as the exemplar of the miraculous power of instruction. Unlike capability and telepathy, then, the power of instruction is presented in a positive light.]

10.2 *Mahābhārata* 12.289.20–21, 24–29b. The power of yoga:

(20) And, O king, just as when a fire, grown even stronger with the wind, quickly consumes the entire earth, (21) so the yogi who has grown strong [by means of the breath], his splendour blazing, mighty, like the sun at the end of the world, desiccates the whole universe. [. . .]

(24) And yogis, endowed with the power of yoga (*yoga-bala*), O Pārtha, enter freely the Prajāpatis, the sages, the gods and the major elements, as Lords. (25) Not Yama, not Angry Antaka, not Death, terrifying in valour: none of these rules over the yogi of unlimited splendour. (26) After attaining power, the yogi may make many

thousands of replicas of himself, O bull of the Bharatas, and wander the earth in all of them. (27) He may indulge the senses, and then practise severe asceticism, and then concentrate [it], like the sun its rays. (28) For the yogi who has power, who rules over bondage, O king, has assuredly obtained the ability to bring about liberation. (29) I have taught you these powers in yoga, O king.

10.3 *Mahābhārata* 12.289.42–6. Power (*bala*) attained through diet:

Yudhiṣṭhira said:

(42) 'After eating what sort of food and mastering what things (? *kāni*), O Bharata, does a yogi attain power? Please explain that.'

Bhīṣma said:

(43) 'The yogi who is committed to eating grains and eating oil-cakes, who is committed to avoiding oily things, may attain power. (44) Eating only plain barley for a long time, O conqueror of enemies, with the self purified, the yogi may obtain power. (45) And practising thus in secret for fortnights, months [or] various seasons, after drinking water mixed with milk the yogi may obtain power. (46) Or having fasted continuously for a whole month, O lord of men, with his self duly purified, the yogi may obtain power.'

10.4 *Pātañjalayogaśāstra* 3.16–57, 4.1, with selected passages from the *bhāṣya*.[21] The powers produced by yoga:

(3.16) Through concentration (*saṃyama*) on the three transformations [there arises] knowledge of the past and future.

Through concentration on transformations of properties (*dharma*s), characteristics (*lakṣaṇa*s) and states (*avasthā*s) yogis attain knowledge of the past and future. Concentration (*saṃyama*) is said to be the triad of fixation (*dhāraṇā*), meditation (*dhyāna*) and *samādhi* [focused] on a single [object].

(3.17) Because of their being placed upon one another, there is confusion of words, meanings and cognitions. Through concentration on their distribution, [there arises] knowledge of the cries of all creatures.

(3.18) Through direct experience of karmic residues (*saṃskāras*), [there arises] knowledge of past lives.

(3.19) [Through direct experience] of cognition, [there arises] knowledge of the thoughts of others.

Through concentration on cognition, i.e. through direct experience of cognition, knowledge of the thoughts of others arises.

(3.20) And that [knowledge of the thoughts of others] does not include those thoughts' supports, because that is not the sphere of operation [of the yogi's concentration].

[For example, the yogi] knows that the cognition he has had is of someone in love, but he does not know the object of that love: the support of the thoughts of another person's mind is not made a support by the yogi's mind. The only support of the yogi's thoughts is the other's cognition.

(3.21) When through concentration on the form of [his] body its form's capacity to be perceived is suspended, then the eye and the light [from its form] are disconnected and [there arises] the power of becoming invisible.

(3.22) An action produces results either quickly or slowly. Through concentrating on it, or from portents,[22] [there arises] knowledge of [one's] death.

(3.23) [From concentration on] friendship, [compassion and joy] strengths [in them arise].

(3.24) [From concentration on their] strengths [there arises] the strength of elephants and other [animals].

(3.25) By casting [on them] the light of [mental] activity, [there arises] knowledge of that which is subtle, hidden or distant.

(3.26) Through concentration on the sun, [there arises] knowledge of the worlds.

(3.27) [Through concentration] on the moon, [there arises] knowledge of the arrangements of the stars.

(3.28) [Through concentration] on the Pole Star, [there arises] knowledge of the movements of the stars.

(3.29) [Through concentration] on the circle of the navel (*nābhi-cakra*), [there arises] knowledge of the arrangement of the body.

(3.30) [Through concentration] on the Adam's apple, hunger and thirst cease.

(3.31) [Through concentration] on the tortoise channel, steadiness [arises].

Below the Adam's apple and on the chest there is a channel in the shape of a tortoise.

(3.32) [Through concentration] on the light in the head, one gets a vision of the adepts.

(3.33) Or through luminous cognition (*prātibha*) [the yogi knows] everything.

'Luminous cognition' is the name of the salvific [cognition], which is the prior form of knowledge born from discrimination.

(3.34) [Through concentration] on the heart [there arises] understanding of the mind.

(3.35) Experience is the identification of the pure intellect (*sattva*) and the self (*puruṣa*) when [in fact] they are completely distinct. This is because [the mind] exists for the sake of other things. Through concentration on [that which exists] for the sake of itself [there arises] knowledge of the self.

(3.36) As a result there arise luminous cognition and [divine] hearing, sensation, sight, taste and smell.

(3.37) Those powers are hindrances when [the yogi is] in *samādhi*; when the mind is active they are perfections.

Those [powers], i.e. those beginning with luminous cognition, when arising in one whose mind is absorbed, are hindrances because they are inimical to the vision of [the self]. When arising in one whose mind is active, they are perfections.

> (3.38) From weakening the causes of the mind's connection [with the body] and from understanding its movements [there arises] entry into someone else's body.
>
> (3.39) From mastery of the *udāna* breath [the yogi] does not come into contact with water, mud, thorns and the like, and [he is able to perform] yogic suicide (*utkrānti*).[23]
>
> (3.40) From mastery of the *samāna* breath, [there arises] burning [of the body].
>
> (3.41) From concentration on the connection between hearing and space, [there arises] divine hearing.
>
> (3.42) From concentration on the connection between the body and space, and from identification (*samāpatti*) with light cotton, [there arises] movement through space.
>
> (3.43) Activity of the mind outside [the body] which is not deliberate is 'the great bodiless [activity]'. It results in the disappearance of that which conceals the light.
>
> (3.44) Through concentration on the gross [forms], the true natures, the subtle [forms], the inherent qualities and the purposefulness [of the elements, there arises] conquest of the elements.
>
> (3.45) As a result [the eight powers of] atomicity and so forth arise, [as do] perfection of the body and immunity to harm from the characteristics of the elements.

Among these [eight powers] are the following. Atomicity (*aṇimā*): one becomes an atom. Lightness (*laghimā*): one becomes light. Greatness (*mahimā*): one becomes great. Reach (*prāpti*): one can touch the moon with even one's finger. Freedom of will (*prākāmya*): unobstructed in one's desires one rises up from or enters into the earth as if it were water. Mastery (*vaśitva*): one controls the elements and things derived from them, and one cannot be controlled by others. Lordship (*īśitṛtva*): one has power over the coming into being, the disappearing and the arrangement of [the elements]. The ability to achieve one's wishes (*yatrakāmāvasāyitva*): one's desire becomes true, such as the desire to arrange the elements and [other forms of] matter. And even if one can, one does not upset things. Why? Because of the desire for the elements to be how they are of another, previous adept with the power of achieving one's wishes.

These are the eight powers (*aiśvaryas*). Perfection of the body will be explained [in the next *sūtra*] and immunity to harm from the characteristics of the elements [is as follows]: the earth does not obstruct the activities of the yogi's body with solid forms, so he can enter a rock; water, [even though it is] wet, does not dampen [him]; fire, [even though it is] hot, does not burn [him]; wind, [even though] it makes [everyone] bow, does not move [him]; his body is concealed in space, even though [space] does not conceal [anything, and] he becomes invisible to even the adepts.

> (3.46) Perfection of the body is beauty, grace, strength and firmness like diamond.
>
> (3.47) From concentration on the means of perception, true nature, egoism, inherent qualities and purposefulness, [there arises] mastery of the senses.
>
> (3.48) From that [there arise] the power of moving as fast as the mind, the ability to exist without using the senses, and mastery over matter.
>
> (3.49) For [the yogi] who is nothing but the perception of the difference between the pure intellect (*sattva*) and the self (*puruṣa*) [there arise] dominion over all things and omniscience.
>
> (3.50) When the seed of all faults is destroyed as a result of a lack of attachment to that perception, isolation (*kaivalya*) [arises].
>
> (3.51) On receiving an invitation from the gods [to enjoy himself with them, the yogi] should not develop attachment or smile, because it would result in the return of things which are undesirable.
>
> (3.52) Through concentration on moments and their sequence [there arises] knowledge born of discrimination.

(3.53) As a result, [there arises] the perception [of the difference] of two equal things without distinguishing [them] according to their species, characteristics or location.

(3.54) Knowledge born of discrimination is salvific [and] acts on everything in all situations instantly.

(3.55) When the pure intellect and the self are equally pure, isolation (*kaivalya*) [arises].

Thus ends the third quarter (*pāda*), on the powers, in Vyāsa's commentary on glorious Patañjali's discourse on Sāṃkhya, his treatise on yoga.

The fourth quarter, on Isolation.

(4.1) The powers are produced by birth, medicinal herbs, mantra, asceticism and *samādhi*.

10.5 *Pāśupatasūtra* 1.20–38. The powers resulting from yoga:

(20) Then yoga begins for him. (21) He gets the abilities of long-distance seeing, hearing, mind-reading and perception. (22) He is omniscient. (23) He can move as fast as the mind. (24) He can assume whatever form he wants. (25) [He can operate] without instruments. (26) He possesses special qualities. (27) He can control anyone. (28) He cannot be controlled by anyone. (29) He can enter anyone. (30) He cannot be entered by anyone. (31) He can kill anyone. (32) He cannot be killed by anyone. (33) He is fearless. (34) He is imperishable. (35) He does not age. (36) He is immortal. (37) He can go anywhere unimpeded. (38) Possessing these qualities he becomes a leader of Lord Śiva's great troop.

10.6 Praśastapāda's *Padārthadharmasaṃgraha* commentary on *Vaiśeṣikasūtra* 8.12.2.1.[24] Yogic perception:

But when they are engaged in yoga (*yukta*), yogis, who are superior to us, by means of minds which are graced by a quality produced by yoga, get the ability to see correctly the true natures of their own selves, [the selves] of others, ether, space,[25] time, air, atoms and minds, of qualities, actions, universals and particulars which are inherent in these things, and of inherence. Furthermore, yogis who are exceptionally engaged in yoga (*viyukta*), as a result of a capability that arises thanks to a quality produced by yoga after the drawing together of four [factors], can perceive things which are subtle, hidden or far off.

10.7 *Mañjuśriyamūlakalpa* Chapter 55, p. 713.[26] The threefold powers:

Now the aspirant (*sādhaka*) who wants to obtain mastery over a ghoul (*vetāla*) should take a corpse whose body is undamaged, bring a sacrificial offering [suitable] for all beings to a cremation ground or a place with one tree or a crossroads or a place with a single *liṅga*, paint a *maṇḍala* at the south face of Lord Śiva, make the sacrificial offering, beautify [the corpse] by bathing it, write a *maṇḍala* with ashes on its middle, make its head face east [and], covered in a white cloth and with a companion wearing white, set up protectors for the directions.

He should sit on the upper chest of the corpse and make an offering of mustard and sesame into its mouth until a jewel emerges from its mouth. He should take that [jewel], put it in his own mouth, make a sacrificial offering suitable for all beings, stand at the south face [of Lord Śiva], take one from among yellow orpiment, red arsenic, collyrium, madder or bezoar, wrap it in an *aśvattha* leaf and repeat [a mantra] until [one variety of] the threefold supernatural powers arises. It gets hot, it smokes [or] it catches fire. If it gets hot he can travel great distances on foot and lives for five thousand years. If it smokes he can subjugate all creatures, become invisible and lives for ten thousand years. If it catches fire he becomes a sorcerer (*vidyādhara*).

10.8 *Parākhyatantra* 14.98–104. Proof of the existence of yogic powers:[27]

(98) Success in yoga, accompanied by the eight [supernatural] properties, [is achieved] through the intensive practice of that [yoga]. By the means taught above for achieving this yogis become possessed of supernatural powers, supreme because of yoga. (99) And they can demonstrate their power in special circumstances before certain special persons when it is demanded by those persons. [Such power] must be accepted [to have existed too] at other times and places and in other men.

(100) Now you may say, '[But] this is just popular belief, [for] why is it not directly observed?'

[To this we reply:] Does everything on the surface of the earth that you have not yourself seen not exist? (101–102) The circle of the earth is a repository of manifold variety: no person can see or hear everything. The non-existence on the earth of wondrous things decided upon by such [a person] cannot be proved.

We know about the consciousness that yogis have because of the power [they have] that exceeds [our] knowledge. (103) Through scripture, too, we know of the state of being a yogi, together with its limitless powers. Such a yogi should play about with his powers for the sake of inspiring faith. (104) Because of faith other seekers after liberation will get initiation. Such a yogi engaged in yoga will also [himself] have faith.

10.9 *Brahmayāmala* 15.13–15, 58–64.[28] Eight varieties of supernatural power:

(13) Now I shall teach the special method of mastering a ghoul (*vetāla*), by which the aspirant gets the eight types of supernatural power, (14) those of the magical sword, bezoar,[29] journeying to the underworld, becoming a sorcerer, magical sandals, magical ointment, raising the dead and invisibility. (15) These supernatural powers [which arise] when the special method of mastering a

ghoul [is accomplished], O goddess, are tantric and powerful.

[The text then describes how and during which lunar phases to choose a suitable corpse (16–18), how to prepare the body (19–23), purify the cremation ground by sprinkling with female generative fluid (24–6), make food offerings and install mantras on the corpse (27–35), and how to perform a fire sacrifice (38–45) which results in the powers of levitation, magic sandals, moving through space and bezoar (45–6). Beautiful visions then arise, culminating in visions of the gods Indra, Viṣṇu and Brahmā, who speak to the yogi, saying 'Come, great hero. Become Indra! Become Brahmā! Become Viṣṇu! Become a sky-rover!' (48–57).]

(58) On hearing them, the great hero must not break his silence, nor abandon the sacrifice, but give a guest-offering of water. (59) Then a great flame rises up from [the corpse's] mouth looking like a thousand suns and seeming to consume the three worlds. (60–61) And then a greedy tongue rises up, pointing towards the aspirant. He should take a sword, razor or knife previously placed to hand and cut off the tongue. The knower of mantras must cut it before it touches him. (62) If he foolishly does otherwise, he is sure to be devoured. He may alternatively have it cut by adepts and brought to him. (63) Once it is in his hand it becomes a brilliant sword. Then, holding it, the knower of mantras flies up into the sky. (64) The hero mounts a flying palace surrounded by [other] flying palaces, and rises upwards on it [and] becomes the lord of the emperors and the master of ten million flying chariots.

10.10 *Skandapurāṇa* 179.28–31. The attainment of yogic perception:

(28) [The yogi] should assume a single posture and, while thinking of the twenty-sixth elemental principle, draw in all his limbs and, motionless, practise meditation.

(29) He should gently make the breath in the trachea flow through the channels. He should remain focused, free from desire because of the practice of meditation (30) until he sees an image of the orb of the moon in his heart. When he has seen the light that exists in his body, mastery of yoga arises [for him]. (31) From regular practice in this way and the appearance of success in yoga, yogic perception arises, which is knowledge of the past, present and future.

10.11 *Vāyavīyasaṃhitā* 2.29.84c–114d. The sixty-four powers:

When even only a fraction of the powers of yoga are experienced, the mind becomes [set] on liberation. (85) I have seen this: it is how liberation arises.

Becoming 1. thin, 2. fat, 3. a child, 4. old, 5. and young, (86) 6. taking the form of various species, 7. having a body made of four [elements] (excepting the earthy part), 8. [and] always smelling sweet, [being] a collection of scents: (87) thus is taught the eightfold earth level, of the *piśāca* [demons].

9. Living in water; 10. disappearing into the earth; (88) 11. being able oneself to drink even the ocean without ill-effects; 12. finding water exactly where one wants in this world; (89) 13. holding a mass of water in one's hands without a pot or such like; 14. if one wants to eat even something tasteless, it immediately (90–91) becomes something delicious; 15. having a body made of three [elements]; 16. having a body which cannot be wounded: this is the wondrous water power, which, in combination with the earth [powers], is sixteenfold.

17. Producing fire from one's body; 18. being free from fear of its heat; (92) 19. effortlessly burning up this world if one wishes; 20. putting fire in water; 21. holding it in the hand; (93) 22. returning something burnt to its original state; and 23. cooking grains and other [food] in the mouth; 24. fashioning one's body from two

[elements]: in combination with the water powers, (94) this is taught as the twenty-fourfold fire [power].

25. Moving as fast as thought; 26. entering instantly into [other] beings; (95) 27. effortlessly carrying mountains and other great weights; 28. becoming heavy and 29. becoming light; 30. holding the wind in one's hand; (96–7) 31. making the ground tremble with taps from the tip of the finger and other such [actions]; 32. creating one's body from one element: the sages teach [this to be] the wind power, which, in combination with the fire powers, is thirty-twofold.

33. Going forth without a shadow; 34. being imperceptible by the sense organs; (98) 35. becoming a sky-rover; 36. connecting with the objects of the senses at will; 37. jumping through space and 38. entering space in one's own body; (99–100) 39. making oneself space and 40. existing without a body: this is taught to be the great sky power of Indra, which, in combination with the wind powers, is fortyfold.

41. Attaining things according to one's wishes and 42. disappearing at will; (101) 43. overcoming everything and 44. seeing all hidden objects; 45. creating things in accordance with one's actions; 46. controlling [others]; 47. having an agreeable appearance; (102) and 48. seeing the cycle of transmigration: this is the lunar power of the mind, which, in combination with the powers of Indra, has more powers [than the sky power].

(103) 49. Cutting and 50. striking, 51. binding and 52. loosening, [and] 53. possessing all beings which live in the thrall of transmigration (104–105) and 54. bestowing grace on all, and overcoming 55. death and 56. time: this is said to be the great ego-based power of Prajāpati, which, [in combination] with the lunar powers, is fifty-sixfold.

57. Creating merely through will; 58. saving and 59. destroying (106) and 60. having personal authority over

everyone; 61. stimulating the minds of all beings; 62. being unlike everyone; 63. creating a new world; (107) 64. causing the auspicious and the inauspicious: this is said to be the power of Brahmā, which, in combination with the powers of Prajāpati, is sixty-fourfold.

(108) It is taught that the power of matter (*prākṛta*), with its subsidiary powers, is superior to this [power], which is of the intellect. That [power of matter] is said to be of Viṣṇu; it is situated in the world. (109) By means of Brahmā, not by the other [powers], may one know that level in its entirety.

So the level of the spirit (*puruṣa*), which has the subsidiary powers, is of Gaṇeśa [and] of the Lord. (110) It is by means of Viṣṇu, not by the other [powers] that anything of that level can be known.

And all of these powers of consciousness are obstacles. (111) They are to be carefully kept in check, by means of the utmost detachment. When the powers such as luminous cognition are impure, for one whose mind is intent upon the subsidiary powers, (112–13) the supreme, imperishable power which fulfils all desires is not perfected. Therefore, he who shuns the powers and indulgences of gods, demons and kings as if they were straw attains the highest perfection of yoga. Alternatively the sage may grant boons or he may wander +the beautiful places+ of the earth. (114) After enjoying powers and indulgences according to his desires, he will attain liberation.

10.12 *Siddhayogeśvarīmata* 29.8–11. The three grades of supernatural power:

(8) Supernatural power (*siddhi*) should be known to be of three kinds: superior, inferior and middling. The superior [powers] are taught to be the attainment of the eight powers beginning with the ability to become as small as an atom, and liberation. (9) [Entering] into the underworld, becoming a sky-rover, invisibility, the

magical pill, the magic wand and the magic waterpot: (10) the middling powers take these and other forms in this system, O goddess. Having lords do one's bidding, (11) drawing people into one's power, rewarding, punishing and having the affection of all people: these and others are the inferior powers.

10.13 *Bhāgavatapurāṇa* 11.15.3–9, 31–6. The eighteen supernatural powers:

The blessed Lord said:

(3) Those who have mastered yoga by means of fixation (*dhāraṇā*) have taught eighteen supernatural powers (*siddhi*s). Of them, eight have me as their primary cause [and] ten arise from the strands of existence (*guṇa*s). (4) The powers of making one's form as small as an atom, huge or light, of obtaining with the senses [whatever one wants], of being able to fulfil one's desires, of sovereignty, i.e. implementing one's power over things that are heard or seen, (5) of dominion (being without attachment to the strands of existence) [and] of having desire cease: I have these eight powers, O lovely lady; they are considered to be innate.

(6) Freedom from the [six] 'waves' [of existence, i.e. cold and heat and so forth] in this body, the powers of hearing and seeing things far away, of moving as fast as thought, of assuming whatever form one wants, of entering another's body, (7) of dying at will, of witnessing the gods sporting together, of accomplishing whatever one wishes, of having one's instructions carried out without obstruction, (8) of knowing the past, present and future, of being unaffected by extremes, of knowing the thoughts of others, of standing firm against fire, the sun, water, poison and so forth, [and] invincibility: (9) these are taught to be the powers that arise through yogic fixation.

Now learn from me which power arises from which type of fixation, and how it happens.

[Verses 10–30 describe various fixations, mainly on the different aspects and manifestations of the Lord, for attaining particular powers, such as becoming small, huge and light (10–12), attaining ultimate bliss (17), understanding the elements (19), omniscience (28) and invincibility (30). Verses 23–4 describe how to enter another's body by visualizing one's self in it and raising the breath to the top of the skull, but without visualization of the Lord.]

(31) All the powers just taught arise for the sage who worships me by means of yogic fixation in this way. (32) For a sage whose senses are conquered, who is controlled, who has mastered his breath and self [and] who holds steady his fixation on me, no supernatural power is hard to obtain. (33) They say that these [powers] are time-wasting hindrances for he who practises the supreme yoga while being brought to perfection by me. (34) One obtains through yoga all the powers [that are obtained] here on earth by means of one's birth, herbal elixirs, austerities and mantras; not by other means does one attain success in yoga. (35) And I, the Lord, am the cause [and] master of all the supernatural powers. I am [the Lord] of yoga, Sāṃkhya, *dharma* and those who expound the Vedic texts. (36) Unconfined, I exist inside and outside the selves of all embodied creatures, in the same way that the elements naturally exist inside and outside living beings.

10.14 *Kathāsaritsāgara* 7.4.45–72. A deceitful Buddhist monk seeking supernatural power:

The minister Buddhivara ('Best of Brains') said, 'Your highness, tell me what service that Buddhist monk did for you.'

The king replied, 'Listen. I shall tell you his story.

'Some time ago in Pataliputra a Buddhist monk called Prapañcabuddhi ('Trickster') would enter my assembly hall every day and give me a box. For a year I kept handing them over as they were, unopened, to my treasurer. One day the box that the Buddhist monk gave me happened to fall from my hand and break in two on the ground. Out of it came a huge jewel, glowing like fire – it was as if the Buddhist monk had revealed to me his heart, which I had not recognized earlier. On seeing the jewel I picked it up and had the other boxes brought in and opened. In each one I found a jewel. Astonished, I asked Prapañcabuddhi, "Why are you giving me jewels like this?"

'At this the Buddhist monk took me aside and said, "At midnight on the next dark of the moon, I am going to use a magic spell (*vidyā*) in a cremation ground outside the city. I want you to come to help, O hero, for supernatural powers are easily obtained when obstacles to their attainment are removed with the help of a hero."

'I agreed and he went away, delighted. After some days the dark of the moon came and I remembered my promise to the monk. When I had performed my daily rituals I got ready for the evening, but it so happened that as soon as I had completed the dusk rites I fell asleep. Immediately Lord Viṣṇu – who is good to his devotees – appeared in a dream riding on Garuḍa with Lakṣmī in his lap and gave me the following instructions:

' "The name of this Prapañcabuddhi is apt, my child: as part of his worship of the *maṇḍala*, he will get you to the cremation ground and offer you as a sacrifice.

' "He wants to harm you: do not do what he tells you to, but tell him to do it first so that you will know what to do.

' "While he is showing you take your chance and kill him there and then. As a result, the magical power (*siddhi*) he seeks will be yours."

'After saying this Viṣṇu vanished and I woke up. I said to myself, "By the grace of Viṣṇu I have learnt that today I have to kill this sorcerer."

> 'When the first watch of the night had passed I took my sword and went alone to the cremation ground. There I saw the Buddhist monk. He had finished his worship of the *maṇḍala* and I went up to him. On seeing me the rogue greeted me and said, "Close your eyes, stretch out your body and lie face down on the ground, O king, and both of us will get the supernatural power."
>
> 'I replied, "You do it first. Show me and then I will know exactly what to do."
>
> 'When he heard this the stupid monk duly lay on the ground and I cut off his head with a blow from my sword. Then a voice came from the sky: "Bravo, king! Today you have made a sacrifice of this sinful monk! The supernatural power which he wanted to get, the power of flight, has now been obtained by you."'

10.15 Hemacandra's *Yogaśāstra* 1.8–9, with selected passages from his *Svopajñavṛtti* auto-commentary. Lesser powers arising in the body and the great powers:

> (8) Phlegm, faeces, [bodily] impurities, touch and all [other bodily excretions become] great healing powers [and] one attains [the power of] experiencing all sensory inputs through a single sense organ: this is the wonderful wild dance of yoga.

Bodily impurity is produced by the ears, teeth, nose, eyes or tongue. All [excreta] such as faeces, urine, hair and nails – those which have been taught and those which have not – become great healing powers as a result of yoga. Alternatively, the various great powers such as the ability to become as small as an atom arise. [. . .]

Rainwater, too, simply by coming into contact with the yogi's body, even if it then goes to somewhere such as a river or a well, removes all diseases. And those who have been rendered unconscious by poison become free from poison merely from the touch of wind that has come into contact with the yogi's body. And food which has been poisoned becomes free from poison when it enters the yogi's mouth. And people who are stricken by great disease from [consuming] poison are cured merely by hearing the yogi's words or seeing him. This is the entirety of the types of medicine from all [the parts of the body]. These are phlegm and other [excreta] in the form of great powers.

Or the great powers are quite different. The transformative capabilities are several and are divided into the power to become smaller than an atom (*aṇutva*), hugeness (*mahattva*) and lightness (*laghutva*), infinite reach (*prāpti*), going where one wants (*prākāmya*), sovereignty (*īśitva*), dominion (*vaśitva*), freedom from obstacles (*apratighātitva*), invisibility (*antarddhāna*) and shape-shifting (*kāmarūpitva*). [. . .]

> (9) These are the glories of the blossoming flowers of the wish-fulfilling tree of yoga: the attainments of magical movement,[30] the power to give curses and blessings, clairvoyance and telepathy.

[. . .] The result is pure knowledge or liberation.

10.16 *Dattātreyayogaśāstra* 75–88. The powers resulting from pure breath-retention:

> (75) At first sweat appears. [The yogi] should massage [himself] with it. By slowly increasing, step-by-step, the retention of the breath, (76) trembling arises in the body of the yogi while he is on his seat. Through further increase [in the duration] of the practice, the frog [power] (*dardurī*) is sure to arise. (77) In the same way that a frog hops across the ground, so the yogi seated in the lotus position moves across the ground. (78) And through further increase [in the duration] of the practice levitation arises. Sitting in the lotus position, [the yogi] leaves the ground and remains [in the air] (79) without a support.
>
> Then peculiar powers arise. The yogi is not troubled whether he eats a little or a lot. (80) His faeces and urine diminish and he sleeps very little. Worms, rheumy eyes, slobber, sweat, body odour: (81) henceforth these never arise for him. Through further increase [in the duration] of the practice, great strength arises, (82) through which he gets the animal power (*bhūcarasiddhi*), the power to overcome animals. A tiger, a buffalo, a wild gayal, an

elephant (83) or a lion: these are killed by a blow from the hand of the yogi.

The yogi looks like the god of love; (84) then a great obstacle can arise for the yogi if he is not careful. Overcome by his beauty, women want to have sex with him. (85) If he has sex, his semen is lost. Through loss of semen, [his] lifespan is diminished and he becomes weak. (86) Therefore, he should carefully carry out his practice and not have sex with women. Through constant retention of semen, a fine odour arises in the body of the yogi, (87–8) so the yogi should make every effort to preserve his semen.

10.17 *Dattātreyayogaśāstra* 99–107. The powers resulting from withdrawal of the senses (*pratyāhāra*):

Amazing powers are then sure to arise for the yogi: clairaudience, clairvoyance and the ability to travel long distances in an instant; (99) eloquence, the ability to do what he wants and the power to make things invisible; turning iron and other metals into gold by smearing them with his faeces and urine; (100) the power of moving through space; through regular practice these and other powers [arise]. Then the wise yogi, in order to gain success in yoga, should think that (101) these are obstacles to the ultimate attainment; the wise yogi should not take pleasure in them. He should never show his powers to anyone (102–3) (although he might perhaps, out of affection, show [them] to one full of devotion). In order to keep his powers secret, he should behave among people as if he were dumb, simple or deaf. If not, he is sure to get lots of disciples (104) and they are bound to ask that lord among yogis about their own various problems. Busy with solving them he will forget his own practice. (105) Neglecting his practice he will then become an ordinary man. So he should not forget his guru's teachings and practise day and night. (106) The action state (*ghaṭāvasthā*) of yoga arises through constant practice in this way. Not practising yoga gets one nowhere; it is not mastered by getting together and talking. (107) So one should make every effort to practise nothing but yoga.

10.18 The *Fawā'id al-fu'ād* of Amīr Hasan Dehlavī.[31] A battle of powers between a Sufi and a yogi:

In this connection Sheikh Nizām al-Dīn told a story:

A yogi came into the town of Ucch to dispute with Sheikh Safī al-Dīn Gāzarūnī. The yogi challenged the sheikh to show any powers that he could not equal. To this the sheikh replied that it was the yogi who was advancing a claim and he should show his own accomplishment first. The yogi rose from the ground into the air until his head reached the ceiling, and then came down to the ground in the same fixed position and invited the sheikh to show his power. The sheikh turned his gaze towards heaven and said: 'O Lord! You have given this power to [one who is] a stranger [to Thee]! Bestow on me also this grace!'

The sheikh then rose from his place and flew away towards the Qibla [i.e. westwards in the direction of Mecca]; from there he flew towards the north and towards the south, and finally came back to his own place and sat down. The yogi was astonished and, laying his head at the sheikh's feet, said: 'I can do no more than rise straight upwards from the ground and come down in the same way. I cannot go to the right and to the left. You turned whichever way you desired. This is true and [from] God: my own [powers] are false.'

10.19 *Khecarīvidyā* 4.1–4. Elixirs that bring about perfection of the body:

(1) And now I shall teach you some very sacred herbal medicines. Without herbal medicines a yogi can never attain perfection.

(2) [Having prepared] a powder of the leaves, flowers, fruits and stem, together with the root, of the plant whose name consists of the highest limb of the mendicant [i.e. muṇḍī] with buttermilk and water, fermented rice gruel and milk, together with honey, sugar and the like, one should give [to the yogi] in separate mouthfuls round essential pills [of the mixture]. +[The yogi attains]+ all together the absence of grey hair, great well-being, great vigour and the removal of debilitating diseases. (3) [His] ears [become like those of] a boar, [his] eyes [become like those of] a bird of prey, and [his] nails [and] teeth [become] like diamonds; [he becomes] young, as fast as the wind, and lives as long as the earth, the moon and the stars.

(4) [If the yogi] should eat powdered bulb of vārāhī with ghee and unrefined cane sugar, [there arise] health and growth. [If he should eat that powder] in buttermilk and water, piles are got rid of. [If he should eat it] in cow's milk, leprosy is got rid of. One should have [the yogi] drink that powder with sugar and the like and sweet water twice a day for two years. [He will become] black-haired, without grey hair or wrinkles, +[and] he gets rid of blackness on the body+.

[Verses 5–14 describe more herbal medicines that get rid of old age and death, including the well-known āyurvedic preparation triphalā and the herb aśvagandhā, as well as preparations made from mercury and sulphur.]

10.20 *Yogabīja* 164–82. Intentional and unintentional powers:

The Lord said:

(164) 'Now, O goddess, I shall teach clearly the result of practice. First diseases disappear, next bodily torpor. (165) Then, its essence equalized, the moon rains [nectar] continuously. With the [help of the] wind, fire completely consumes one's bodily essence. (166) Many sounds arise; the body becomes soft. (167) Having

overcome torpor [produced by] the earth and other elements, a man may go forth as a sky-rover. He becomes omniscient, can assume any form at will [and] is as fast as the wind. (168) He plays in the three worlds. All the supernatural powers arise. When camphor is melting, what solidity is found in it? (169) When egoism has dissolved, how can there be hardness in the body? Omniscient, omnipotent, free, with cosmic form, (170) the yogi becomes liberated while alive [and] wanders the world at will.'

The goddess said:

(171) 'Whatever activities [there may be in the world], they are for the purpose of liberation, O Śaṅkara. What do the supernatural powers do when the essence of consciousness is without differentiation? (172) Please get rid of this doubt of mine, O holy Lord.'

The Lord said:

(173) 'What you have said is true, O beautiful lady. I shall explain. Listen. There are two sorts of supernatural powers in the world, intentional (*kalpita*) and unintentional (*akalpita*), good lady. (174) The powers that are mastered by directed practices such as alchemy, herbal medicines, ritual, deadly spells and physical techniques are said to be intentional. (175) Those impermanent [and] weak powers which arise from directed practice can arise in the same form even without directed practice, spontaneously. (176) The great powers such as freedom (*svātantrya*) which arise in one who is solely focused on the yoga of his self are taught to be devoid of intention. (177) Perfect, eternal, powerful, taking whatever form one wishes and produced by yoga, they arise after a long time in those who are free from latent impressions. (178) Appearing as a result of the great yoga on the unchanging level of the supreme self, they are auspicious. Constantly shining forth with no purpose, they are a sign of one who is perfected through yoga. (179) In the same way that lots of places of

pilgrimage are seen by pilgrims on the way to Varanasi, so are supernatural powers seen on [the way to] liberation. (180) They arise completely of their own accord in one who is free [from concern] for gain or loss. The many powers that arise on the path of yoga are like this. (181) In the same way that gold is verified by assayers, one recognizes from [his] supernatural powers the perfected yogi who is liberated while alive. (182) An otherworldly quality is sure sometimes to be seen in him. Thus have I taught you the mark of one who has been perfected by yoga, O goddess. One should know the man devoid of supernatural powers to be in bondage.'

10.21 *Lallāvākyāni* 38. Fraudulent powers.

Stopping water [from flowing] or cooling fire
or, similarly, travelling by foot in the sky,
or, similarly, milking a cow made of wood:
in the end, all this is fraudulent display.

10.22 *Śārṅgadharapaddhati* 4505–7. The greatness of the yogi:

(4505) The first signs of progress in yoga are firm resolve, good health, absence of cruelty, a good odour, urinating and defecating in small amounts, beauty, clarity of complexion and a pleasant voice. (4506) People become devoted, praises are sung in his absence and creatures do not fear him: these are the ultimate signs of success. (4507) He who is not troubled by extremes such as cold and heat and has no fear of other things has attained success.

10.23 *Amanaska* 1.36–40, 82–6.[32] The powers attained through increasing durations of dissolution:

(36) Through meditative dissolution (*laya*) lasting the blink of an eye the yogi is sure to make contact with, and reside in, the ultimate reality (*paratattva*) over and over again. (37) In the yogi who is established in

dissolution for six blinks of an eye, relief from heat, sleep and unconsciousness arise repeatedly. (38) And through dissolution lasting the length of time it takes to make one inhalation [i.e. two seconds], *prāṇa* and the other [four principal bodily] winds flow in their own respective places as a result of the restraint of the flow of the breath. (39) And through dissolution for [the time it takes to make] an inhalation and exhalation [i.e. four seconds], *kūrma*, *nāga* and the other [three minor bodily] winds stop functioning and, being in the bodily elements, they arrest their [transformation]. (40) And through dissolution for [the time it takes to make] four breaths [i.e. eight seconds] the nourishing fluids [produced from the digestion of food] in the seven bodily constituents, together with the breaths, evenly nourish the constituents.

[Verses 41–81 describe further attainments that arise as a result of temporal increases in the duration of dissolution, including tirelessness (41: 24 seconds), the disappearance of sexual desire (44: 192 seconds), the awakening and raising of Kuṇḍalinī (45–8: 6, 12, 24 and 48 minutes), knowledge of his true self (52: 6 hours), extrasensory perception and omniscience (52–61: 12 hours to 8 days), and so on up to twenty-four years.]

(82) [The yogi] who remains in dissolution continuously for twenty-four years attains mastery over the goddess (*śakti*) element [and] becomes absorbed in the goddess element. (83) He sees the whole universe like a pearl in his hand and he perceives the form of his own body as it truly is. (84) He is seen in the world in a body, doing the rite of the elements. He performs the rite of the elements in order to achieve *samādhi* in the goddess element. (85) Through practising dissolution in this way with gradual increments, yogis enjoy supreme bliss, like Bhuśuṇḍa and other great souls. (86) Even in the great universal dissolutions of Brahmā, Viṣṇu and Śiva, yogis enjoy supreme bliss, like Bhuśuṇḍa and other great souls.

10.24 *Siddhasiddhāntapaddhati* 5.32–41. The powers produced in each year of yogic mastery:

> (32) The yogi established in the self acts autonomously [and] playfully. He is free from old age and death. Unkillable by gods or demons, he sports like Bhairava. (33) Established thus, he gradually and easily obtains all the powers that are hard to master. The Lord has spoken the truth.
>
> (34) In the first [year] [there arises the power] of freedom from disease, [and] he becomes dear to all people. They constantly yearn to see him, the one who has attained the self. (35) In the second [year] [all] his aims are accomplished and he can speak to all [creatures]. In the third [year] he gains a divine body and is not troubled by wild beasts [such as] tigers. (36) In the [fourth] year he is freed from hunger, thirst, sleep, cold and heat. He is sure to become a divine master of yoga and obtain long-distance hearing. (37) In the fifth year [there arise] mastery of speech and the ability to enter other people's bodies. In the [sixth] year he cannot be injured by weapons, and thunderbolts do not trouble him. (38) In the seventh [year he becomes] as swift as the wind, has the ability to levitate, and can see things from afar. In the eighth year he attains the powers of becoming as small as an atom and so forth. (39) In the ninth [year] his body becomes [as hard as] a diamond and he can move through space and the directions. In the tenth [year] he can race wherever he desires faster than the wind. (40) In the eleventh year he becomes omniscient and acquires [all] the supernatural powers. In the twelfth [year] he becomes equal to Śiva himself, the creator and the destroyer. (41) Truly the accomplished master is worshipped in the three worlds like the blessed Bhairava. Thus, in twelve years the master yogi attains great power through the potency of the feet of the true guru. In this there is no doubt.

10.25 *Arayish-i mahfil* ('The Adornment of the Assembly'), pp. 39–40.[33] The powers of the yogis:

> [The yogis] spend their time day and night in recalling their God to memory, and, by holding in their breath for a long time, live for hundreds of years; by reason of their strict austerities (*riyaḍat*) [i.e. yoga], their earthly garment [i.e. their body] is so light that they fly in the air and float on the water, and by the power of their actions, they can cause their souls to flee away whenever they please, assume whatever form they like, enter the body of another person, and tell all the news of the hidden world; from putting copper in ashes, they can turn it into gold, and by the power of their magic, fascinate the hearts of the whole world; they can make a sick man, on the point of death, well in one moment, and can instantaneously understand the hearts of other people, and their custom is to have no cares or acquaintances; it is true that 'the jogi [i.e. yogi] is no man's friend'; and although in magic and sorcery, alchemy and chemistry, Sannyasis have great skill, still the art of the Jogis in these matters is more widely famous.

ELEVEN
Liberation

The final chapter of this book presents accounts of the final stage of yoga, known variously as *mukti* or *mokṣa* ('liberation'), *kaivalya* ('isolation') and *nirvāṇa* ('extinction'). As we saw also to be the case with *samādhi* (Chapter 9), there is no clear consensus across texts as to liberation's defining characteristics, and descriptions of it are often poetic, symbolic or apophatic (i.e. pointing to what it is not). *Amaraughaprabodha* 70 notes, with reference to liberation while living (*jīvanmukti*), that such states are 'impossible to describe' (**11.2.4**), because they pass beyond the boundaries of normal cognition, and even beyond binaries of life and death. And it is because of the extreme difficulty of conveying the nature of *nirvāṇa* to others that the Buddha initially decided against teaching: nobody, he declared, would understand (**11.1.1**).

Given such difficulties, it is unsurprising that we should also encounter significant doctrinal variation regarding the nature of liberation. Bhaṭṭa Rāmakaṇṭha's *Paramokṣanirāsakārikāvṛtti* (**11.1.6**) is a sustained criticism of twenty 'false views' of liberation from the point of view of the Śaivasiddhānta. As Watson et al. point out, alongside its presentation of Saiddhāntika perspectives on liberation, the text is especially interesting for 'the snapshot it provides of the religio-philosophical landscape of tenth-century India'.[1] What becomes overwhelmingly clear from the text is that, at the time, there was no consensus on what constituted liberation, nor indeed on the status of exactly what or who was to be liberated. To take just a few examples, in theistic systems the goal could be union with God (in which aspirant and deity are one), being an attendant on God or becoming superior to God, as well as the ('correct') Saiddhāntika view of liberation in which the soul realizes its own innate, qualitative identity with – but numerical distinction from – God. In non-theistic systems, the self might be preserved in liberation (Sāṃkhya), or dissolved (Advaita Vedānta), or there may not even be a self to begin with (Buddhism).[2] And as we shall see below, in some systems liberation may only be possible at death while in others one may be liberated while living.

This rather bewildering array of ideas about liberation suggests an interesting counterpoint to a particular perspective on (Indian) spirituality that is characteristic of perennial philosophy and the New Age.[3] This view, which holds considerable currency in contemporary globalized yoga, proposes that the paths to the ultimate goal are many, while the goal itself is one, and common to all the world's religious and spiritual traditions.[4] However, what we see in the *Paramokṣanirāsakārikāvṛtti* – and in this chapter as a whole, in fact – is that even in the (relatively) limited context of Indian religion, the goals are also many. Indeed, restricting the argument to the history of Indian yoga, we might further venture that, with the consolidation of *haṭha*-inflected eightfold yoga as a shared technique across a variety of metaphysical and doctrinal traditions from the seventeenth century, we see a situation in which one path leads to many goals.

While yoga is by no means the only method to attain liberation across Indian religious traditions, it is often a privileged one. In the earliest known tantra, the *Niśvāsatattvasaṃhitā*, it appears that yoga may constitute an independent path to liberation.[5] In Hemacandra's *Yogaśāstra* (1.15) liberation is said to be the foremost among the four goals of life, and yoga its means. And *Yogabīja* 32 notes that even the gods cannot attain liberation without yoga (see **1.2.7**).

Liberation and Casting off the Body

As was noted in the main introduction, around 500 BCE new groups of extra-Vedic religious practitioners, collectively known as Śramaṇas ('strivers'), began to emerge in northern India, teaching methods of final liberation from endless, *karma*-driven suffering and rebirth, practices which subsequently became known as 'yoga'. The most well known of these Śramaṇa groups are the Buddhists and the Jains. In the *Ariyapariyesanā Sutta*, the Buddha presents liberation (*nirvāṇa*), which permanently discontinues the cycle of rebirth, as the supreme security from the bondage of birth, ageing, sickness, death, sorrow and defilement (11.1.1).

References to yoga as a means of casting off the body to attain liberation may be found in early Brahmanical texts. For instance, at *Mahābhārata* 12.47.1, Janamejaya questions Vaiśampāyana about how Bhīṣma cast off his body while lying on his bed of arrows, and asks 'What yoga did he practise?' Similarly, both Droṇa (7.165.35–40) and Bhūriśravas (7.118.16–18) cast off their bodies by means of yoga. In the *Bhagavadgītā*, which is part of the *Mahābhārata*, Kṛṣṇa teaches that at the time of death one may reach the ultimate destination by practising yoga of the body, mind and breath, uttering *oṃ* and thinking of him (8.12–13). A comparable early literary reference appears in Kālidāsa's *Kumārasambhava* (1.21), when Satī is said to have abandoned her body through yoga when offended by her father's treatment of Śiva.

The *Pātañjalayogaśāstra* uses the term isolation (*kaivalya*) to indicate the highest goal of yoga. The 'isolation' in question is of the spiritual principle (*puruṣa*) of Sāṃkhya (defined as 'that which sees') from the material principle (*prakṛti*) and its three constituent qualities (*guṇa*s) by means of discrimination (*viveka*). The result of the flow of discerning cognition is omniscience (3.54). Karmic seeds are burnt up and the self 'is illuminated by only its own true form' (11.1.3). The yogi even becomes detached from pure consciousness, resulting in a *samādhi* known as the 'Cloud of Virtue' (*dharmameghasamādhi*) (see 11.1.4). In a passage included in this chapter, Vijñānabhikṣu, commenting on *Pātañjalayogaśāstra* 1.1–3, is of the opinion, however, that liberation arises from both *samādhi* with cognition (*saṃprajñāta samādhi*) and *samādhi* without cognition (*asaṃprajñāta samādhi*) (11.1.5). The yoga of the *Pātañjalayogaśāstra* entails a radical effacement of individual existence, described disapprovingly by the *Paramokṣanirāsakārikā* as the 'destruction of the self' (11.1.6), a vision which the commentator, Rāmakaṇṭha, implies later (57ab) is shared by the Buddhists.

What these accounts have in common is the notion that liberation is something that happens when one leaves the body at the time of death (*videhamukti*). And from early on yoga is identified as a means of obtaining this liberation at death, as we have seen with the *Mahābhārata* and the *Kumārasambhava*, and as also appears to be the case with regard to the Buddha's final liberation at the moment of death (*mahāparinirvāṇa*).[6] However, more than a millennium after the *Mahābharata* and the life of the Buddha, and about 500 years after the composition of the *Kumārasambhava* and the *Pātañjalayogaśāstra*, a new idea begins to gain popularity, which posits that one need not actually die in order to attain liberation.

Liberation while Living

The category of liberation while living (*jīvanmukti*, 11.2) is an important and contested one in post-medieval Indian thought. Although, as the Advaitin author Vidyāraṇya points out in his *Jīvanmuktiviveka*, living liberation is foreshadowed in both the revealed and traditional texts (*śruti* and *smṛti*) of the Vedic religion (see 11.2.7), sustained discussion of the topic only begins around the time of Śaṅkara (eighth to ninth century CE), largely in the context of non-dual (*advaita*) Vedānta (see 11.2.1), but also in other areas, such as the non-dual tantric Trika traditions.[7] In the eleventh century the non-dual *Mokṣopāya* (later known as the *Yogavāsiṣṭha*) 'celebrated and help[ed] to popularize the concept of *jīvanmukti*', and by the seventeenth century it was a topic of discussion in every school of thought within Hinduism.[8]

Given Advaita's view that liberation arises from the knowledge that the phenomenal world (including one's body) is not real, embodied liberation poses no contradiction.[9] However, for other schools of Vedānta which rejected non-dualism, *jīvanmukti* was not considered to be a legitimate concept, insofar as the inevitable bondage to materiality (*prakṛti*) entailed by the embodied state prevents the full knowledge of God, which is only possible after death.[10] For the Mīmāṃsaka author Maṇḍanamiśra, liberation while living may occur for the advanced practitioner (*sādhaka*) who possesses stable insight, but who has not yet reached the final goal, and for whom the effects of *karma* are therefore still in motion (*Brahmasiddhi* 130–31). In contrast, the body of the perfectly realized practitioner (*siddha*) who is free from *karma* and its effects may instantly collapse (ibid.). So while Maṇḍanamiśra's view does not reject the possibility of living liberation, it presents it as an intermediate stage, inferior to the ultimate goal of liberation.[11] Maṇḍanamiśra's notion is vigorously rejected by the Advaitin author (and commentator on the *Pātañjalayogaśāstra*) Vācaspatimiśra, who, following Śaṅkara, argues that the mental and conceptual nature of realization cannot negate another merely mental concept (the body) and that the realization of Brahman and continued life in the body are therefore compatible.[12]

In the context of the dualistic, Sāṃkhya-oriented *Pātañjalayogaśāstra*, *jīvanmukti* is also a difficult and contradictory notion. The idea of liberation in life can be traced back to the *Sāṃkhyakārikā* itself, although it is not named as such there and remains a cryptic idea (cf. Rukmani 2005: 68). In the *Pātañjalayogaśāstra* the commentary to 4.30 notes with regard to the 'Cloud of Virtue' *samādhi* that the wise man is liberated while living (11.1.4). However, the continued presence of the *jīvanmukta*'s body in the liberated state is philosophically problematic on account of the two stages of *samādhi* (with and without cognition, 9.1.3), and because the modifications must be entirely abolished before the highest wisdom manifests – facts which did not escape the text's commentators, and which ultimately made living liberation an unsustainable notion within Pātañjala yoga.[13]

In a passage included in this chapter (11.1.2) the *Mahābhārata* describes one who has attained yoga (*yukta*) as like a man who climbs a stairway with a bowl full of oil and does not spill a drop even when threatened by men with swords. Even though, in this 'everlasting Vedic teaching', the *summum bonum* of yoga is called isolation (*kevala*) and entails the abandonment of the body, the metaphor of the equanimous, unperturbable yogi appears to leave room for a state in which the yogi continues to exist as a cognizant entity in the world even after the accomplishment of yoga, perhaps prefiguring later theorizations of liberation-in-life.

Other texts on yoga included in this chapter also express the ontological contradictions of living liberation. The realized yogi is alive, at least in a biological sense, but, as *Yogabīja* 56–8 puts it, he has already died (11.2.3). *Śivasaṃhitā* 5.223 similarly urges the yogi to 'die in his body' while it is still alive (11.3.9). In the world of the liberated yogi, dichotomies of life and death do not apply and, indeed, noting the conventional understanding of life as consciousness and death as lack of consciousness, the *Amaraughaprabodha* states that, for the undead *jīvanmukta*, consciousness and its absence are the same (11.2.4).

However, this ontological and cognitive no-man's-land need by no means entail the cataleptic inertia of an unperceiving body, although it may resemble it (the yogi in *samādhi*, as noted in Chapter 9, is sometimes described as being insensible like a piece of wood, e.g. 9.2.3). Especially in tantric-oriented texts, the liberated yogi is not only fully cognizant but able to fulfil all his desires by virtue of the powers (*siddhi*s) that he has accumulated. Eternally young, he roams the universe sporting in the three worlds (11.2.3), having sex with divine women (11.2.4), omniscient and omnipotent (11.2.5).

In these texts the enjoyment of *siddhi* is, however, only one option for the yogi, the other being final, disembodied liberation such as we have noted in the context of the *Mahābhārata* and early Buddhism. For example, the *Mṛgendratantra* notes that the yogi who is 'a substrate of miraculous action' may abandon his body when his chosen moment arrives (11.1.7). The *Jñāneśvarī* similarly notes that one who is not interested in the special powers like those of the miraculous, sky-walking yogi may opt instead to dissolve the elements of the body and 'merge with the interior of heaven' (11.1.10). A similar choice is offered by the *Dattātreyayogaśāstra* (124c–31b) in which the yogi may cast off his body or, if it is dear to him, wander the worlds exercising his supernatural powers. This equivalence in value accorded to what might initially appear contradictory paths is particularly characteristic of tantric Śaiva texts, in which magic and soteriology are placed on the same plane, and in which 'liberation (*mukti*) and the enjoyment of supernatural powers (*bhukti*) are both goals to be attained through the same means'.[14] Such equivalences may also represent a synthetic compromise born of the impulse to ease the ancient tension between the life of the renouncer ascetic and that of the worldly householder.[15]

From a Jain perspective, Hemacandra notes that embodied liberation, while indeed bestowing the god-like qualities of omniscience, etc., may be used in order to teach the *dharma* with supernatural efficacy, and thereby also lead others to liberation (11.1.8). This is, of course, similar to the Buddhist ideal of the *bodhisattva*, a figure who delays final, disembodied liberation in order to help unenlightened beings towards *nirvāṇa*. A comparable orientation can also be seen in the *Khecarīvidyā*, where the yogi may, 'for the good of the universe', decide against abandoning his body (11.3.7). The *Jogpradīpakā* similarly urges the devotee to reject final, disembodied liberation and to always remain in his body as a servant of the Lord (11.1.11). Religious traditions may also have a practical motivation to endorse the truth and validity of *jīvanmukti*, in that without the continued, embodied existence of enlightened beings there would be nobody to teach the experience authoritatively to others, nor to act as a role model for those who aspire to that state. As Mumme puts it, '[t]he various traditions that aim at liberation would be reduced to the blind leading the blind'.[16]

Cheating Death, Entering Another's Body and Yogic Suicide

The translations in the final section of this chapter concern the ways in which the yogi can recognize the signs of approaching death, and then either eject the vital energy from his body through *utkrānti* ('yogic suicide') or take measures to cheat death (including taking possession of another body) and go on living as a *jīvanmukta*.[17] For the yogi intent on eluding death, recognizing *ariṣṭa*s, its portents, and knowing what action to take obviously become of utmost importance, which is why lists of *ariṣṭa*s, sometimes very extensive, are found in a vast range of texts from at least the *Mahābhārata* onwards. Prognostications based on the flow of the breath and the shape of one's shadow are particularly common. A passage from the *Pātañjalayogaśāstra* translated here (11.3.3), describes the signs of approaching death in oneself (e.g. an absence of light when the eyes are closed) and in others (e.g. the sudden apparition of dead relatives).[18]

A key procedure in the attainment of liberation is a practice known as *utkrānti* ('yogic suicide') in which the yogi's vital energy is propelled from the body, leaving it lifeless. Such practices are attested in the *Mahābhārata* (12.305.1–7); a passage included in this chapter describes the egress of the yogi through various parts of the body, from the feet to the head, each of which points leads to a different divine destination (11.3.1). Another section of the *Mahābhārata* included here describes the spectacular, flaming exit of King Ikṣvāku and a Brahman through their palates and into union with Brahmā (11.3.2). Comparable methods of yogic suicide are prevalent in tantric texts. Also included in this section are passages from the *Parākhyatantra* and the *Mālinīvijayottaratantra*, both of which outline yogic methods of exiting the body and ascending to the realm of Śiva (11.3.5 and 11.3.6), in spite of such methods being later condemned within Śaiva tantrism as based on an erroneous duality of body and spirit.[19] Similar methods, described in terms of the ascent of Kuṇḍalinī, are taught in the *Khecarīvidyā* and the *Jñāneśvarī* (11.3.7 and 11.1.10).[20]

As with liberation methodologies more generally, yogic methods of ejecting the vital principle out of the body do not only lead to states of disembodied liberation. The yogi may transfer his consciousness out of his own body and into the body of another, thus allowing him to live on in an embodied state in a reanimated corpse or, in certain cases, in a living individual. Such 'entry into another body' (*parakāyapraveśa*) allows the yogi to migrate from body to body and thereby to cheat death indefinitely. Transference of the vital energy of the individual is in evidence in the *Mahābhārata*, such as when Vidura uses yoga to enter the body of Yudhiṣṭhira, thereby strengthening him (15.33.26–8). The entry of one's mind into another body (*cittasya paraśarīrāveśaḥ*) is listed as one of the special powers in *Pātañjalayogaśāstra* 3.38 (10.4), and the commentator Vijñānabhikṣu notes that this process is accomplished along a particular subtle channel.[21] Similarly, the *Bhāgavatapurāṇa* includes entering another's body among its list of eighteen special powers, and provides instructions on how to accomplish this through the medium of the breath (10.13). Entering the bodies of others is also a common motif in fictional accounts of yogis.[22]

In his *Yogaśāstra* Hemacandra describes in detail the procedure for entering another body, by which the yogi can live 'as if liberated' (11.3.10). He stipulates that it must be a dead body on account of the sin that would be accrued by the inevitable death of the inhabitant of a living body (5.272). However, as Smith points out, Hemacandra's prohibition does not prevent him from providing detailed instructions on the possession of a living body in his auto-commentary, the *Svopajñavṛtti*, including a technique for fatally obstructing its owner's life force.[23]

Also included in this section are the *Jogpradīpakā*'s instructions for entering a dead body (**11.3.12**); a passage from the *Ḥawż al-ḥayāt* (**11.3.13**), which describes some of the risks that the yogi himself runs in moving between bodies; and the famous account from the pre-eminent hagiography of Śaṅkara, the *Śaṅkaradigvijaya*, in which Śaṅkara enters the body of the dead king Amaruka in order to gain carnal knowledge, and thus win a debate on sexual love without defiling his own body (**11.3.4**).

Chapter Contents

11.1.10 *Jñāneśvarī* 6.293–306. The dissolution of the body, the final ascent of Kuṇḍalinī and the fruit of the tree of yoga.

11.1.11 *Jogpradīpakā* 940–41. A servant of the Lord never accepts liberation.

11.2 Living Liberation (*jīvanmukti*)

11.2.1 Śaṅkara's *Brahmasūtrabhāṣya* 4.1.15. The body of the knower of Brahman.

11.2.2 *Mokṣopāya* 1.2.14–15, 2.14.31–5. Living liberation and the characteristics of great minds.

11.2.3 *Yogabīja* 4–9, 54–9, 164–70, 183c–187d. Death, liberation and the signs of success.

11.2.4 *Amaraughaprabodha* 69–72. Liberation while living as *rājayoga*.

11.2.5 *Amṛtasiddhi* Chapter 30. The characteristics of liberation while living.

11.2.6 *Śārṅgadharapaddhati* 4591–7. Bodiless liberation (*videhamukti*).

11.2.7 *Jīvanmuktiviveka* 1.3.2, 1.3.4, 1.4.1–7. Revealed and traditional texts prove the existence of living liberation.

11.3 *Ariṣṭa*s, Cheating Death, Entering Another's Body, Yogic Suicide

11.3.1 *Mahābhārata* 12.305.1–7. The bodily locations for ascent to various realms through yogic suicide.

11.3.2 *Mahābhārata* 12.193.15–25. Ikṣvāku and a Brahman exit their bodies.

11.3.3 *Pātañjalayogaśāstra* 3.22. *Ariṣṭa*s, the signs of approaching death.

11.3.4 *Śaṅkaradigvijaya* 9.101–9. Śaṅkara entering the dead body of King Amaruka.

11.3.5 *Parākhyatantra* 14.104–6. Performing yogic suicide when bodily powers fail.

11.3.6 *Mālinīvijayottaratantra* 17.25–8. Yogic suicide when bodily experience becomes repulsive.

11.3.7 *Khecarīvidyā* 3.43c–55b. Cheating death and abandoning the body.

11.3.8 *Śārṅgadharapaddhati* 4598–612. Recognizing the signs of approaching death in order to cheat it.

11.3.9 *Śivasaṃhitā* 2.47, 2.52–5, 5.48, 5.52–4, 5.213, 5.223. Liberation.

11.3.10 Hemacandra's *Yogaśāstra* 5.264–73, with selected passages from the *Svopajñavṛtti* auto-commentary. Entering the body of another 'as if liberated'.

11.3.11 *Jogpradīpakā* 773–9. The observance for cheating death.

11.3.12 *Jogpradīpakā* 797–804. Casting off the old body and taking on a new one.

11.3.13 *Ḥawż al-ḥayāt* 7.13–15. Entering the body of another, living or dead.

11.3.14 *Tirumandiram* 1910–22. What to do with the yogi's body after death.

11.1
Liberation

11.1.1 *Ariyapariyesanā Sutta* (*Majjhimanikāya*). *Nirvāṇa*:

Then, O monks, being myself subject to birth and having understood how wretched it is to be subject to birth, seeking the unborn, peerless, utter peace that is *nirvāṇa*, I obtained the unborn, peerless, utter peace that is *nirvāṇa*.

[The same formula is then repeated for old age, disease, death, sadness and impurity.]

Then the knowledge and realization arose in me that my liberation was unshakeable, that this is my last birth, that I will not now be reborn again. Then, O monks, this occurred to me: this condition that I have obtained is profound, rare, difficult to understand, peaceful, complete, beyond the scope of reason, subtle [and] knowable [only] by the wise. But people here delight in attachment, are devoted to attachment, are made happy by attachment. Moreover, for people who delight in attachment, are devoted to attachment, are made happy by attachment, it is hard to see this condition, which is dependent origination from an ascertained cause, hard to see this condition which is the cessation of all aggregation, the abandoning of all attachments, the end of craving, detachment, cessation, *nirvāṇa*. And furthermore, if I were to teach the *dharma*, other people would not understand me, I would get tired, I would be vexed.

11.1.2 *Mahābhārata* 12.304.18–26. The marks of one who has attained yoga:

Yājñavalkya said:

(18) O great king, one should reflect upon the marks of one who has attained yoga (*yukta*). The mark of tranquillity is that he sleeps happily, as if content. (19)

> The wise say that one who has attained yoga is like a lamp full of oil burning in a windless place, its flame steady and upright. (20) The mark of one who has attained yoga is that, like a rock struck by raindrops, he cannot be made to move. (21) The sign of one who has attained yoga is that he does not flinch when the sounds of conch shells and kettledrums [and] various types of singing and music are performed. (22–4) One should reflect upon the signs of the sage who has attained yoga thus: rising up with his mind focused as a result of the steadiness and stillness of his senses, he is exactly like a man who, holding in his hands a bowl full of oil, climbs a stairway while being threatened by men with swords in their hands, [but] having controlled himself out of fear of them does not spill a drop from the pot. (25) The man who has attained yoga sees Brahman, which is the supreme imperishable, located in the middle of the great darkness looking like a fire. (26) By means of this he reaches isolation (*kevala*) having abandoned the body, which is not a witness. This, O king, is the ancient everlasting Vedic teaching.

11.1.3 *Pātañjalayogaśāstra* 3.55. Isolation (*kaivalya*):

For one who has attained knowledge produced by discrimination or for one who has not,

> (3.55) Isolation occurs when the intellect and the self are equally pure.

When the pure intellect (*buddhisattva*), cleansed of the impurities of passion (*rajas*) and inertia (*tamas*), becomes concerned only with the cognition of its difference from the self, and its seeds of [further] affliction are burnt up, then it is as if it has become equally as pure as the self. [And] then there is the purity that is the absence of the experience [wrongly] attributed to the self. In this state isolation arises whether one has powers or not, whether one has knowledge produced from discrimination or not. Because for him in whom the seeds of further affliction have been burnt up, when knowledge arises there is no need of anything more. The power and knowledge produced by *samādhi* as a result of purity of the intellect have already been mentioned. But in reality it is through knowledge that wrong understanding ceases.

When it has ceased there are no further afflictions. As a result of the absence of afflictions there is no fruition of *karma*. And in this condition the *guṇas* [*sattva*, *rajas* and *tamas*], which have done their job, do not come to the self in visible form again. That is the isolation of the self. Then the self is illuminated by only its own true form, unsullied and isolated.

11.1.4 *Pātañjalayogaśāstra* 4.29–34. Isolation (*kaivalya*):

> (4.29) The 'Cloud of Virtue' *samādhi* (*dharmameghasamādhi*) arises for he who has complete discriminatory cognition and is not interested in even pure consciousness.

When this Brahman is not interested in even pure consciousness then he has no desire for anything. For he who is detached from even that, complete discriminatory cognition arises. As a result of the destruction of the seeds of latent impressions no other thoughts arise in him. Then the *samādhi* called 'Cloud of Virtue' arises for him.

> (4.30) As a result of that, afflictions and actions cease.

As a result of attaining [the 'Cloud of Virtue' *samādhi*], afflictions such as ignorance are destroyed down to their roots. And good and bad karmic residues are destroyed down to their roots. When the afflictions and actions have ceased, the wise man is liberated while he is living. How? Because mistaken cognition is the cause of existence. For nobody who has got rid of mistaken cognition is ever seen by anyone to be [re]born.

> (4.31) Then, because the knowledge from which all covering impurity has been removed is infinite, what remains to be known is insignificant.

Knowledge free from all the coverings of afflictions and actions is infinite. Infinite pure knowledge (*jñānasattva*) is suppressed [and] covered by the concealing [*guṇa* of] darkness (*tamas*); it is sometimes activated [and] made manifest by [the *guṇa* of] passion (*rajas*), [and] then becomes capable of [truly] perceiving. Once that has happened, when it is freed of all obscuring impurities it becomes eternal. Because knowledge is infinite, what remains to be known is trivial, like a firefly in the sky. In this context the following has been said:

'A blind man pierced a jewel, a fingerless man strung it, a man without a neck put it on [and] a man without a tongue praised it.'

> (4.32) As a result of that, the *guṇa*s achieve their aim and stop their sequence of transformation.

As a result of the [*samādhi* called] 'Cloud of Virtue' the *guṇa*s achieve their aim and their sequence of transformation is stopped. For, when they have effected experience and deliverance, and their sequence is complete, they cannot bear to remain even for an instant.

Now what in fact is this sequence?

> (4.33) The opposite of the moment, the sequence is to be understood at the very end of the transformations [of the *guṇa*s]. [. . .][24]

Isolation is said to arise when the sequence of functions of the *guṇa*s ends. Its true form is determined thus:

> (4.34) Isolation is the involution of the *guṇa*s, which are free from any aim for the self; alternatively it is being established in one's own form [which is] the power of consciousness.

Isolation is the involution of the *guṇa*s, which consist of effect and cause, when they have effected enjoyment and deliverance, [and] are free from any aim for the self; furthermore, [isolation] is being established in one's own form as a result of not being connected with the pure intellect, i.e. it is the self's isolated power of consciousness. When that [power of consciousness] remains thus for ever, that is isolation.

11.1.5 *Yogasārasaṃgraha* of Vijñānabhikṣu, commentary on verses 1–3. *Samādhi* and liberation:

> And the following is said in a traditional scripture: 'Liberation is being established in one's true form after giving up existing otherwise.' On this subject, the yoga [of *samādhi*] with cognition brings about liberation, because it cuts away the afflictions and so forth by revealing the true reality. And that the yoga [of *samādhi*] without cognition [also brings about liberation] by burning away all the residues of mental fluctuations and by overcoming activated [*karma*] has been taught by us in the *Vārttika*. We shall explain it in brief below. In

> the context of the auxiliaries of yoga and knowledge (*jñāna*), devotion (*bhakti*), action (*karma*) and so forth there is a secondary application of the word yoga, because they are means of accomplishing yoga and methods of attaining liberation.

11.1.6 *Paramokṣanirāsakārikā* 55, 56, 58a, 58b, with the *vṛtti* of Bhaṭṭa Rāmakaṇṭha. The deficiency of the Sāṃkhya isolation and the superiority of the Śaivasiddhānta view:[25]

[Sāṃkhya:] Surely even your scriptures teach that the soul can attain Isolation through the destruction of *karma*; how can that be?

[Sadyojyotiḥ] states:

> (55) Isolation is possible of the bound soul in the world of Aṅguṣṭhamātra by the destruction of *karma* through knowledge, yoga, renunciation (*saṃnyāsa*) or consumption.

['In the world of Aṅguṣṭhamātra' means:] in the world of *kalā*, [i.e.] the place of residence of those having such names as Aṅguṣṭhamātra. ['Through knowledge, yoga, renunciation or consumption' means:] 'through knowledge', whose content is the discrimination of the soul from primal matter, 'through yoga' consisting in the conquest of the mind, effected by the [six] constituent parts [of yoga] beginning with withdrawal of the senses, or 'through renunciation' of action in which all action is offered to the Lord [with the words] 'All this is for the Lord', which results in discrimination [of the soul] from primal matter, 'or' simply 'through consumption' of the fruits of the [*karma*]. There alone [i.e. at that level of the universe], as a result of the destruction of all actions [by one of these four means], isolation which produces complete cessation of the state of being an experiencer is possible, but not in your 'liberation'.

[Objection:] Surely that very isolation [which you have just described] is our liberation?

[Sadyojyotiḥ] replies:

> (56) And that [isolation], which when it arises [from destruction of *karma*] is full of impurity, proclaimed [by you] as the [ultimate] fruit, is [in fact] destruction of

> the self, because of the destruction of the qualities of knowledge and action [in that state]. For there is thus rather reabsorption into a material cause for you, so [you] make this same great mistake [as the Vedāntins and the Pāñcarātrikas in the preceding two sections].

Whatever kind of isolation [you] propose as liberation, that too [taken as] the fruit is clearly, on the contrary, simply destruction of the self, because, since impurity [still] exists for selves [in that state], there is not even partial knowledge and power to act, as in the state of one devoid of all faculties. For liberation for you too [as well as for Pāñcarātrikas and Vedāntins] is [effectively] reabsorption into *avyakta* (the unmanifest), which is the material cause of the *guṇa*s. [. . .]

[The value of the teachings of other traditions]

[Objection] [. . .] Since absolutely all of the traditional teachings regarding liberation are, as has been taught above, refuted [by valid means of knowledge] and mutually contradictory, are they simply invalid?

[Sadyojyotiḥ] says not:

> (58a) Other [traditions apart from Śaivasiddhānta] are deficient in [their ability to see all] reality.

For not every means of knowledge need reveal everything. Thus other [teachings] too are certainly means of knowledge, in that they reveal a small [range of] objects, just as direction, perception etc. [are means of knowledge despite revealing only a small range of objects]. [Sadyojyotiḥ] says why they reveal [only] a very small [range] of objects:

> (58b) Because they do not teach higher [levels of the universe], [namely] *rāga* and the like.

11.1.7 *Mṛgendratantra Yogapāda* 61c–63b, 66, with the *vṛtti* of Bhaṭṭa Nārāyaṇakaṇṭha. Realizing the innate nature of Śiva and final beatitude:[26]

> (61c–63b). If he practises correctly in this way, visualizing no [iconic] form, then, thinking nothing, he experiences the unfolding of his own nature as all-encompassing vision and action, full of bliss and eternal. Once he has attained this, he is never touched again by the suffering

> that perpetuates the pernicious [condition of transmigratory existence].

If the yogi practises correctly in this way, succeeding by virtue of the great purity of his discipline in doing the aforesaid yoga method without imagining any icon, then thinking no thought, coming through the cessation of all mental activity to rest in nothing but his own identity, an identity that is as tranquil as a waveless ocean, he experiences the unfolding of his innate nature. It expands and becomes infinite. The sense is that he becomes such that his innate nature functions freely and without obscuration. The text describes this innate nature as consisting of all-encompassing vision, knowledge of everything, and [all-encompassing] action, where action means the transformation of material things.

This is the nature of Śiva himself as taught in the Āgamas:

'In Śiva [these powers of] knowledge and action are said to be all-encompassing, pure and absolute.' This nature, which, furthermore, is beautiful with incomparable joy and unending, becomes manifest to the yogi who does this practice. If he attains it he [never again] experiences that contact with suffering which is transmigratory existence, which perpetuates the mischief of birth, death and all that they entail. As Avadhūtaguru has said:

'As [base] metals become gold by means of quicksilver, so those who are inspired by his doctrine can never be reborn.' [. . .]

> (66) Through the practice of this [yoga] he roams the worlds of his choice radiant with the massed rays of the divine perfections. Then when the moment comes he puts aside his sense-free body and dwells only in his own identity, a substrate of miraculous action.

11.1.8 Hemacandra's *Yogaśāstra* 11.24–30, 48, 57–61. Embodied and disembodied liberation as a result of the highest two meditations:

> (24) Then he wanders around the world as a deity, a god, omniscient, all-seeing, endowed with countless qualities, bowed down to by gods, demons, men and snake-people (*nāga*s). (25) With the moonlight of his words he opens the lotuses that are beings fit for

liberation. In an instant he uproots mistaken understanding of the external and inner objects of experience. (26) Merely by taking his name the sorrow born of beginningless transmigration suffered by the souls of those who are fit for liberation is instantly and completely destroyed. (27) Through his power a billion gods, men and other beings gathered to worship [him] will fit into an area one league across. (28) Gods, men, animals and other beings understand his teachings on *dharma* in their own respective languages. (29) Through his power terrible diseases are cured up to 100 leagues away, like heating diseases around the world when the cool ray of the rising moon [shines on them]. (30) Pox, plague, famine, flood, drought, unrest and hostility do not happen when he is about, like darkness when the sun [is shining].

[Verses 31–47 continues the account of the miraculous attributes, effects and powers of the liberated yogi.]

(48) He who does not possess the *karma* called 'The Name of the Saviour' also attains perfect abstraction through the power of yoga, and, while living, teaches the world. [. . .]

(57) After attaining, in the time it takes to pronounce the five short vowels (*a*, *i*, *u*, *ṛ* and *ḷ*), a condition of constancy like that of Mount Meru, [the yogi] simultaneously casts off all [*karma*s related to] experience, lifespan, name and lineage. (58) Having abandoned in this world the physical, luminous and karmic bodies, which are the root causes of transmigration, [the yogi] goes directly and immediately to the summit of the universe. (59) His motion is not upwards [beyond the universe], because there is no medium for him to move in, nor is it downwards, because he is weightless, nor is it sideways, because there is no physical activity or incitement of others to act. (60) The motion of the adept is upwards because he is light like smoke, free from attachment like a bottle-gourd [which, when clean of mud, rises to

the surface from under the water] and free from bondage, like a castor-oil seed [when its pod has burst]. (61) Having attained the happiness which has a beginning [but] no end, which is unequalled, which is free from suffering [and] which is born of one's own nature, one understands pure wisdom and rejoices, liberated.

11.1.9 *Dattātreyayogaśāstra* 124c–131b. Liberation through *samādhi*:

(124c) Then, having perfected meditation without attributes, [the yogi] should practise *samādhi.* (125) In just twelve days he attains *samādhi.* By holding the breath the wise [yogi] is sure to become liberated while alive. (126) *Samādhi* is the condition of identity of the individual and universal selves. If [the yogi] has the desire to cast off [his] body [and] if he wants to cast it off himself (127) [then] he should abandon all actions, good and bad, and dissolve [his self] into the supreme Brahman. And if [he does not want] to cast off his body, if it is dear to him, (128) then he should wander about all the worlds endowed with the powers of becoming infinitesimal and so forth. He might, should he so want, become a god and wander about in heaven. (129) Or, should he so want, he might in an instant become a man or a spirit. Or he might want to become an animal: a lion, a tiger, an elephant or a horse. (130) The wise yogi thus wanders at will as a great lord (*maheśvara*).

11.1.10 *Jñāneśvarī.* 6.293–306. The dissolution of the body, the final ascent of Kuṇḍalinī and the fruit of the tree of yoga:[27]

Dissolution of the Body

(293) Listen, [where] the light of the goddess (*śakti*) disappears, there the form of the body vanishes. Then it hides in the eyes of the world. (294) Otherwise [the body] is still as in the beginning, with members, but as if woven of wind, (295) or [like] the inner [hollow] of a

banana tree, standing after having discarded its cover, or a part of the sky, separated [from it]. (296) When the body becomes like that, then it is called 'sky-walking'. When this state is reached, the body brings about miracles. (297) See, [when] the practitioner (*sādhaka*) walks away, [where] the line of [his] footsteps remains behind, there, in that very place arise [yogic powers like] smallness, etc.

(298) But what [of] it for he [who is not interested in *siddhis*]? – Listen, Dhanañjaya, to how the group of three elements in the bodies inside the body disappears: (299) water makes earth dissolve, fire absorbs water, wind hides fire in the heart, (300) afterwards [wind] itself remains alone, but by imitating [the shape of] the body. Then that, too, leaves in order to merge with the interior of heaven.

(301) At that time the term 'Kuṇḍalinī' disappears, she then gets the name 'Mārutī' ('Belonging to the Wind'), but [her] status as the goddess (*śakti*) remains until she will merge into Śiva.

[Kuṇḍalinī in the Aperture of Brahman]

(302) Then she leaves Jālāndhara, bursts through Kakārānta [and] becomes established in the fortress of heaven. (303) There, immediately putting the feet on the back of the syllable *oṃ*, she leaves behind the stairs of Paśyantī. (304) Afterwards, together with the *tanmātra* and the half[-*mātrā*], in the interior of space, she seems to be filling [herself] into an ocean like a river.[28] (305) Then coming to rest in the aperture of Brahman, spreading the arms of the feeling of 'I' [and] rushing to the *liṅga* of the highest self, she clings [to its] body. (306) Then the curtain of the gross elements disappears, and the two (*paramātmā*/Śiva and the goddess) strike together. There in that union she merges with heaven.

11.1.11 *Jogpradīpakā* 940–41. A servant of the Lord never accepts liberation:

> (940) The Lord gives people four [types of] liberation, but a servant [of the Lord] never accepts liberation. The lord is to be worshipped [and] I am the worshipper: that is what I shall always do. (941) He who worships the feet of the lord with devotion never accepts [any of] the four types of liberation. Keep the condition of being a servant which you have by remaining in the body.

11.2

Living Liberation (*jīvanmukti*)

11.2.1 Śaṅkara's *Brahmasūtrabhāṣya* 4.1.15. The body of the knower of Brahman:

> Moreover, there is no dispute over whether or not he who knows Brahman retains his body for some time, for how can the knowledge of Brahman experienced in the heart of one person be refuted by someone else?

11.2.2 *Mokṣopāya* 1.2.14–15, 2.14.31–5. Living liberation and the characteristics of great minds:

> (1.2.14) In those embodied people who are liberated while living, latent impression (*vāsanā*) does not bring about rebirth [and] does not defile the body, just as the action of rotation [does not defile] a wheel. (15) Those whose latent impressions are pure and who [will not] partake of the calamity that is [re]birth are called 'those who have understood what is to be understood', 'liberated while living' and 'great minds'.
>
> (2.14.31) The mind has Brahman as its constant support [and] has reached a condition of great splendour. It does not set nor does it rise; like the sky it is expansive. (32) It

neither casts off nor takes on anything; it is neither disturbed nor peaceful; merely observing the universe like a witness, it stays in the self. (33) It does not stop, nor does it settle on anything internal or external; it is not inactive, nor does it become immersed in action. (34) It cares not for things that have gone, nor does it concern itself with things that have come. It appears neither shaken nor too unshaken, like the ocean. (35) With minds like this, the great-souled, great-hearted yogis wander about this world liberated while living.

11.2.3 *Yogabīja* 4–9, 54–9, 164–70, 183c–187d. Death, liberation and the signs of success:

The goddess said:

(4) All living beings, through pleasures and sufferings, are caught in the web of delusion. Please say, Lord Śaṅkara, how they can get liberation. (5) Great Lord, you have explained various paths. You who are the best of yoga experts, speak now about the path which brings liberation.

The Lord spoke:

(6) This path brings all supernatural powers and cuts through the web of delusion. It destroys birth and death, old age and disease, and brings happiness. (7) Out of love, O queen of the gods, I shall next teach you the supreme way of Śiva by which bound [souls] are liberated.

(8) The supreme state, emancipation (*kaivalya*), cannot be obtained through the various [other] paths. It can only be achieved by the path of the adepts. This is the word of Śiva. (9) Those whom the many hundreds of [subjects] like logic, grammar and so on have made fall into the snare of book-learning are deluded by wisdom. [. . .]

(54) The best of yogis takes on whatever form he desires, is his own master, does not grow old or die, and playfully sports wherever he wants in the three worlds. (55) The yogi who has conquered his senses possesses

inconceivable power and can assume and cast off various outward appearances at will. (56) Why do you ask about his death, O you whose face is like the moon? He will not die again, thanks to the power of yoga. (57) He has died already: how can the dead die? He lives + . . . + where everyone dies. (58) Where the foolish live, he always dies. There is nothing that he must do [and] he is not tainted by what he has done.

(59) One who is liberated while living (*jīvanmukta*) is always healthy and free from all faults. [. . .]

(164) I shall now teach you clearly the result of practice, O goddess. Diseases disappear first, then bodily inertia. (165) Next, its taste having become uniform, the moon rains forth [nectar] ceaselessly. The fire, with the wind, completely consumes each of the constituents of the body. (166) Various sounds arise [and] the body becomes supple. (167) Having conquered inertia [born from] earth and the other elements, a man may move forth as an aerial being (*khecara*). He becomes omniscient, able to assume any form at will and as fast as the wind. (168) He plays in the three worlds; all the supernatural powers (*siddhis*) arise in him. When camphor melts, no solidity is found in it. (169) When egoism is dissolved, how can there be solidity in the body? Omniscient, omnipotent, free [and] assuming all forms, (170) the yogi becomes liberated while alive and wanders about the world at will. [. . .]

It is only he whose body is ageless and undying who is liberated while living (*jīvanmukta*). (184) When they die, do creatures like dogs, cocks and worms attain liberation as a result of the loss of their bodies, O beautiful lady? (185) The breath does not move out [of the body of he who is liberated while living]: how can [his] body be lost? The freedom (*mukti*) which results from the loss of the body is not called liberation (*mukti*). (186) The body becomes Brahman, just as salt becomes water. When [the yogi] becomes undifferentiated then he is said to be liberated (*mukta*). (187) Bodies and senses are made of consciousness; when they become undifferentiated then [the yogi] is said to be liberated.

11.2.4 *Amaraughaprabodha* 69–72. Liberation while living as *rājayoga*:

(69) Saying 'I am mine', one should visualize the stream of the nectar of immortality. They say that consciousness is life and absence of consciousness is death. (70) When consciousness and its absence become the same it is called, in this text, liberation while living (*jīvanmukti*), the true essence of the natural state of which is impossible to describe. (71) Nobody lives and nobody will die after reaching the state of *rājayoga*, which is beneficial to all beings. (72) The king of yogis can do anything he thinks of, or, if he wishes, not do it. He can be naked in caves or wear divine garments or wear a loincloth; he can enjoy sexual pleasure with a divine woman or be celibate; he can be intent on living off alms or indulge himself in pleasures: his activities are completely unrestricted and he removes all sufferings.

11.2.5 *Amṛtasiddhi* Chapter 30. The characteristics of liberation while living:

(1) Then when the wind in all the stations pierces the knot of Rudra, the mind [becomes] brilliant, adorned by the moment of fruition. (2) When the mind has one form, different from the luminous, the sound of kettledrums arises in the abode of the adepts. (3) When, as a result of the union of the body, voice and mind, [there arises] perfection of [those] three, then know [that to be] the great perfection (*mahāsiddhi*), which gives the reward of liberation while living (*jīvanmukti*). (4) Then the lord of yogis is able to enter *samādhi* at will. Then the celebrated great *samādhi* [arises], O wolf-belly. (5) Then the blissful, omniscient, all-seeing yogi is to be praised by all beings. He has attained yoga in the three worlds. (6) His

movement is always unimpeded; his sight and hearing are unimpeded; his great bliss is unimpeded; he abounds in unimpeded knowledge. (7) The yogi has the power of total dominion, is the seat of infinite knowledge, all-powerful, accompanied by the great adepts, a store of all accomplishments. (8) The lord of yogis does not burn in fire or drown in water, he is invincible in all the worlds; he is without attributes.

(9) As a result the yogi consists of everything, all the elements, is the seat of all knowledge and is constantly worshipped in all the worlds. (10) When happy he may save worlds, angry he destroys success. For the lord of yogis, perfected by knowledge, terrifies the gods. (11) Having playfully broken the revolving wheel of transmigration, the cage of the three worlds, the yogi goes forth blissful, all-powerful. (12) In this way adept yogis sport for hundreds, thousands, hundreds of thousands of years on mountain tops and in caves. (13) With no care for external perception they are intent on *samādhi*. Yogis who have the eye of wisdom stay in deserted places. (14) They remain like this [and] can be seen engaged in their task. Know the adepts who take the form of conquerors (*jina*s) to be liberated while living.

Thus ends the Inquiry into the Characteristics of Liberation while Living.

11.2.6 *Śārṅgadharapaddhati* 4591–7. Bodiless liberation (*videhamukti*):

Now the teaching on bodiless liberation:

(4591) When a sign of approaching death is seen in the first part of the day, or the last part of the day, or the middle of the day, or at some other time, or in part of the night, (4592) the knower of yoga, he who has knowledge, should cast off the fear of death and practise yoga at that same time in order to achieve bodiless liberation. (4593) The wise man should sit in the lotus position, his shoulders even, restrain his *prāṇa* breath and not touch his

> [upper] teeth with his [lower] teeth. (4594) With his eyes shut he should use his intellect to close the nine doors and make the syllable *oṃ* his bow, the quality (*guṇa*) of purity (*sattva*) the string, (4595) [and] his self the arrow. [The arrow] covered with the sense organs and other [faculties], situated in the heart lotus and propelled by impulses from the *prāṇa* breath and the mind, (4696) then, by way of the tenth door, reaches the goal and, joined with the thirty-six elements, dissolves in the supreme self. (4597) Then it attains the infinite, the supreme [element of] space, which is beyond the range of the senses and cannot be described by the intellect.

11.2.7 *Jīvanmuktiviveka* 1.3.2, 1.3.4, 1.4.1–7. Revealed and traditional texts prove the existence of living liberation:

> (1.3.2) It is said that the condition of the mind of a living man, which is characterized by being an agent, being an experiencer, happiness, suffering and so forth, is a fetter because it has the form of affliction. Removing that [fetter] is liberation while living [. . .] (1.3.4) Just as the fluidity of water is overcome by mixing it with earth, or fire's heat [is overcome] by jewels, mantras and so on, so all the fluctuations of the mind can be overcome by the practice of yoga.
>
> (1.4.1) Sayings from the revealed and traditional texts prove the existence of liberation while living. (2) They are found in the *Kaṭha Upaniṣad* and other [texts. E.g.] '[. . .] and [once] freed one is set free' [*Kaṭha Upaniṣad* 5.1]. (3) When one is completely freed from visible bondage, such as desire while one is alive, at death one is completely freed from future bondage.
>
> Even before realization, by cultivating tranquillity and self-restraint one is liberated from desires and so forth [that have not yet arisen]. Nevertheless, in that case, desires and so forth that have already arisen still [must be] suppressed through effort.

(4) In this case, however, simply because mental fluctuations do not arise, [desires and so forth] do not occur, which is why we say 'completely'. And at the final dissolution of the world and at death one [who is not completely liberated] is freed [only] for a while from the bondage of reincarnation. In this case, we said 'complete' to indicate total liberation.

(5) In the *Bṛhadāraṇyaka* [*Upaniṣad* 4.4.7] we read, 'When all desires residing in his heart are set free, then the mortal becomes immortal (*amṛta*) [and] reaches Brahman here and now.'

(6) And in another revealed text [we read]: 'He has eyes, [but] he is as if without sight. He has ears, [but] he is as if without hearing. He has a mind, [but] is as if without a mind' [quoted in *Brahmasūtrabhāṣya* 1.1.4]. Similar examples [can be found] elsewhere.

(7) Here and there in the recollected texts, one who is liberated while living is called 'he whose wisdom is steady', 'devoted to God', 'beyond the qualities', 'Brahman', 'beyond caste and order' and so on.

11.3

Ariṣṭas, Cheating Death, Entering Another's Body, Yogic Suicide

11.3.1 *Mahābhārata* 12.305.1–7. The bodily locations for ascent to various realms through yogic suicide:

Yājñavalkya said:

(1) In the same way, O king, listen carefully to [the description of] a yogi ascending. For one who ascends by way of the feet, the destination is the place of Viṣṇu. (2) We have heard that [one who ascends] by way of the lower legs reaches the Vasu gods. By way of the knees

one reaches those fortunate [gods] the Sādhyas. (3) Ascending by way of the anus one reaches the place of Mitra. By way of the buttocks one reaches the earth, Pṛthivī. By way of the thighs one reaches Prajāpati. (4) By way of the sides one reaches the Marut gods. By way of the nostrils it is the moon [that one reaches]. They say that by way of the arms it is Indra [that one reaches]. (5) From the neck one reaches that supreme man, Nara, who is the best of sages. By way of the mouth one reaches the Viśve Devas and by way of the ear the directions. (6) By way of the nose [one reaches] the wind and by way of the eyes it is the sun [that one reaches]. By way of the eyebrows [one reaches] the twin gods, the Aśvins, and by way of the forehead the ancestors. (7) And by way of the head one reaches Brahmā, the lord who is the foremost of the gods.

These locations for ascent have been taught [to you], O Lord of Mithila.

11.3.2 *Mahābhārata* 12.193.15–25. Ikṣvāku and a Brahman exit their bodies:

(15) Then, O king, [Ikṣvāku and the Brahman,] both at the same time, withdrew [their senses] from their sense organs according to the precepts. (16) They fixed their *prāṇa*, *apāna*, *udāna*, *samāna* and *vyāna* breaths in their minds, then put their minds in their *prāṇa* and *apāna* breaths. (17) Then, by means of their minds, they gently held the two breaths, which had been brought together there, at the tips of their noses, [then] below their brows and [then] between their brows. (18) With their gazes steady thanks to their motionless bodies, the two of them, absorbed, their selves mastered, brought their selves into their heads. (19) Then a huge flame of light burst upwards through the palate of the great-souled Brahman and went to heaven. (20) At this a great cry of 'Hā! Hā!' rang out in all the directions. Then, while being praised, that light entered Brahmā. (21)

> Then, O king, [Brahmā], the Grandfather, went up to that light, which was a person the size of a *prādeśa* [the span between the thumb and forefinger], and said 'Welcome!' (22) Then he spoke more sweet words to him: 'Mantra-reciters and yogis get the same [ultimate] reward: in this there is no doubt. (23) But while yogis, too, receive as a reward the direct vision [of me], for mantra-reciters is enjoined the specific reward of [my] coming forward to greet them.' (24) Then, when Brahmā said 'Live in me!' and returned to his meditation, the Brahman, free from suffering, entered his mouth. (25) The king, too, then entered Lord Brahmā, the Grandfather, using exactly the same method as the great Brahman.

11.3.3 *Pātañjalayogaśāstra* 3.22. *Ariṣṭa*s, the signs of approaching death:

> (3.22) Or from the signs of approaching death [the yogi may know when he will die].

A sign of approaching death can be of three kinds: pertaining to oneself, to [other] beings or to the gods. Of these [the sign] pertaining to oneself is when one does not hear a sound in one's body when one blocks one's ears or when one does not see a light when one closes one's eyes. And [the sign] pertaining to [other] beings is when one sees the messengers of Yama, the god of death, or suddenly sees dead ancestors in front of oneself. And [the sign] pertaining to the gods is when one suddenly sees heaven or the adepts or when one sees everything inverted. By this one knows that death is at hand.

11.3.4 *Śaṅkaradigvijaya* 9.101–9. Śaṅkara entering the dead body of King Amaruka:

> (101) Saying these fine words, which removed the terror of existence, he whose fame must be told [i.e. Śaṅkara], went to a mountain peak inaccessible on foot and spoke once again: (102) 'Now see this fine cave, the broad flat rock in front of it and the pool nearby with clear water,

its banks beautiful with trees bent over by the weight of their fruits. (103) O you of faultless qualities, stay here and carefully guard this body [of mine] while I learn the art of the god of love in a body suitable for that purpose.' (104) After instructing the disciples thus, with his formidable yoga power the great ascetic cast off his body in the cave [and] with his subtle body entered the body of the [dead] king. (105) The master of yoga, drawing his breath [up] from [his] big toe, went out from the aperture in his head and, his mind focused, slowly penetrated the dead [king] by way of the aperture in his head, reaching as far as his toes. (106) The body of the dead king gently quivered in the region of his heart, then one eye opened gradually and then he sat up just as he had before. (107) First the lustre returned to the body's face, then breath came faintly from its nose, next its feet started to move, after that its eyes flickered and then it stood up, its strength restored. (108) On realizing that their lord's life had returned, [his] wives with their loud cries of joy and happy lotus-faces resembled lotus flowers in a lake opening at the rising of the sun to the cries of Siberian cranes. (109) Seeing the fair-eyed ladies' great joy and the revived king the senior ministers were delighted. They blew conch shells and beat cymbals, tambourines and kettledrums, whose sounds immediately deafened heaven and earth.

11.3.5 *Parākhyatantra* 14.104–6. Performing yogic suicide when bodily powers fail:[29]

(104) And he should perform yogic suicide (*utkrānti*) by means of yoga when his [bodily] powers fail. By enunciation of the mantra Sadyojāta, ending with *huṃ phaṭ*, for as many as 8,000 times he certainly achieves yogic suicide. By performing [this] he splits + . . . +. (105–6) Once he has achieved yogic suicide, he who understands what is taught becomes joined with Brahman. Thus the

one who understands the performance of yoga achieves the eternal union (*yoga*).

11.3.6 *Mālinīvijayottaratantra* 17.25–8. Yogic suicide when bodily experience becomes repulsive:

(25) When [the yogi] considers all or rather [its] experience to be repulsive, he abandons his body and proceeds to the eternal state. (26) Then he should perform in reverse the mantra-installation that has already been taught and which is as splendid as the fire at the end of time, with [each syllable] inside the two [mantras] *skṛk* and *chindi*. (27) [Then] after performing the fire-fixation, which heats all of the vital points, he should fill the body with air from the big toe to the top of the head. (28) Then, drawing up that [i.e. the breath] he should lead it from the big toe to the cranial aperture. The knower of yoga should sever all the vital points with this mantra.

11.3.7 *Khecarīvidyā* 3.43c–55b. Cheating death and abandoning the body:[30]

[Cheating Death]

If [the yogi] is keen to deceive death, [then], knowing the apportionment of [the locations of] death, (44) while death is approaching him he should happily remain there [in the skull]. Below the bolt of the gateway of Brahmā is the cause of bodily death; (45) in the region above there, O goddess, there is no opportunity for death. When [the yogi] sees that [the time of] his death has passed, O goddess, (46–7) then he should break the bolt [of the gateway] of Brahmā and lead the goddess [back] to the Base centre. [Re-]placing his vital principle (*jīva*), which has been [re-]produced from the body of the goddess [Kuṇḍalinī], together with the sense organs in their respective [places of] action, he should live happily and healthy. By this yoga, O goddess, [the yogi] can cheat an imminent death.

[Abandoning the body]

(48–51) If the supremely content [yogi] desires to abandon [his] mortal body then he should unite Śiva, who is in the place of Brahmā, with the goddess, pierce the void and enter the rock of Brahmā. He should place the ether element in the great ether, the air element in the great wind, the fire element in the great fire, the water element in the great ocean, the earth element in the earth, the mind in the supportless space [and] his sense organs in the elements from ether to Prakṛti. Thus abandoning transmigratory [existence and] dependent only on the ultimate reality, (52) untouched by the five elements, the mind and the sense organs, [the yogi] breaks the orb of the sun and, absorbed in Śiva, [who is] the serene abode of the ultimate reality, he becomes like Śiva. (53) Not in ten billion aeons will he return again. If for the good of the universe he does not abandon [his] body, (54) then he abandons it at the end of the dissolution of the universe and abides only in his own self.

This is *khecarīmudrā*, which bestows dominion over the sky-rovers (*khecaras*) (55) [and] destroys birth, death, old age, sickness, wrinkles and grey hair.

11.3.8 *Śārṅgadharapaddhati* 4598–612. Recognizing the signs of approaching death in order to cheat it:

Now the Cheating of Death:

(4598) 'Liberated while living, I wander the three worlds with a body': if the yogi desires this, [he] should listen to me. (4599) Death never waits for the body of anyone, so the yogi must take pains to protect his body. (4600) The yogi must continually and carefully reflect upon the signs of approaching death; as a result of doing so death, having been recognized, does not harm him because of a trick [that he uses].

(4601) Having learnt that death [is at hand, the yogi] should duly resort to the place of dissolution and practise yoga so that death is unsuccessful with regard to him. (4602) Sitting in the adept's posture (*siddhāsana*), he should fill the body with the *prāṇa* breath, use his intellect to create a firm staff and block the ten doors. (4603) He should apply *khecarīmudrā*, *jālandhara* on the neck, the root lock (*mūlabandha*) on the *apāna* breath and *uḍḍīyāna* on the stomach. (4604) Using winds at the Base to elevate the snake goddess, the auspicious piercer of the five *cakra*s, who is situated below, inside the Suṣumnā, (4605) he should lead her to the vital principle which resides in the heart and [make her] travel [upwards] joined with the intellect and the mind until she is dissolved in the nectarean Śiva in the thousand-petalled lotus.

(4606) After she has drunk the nectar produced at the moon, he should visualize her sprinkling and flooding the whole body with it from the Base [upwards]. (4607) Then, together with her, the yogi should become one with Śiva. Now made of great bliss, he should cast off the activities of the mind. (4608) After that, when he is imperceptible, without appearance, free from the notion of 'I', without any conception of the body, how can death harm him? (4609) That is death, that is Śiva, that is everything and nothing. Who is harmed by whom? In that [state], nobody dies. (4610) Then, when the time of death, who roams around, has passed, the yogi, awakened, becomes conscious, as if arisen from sleep. (4611) In this way the yogi becomes an adept, having, by means of amazing bravery, duly deceived death, by whom transmigration is effected. (4612) Then that yogi wanders at will all alone in the three worlds, observing the strangeness of transmigration, free from the notion of 'I'. [. . .]

11.3.9 *Śivasaṃhitā* 2.47, 2.52–5, 5.48, 5.52–4, 5.213, 5.223. Liberation:

(2.47) Knowledge is more than capable of eradicating the delusion that arises together with desires. Were such knowledge to arise, it would be the means to liberation.

(2.52) Only when the body acquired through *karma* is the means to *nirvāṇa* does having a body bear fruit. (53) The garland of desires that exists in connection with the vital principle (*jīva*) is similar to the misunderstanding that a living being has in its observance of what it should and should not do. (54) If an aspirant to yoga wants to cross the ocean of *saṃsāra*, he should behave according to his caste and stage of life, unattached to the fruits of his actions. (55) People who are attached to the objects of the senses and seek pleasure from them are prevented from reaching *nirvāṇa* + by words + and abide in sin. [. . .]

(5.48) Now I shall describe the great experience of the liberated man, on knowing which even the sinful aspirant attains liberation. [. . .]

(5.52) Having used this method to cast off his old body and so forth and to receive a divine body, the yogi should do what I am about to describe. (53) Seated in the lotus posture and away from human company, he should block the two *vijñāna* (?) channels with his fingers. (54) Perfection then manifests itself, blissful and pure. One can become an adept by means of this, so great effort should be put into it. [. . .]

(5.213) What is bondage? Who is liberated? The yogi always sees unity. He who does this continually is liberated. In this there is no doubt. He alone is a yogi, devoted to me, worshipped in all the worlds. [. . .]

(5.223) He who does not now quickly die in his body while it is unchanging and alive, lives for the enjoyment of the objects of the senses. In this there is no doubt.

11.3.10 Hemacandra's *Yogaśāstra* 5.264–73, with selected passages from the *Svopajñavṛtti* auto-commentary. Entering the body of another 'as if liberated':

Piercing (*vedha*) [of other beings with one's life force]

(264) Filled by means of inhalation, the downward-facing heart lotus opens up, and, awakened by means of

breath-retention, its flow becomes upwards. (265) Then, having extracted it by means of exhalation, [the yogi] should draw the breath from the heart lotus and, having pierced the knot in the upward-flowing path, lead it to the citadel of Brahmā [in the skull]. (266) The yogi eager [to practise piercing] should enter *samādhi*, make [the breath] exit the aperture of Brahmā [at the top of the skull] and very gently perform piercing on tufts of cotton made from the Arka plant. (267) After repeatedly practising on them, [the yogi] should tirelessly, regularly and single-mindedly perform piercing on jasmine buds and the like. (268) Then, when his practice is consistent, he should perform a thorough piercing on perfumed substances such as camphor, aloe and *kuṣṭha* (?) using the Varuṇa breath.[31] (269) Then, when he has achieved his aim and become skilled at uniting the breath with these [substances], the diligent [yogi] should perform piercing on the bodies of very small birds. (270) After practising [on them] the resolute and single-minded [yogi], his senses conquered, should do it on the bodies of moths and bees, and [then] deer. (271) Entering [and] exiting from men, horses and elephants: thus should he perform transference, even progressing to clay and stone images.

The remainder of this passage follows, summarizing what has been said.

(272) In this way [the yogi] may enter dead bodies by means of the left nostril. Entering living bodies, however, is not taught out of fear of sin.

'Out of fear of sin': for entering a living body would result in the destruction of the life-breath (*prāṇa*) of another [being] and that sin, like [sins] such as causing injury with weapons, must not be prescribed. And it is not possible to enter the body of another living being without harming them. As it says [in the scripture]:

(1) 'After exiting through the aperture of Brahmā, entering through the passage of the lower wind (*apāna*) and resting at the navel lotus, [the yogi] should go to the heart lotus by way of the central channel

(*suṣumnā*). (2) There [the yogi] should restrict the movement of the *prāṇa* breath in that [body] with his own breath until the embodied self moves forth from the body, devoid of activity. (3) In the body that has been abandoned by means of this [technique] the actions of the senses of the knower of yoga become manifest and he engages in all undertakings as if in his own body. (4) The wise [yogi] should enjoy himself in the other's body for half a day or a day and then by the same means re-enter his own body.'

The result of entering others' bodies is taught:

> (273) Through the power attained by gradually practising entering others' bodies in this way, the wise [yogi] behaves how he likes, untainted, as if liberated.

11.3.11 *Jogpradīpakā* 773–9. The observance for cheating death:

Now the observance for cheating death is taught.

> (773) Fix the gaze on the point between the eyebrows and repeat the mantra *oṃ*, by means of which the yogi may attain great age; by mastering this he loses the fear of death. (774) Inhale through Piṅgalā, hold the breath firmly for as long as possible and exhale. By means of this practice one's lifespan is increased. (775) Bring the lunar breath into the solar breath; reverse the lunar [breath] and mix the sun with it. The yogi who by means of this practice holds the moon in the day and the sun in the night wards off death. (776) By keeping the moon and sun equal one can raise the nectar of immortality and taste it. Jayatarāma keeps the unstruck sound in the orb of the sky [in the head] and wards off death. (777) First, sit firmly in the adept's pose (*siddhāsana*) and draw up the *apāna* breath. Practise repeated breath-control and bring the *prāṇa* to the middle of the chest. (778) Next stop all the breath which has come halfway up in the navel, then put it in the Suṣumnā, break death and enter *samādhi*. (779) Jayatarāma has easily accomplished *samādhi* by means of the practice which wards off death, having mastered it according to the guru's words.

11.3.12 *Jogpradīpakā* 797–804. Casting off the old body and taking on a new one:

Now, entering another's body.

(797) When the yogi completely masters yoga he obtains unobtainable powers. By means of the snake technique he may go wherever he wants. (798) The breath comes completely under his control and none of the channels remains hidden. No activity of the mind is concealed whenever it is operating. (799) The entire body becomes divine and nothing is concealed. Know that the vital principle, which has the form of breath, goes wherever the breath goes. (800–801) The yogi who understands this teaching can enter another's body. If he wishes he can immediately enter any dead body that he sees, having learnt the method through the grace of his guru. He should move all the breath together with the mind, bring it to the throat and hold it there. (802) He should repeat the mantra as many times as he has been taught by his guru, make his mouth like a crow's beak and put his *prāṇa* in the mouth of the dead body. (803) The dead body gets up and runs about; the previous body becomes dead. And whatever he needs to know leaves his old body and is taken on by the [new] body. (804) The resolute [yogi] learns how to enter another's body from the words of his guru. Jayatarāma cast off a worn-out body and took on a new one.

11.3.13 *Ḥawż al-ḥayāt* 7.13–15. Entering the body of another, living or dead:[32]

(13) One who wishes to enter the body of another, whether living or dead – if it is dead, his body dies, but he returns to it after abandoning it [the possessed body]. And if he finds that his body has become corrupt, he cannot return to it, but he remains in it [the other body] so long as there is a place for him. If it is someone living [whose body he possesses], he does not die, but he remains as one suspended between two states. If the one whose body he enters is weak, that is, internally, he will

be overcome; if he [the owner of the body] is strong, he will be unable to enter it except by [the owner's] heedlessness. These things are well known among them; there are stories and testimonies to this among them, yet this is not attained except by verifying what we have mentioned in this book. Abandoning sexual intercourse is essential.[33]

(14) It is proper that one meditate in the seven bodily locations and on the seven diagrams, and speak their words, or all the meanings of these words, in the heart. Thereupon he sees it as something white, which all at once emerges, as it were, from his body, with this thought. Then he ascends above the seven heavens, and by so doing he continually attains senses other than these external senses. By means of these he witnesses hidden things, just as he witnesses perceptible things with the external senses. Thereafter he loses consciousness, and he awakens, so that he is firmly rooted in them [the hidden things], and he returns. Waking and sleep, death and life, are the same for him, and he becomes purified of gross instruments.[34]

(15) If one wishes to enter a dead body, and so forth, let him meditate on it in its seven previously mentioned bodily locations and previously mentioned diagrams, with their forms and colours. Let him speak the words while in this meditation. He will become unconscious, the dead body will come to life, move, eat and drink; if it was articulate, it will speak. When he returns to his body, the dead [body] becomes as it was.

11.3.14 *Tirumandiram* 1910–22. What to do with the yogi's body after death:[35]

(1910) If the timeless sage's body is burnt in fire, the entire country will suffer from that fire for ever. If it is eaten by dogs and foxes, wars will erupt and the entire land will fall prey to dogs and foxes. (1911) If the fire engulfs the body of a sage who has stopped thought, it is equal to setting fire to the Lord's temple; the rains will drop not on earth; famine will be on the land; countless kings will lose their kingdoms. (1912) It is religious merit to bury [such sages]. If it is burnt by fire there will be diseases in the country. If it is left to decay on the soil the beauty [of the land] will be spoilt. The entire earth will descend into chaos because of fire engulfing [it]. (1913) When the timeless sage attains grace, if his body is provided with a chamber and set in it, the handsome kings and the people inhabiting the ancient earth will obtain the grace of everlasting bliss. (1914) Make a clean hole nine spans deep, spread the earth to five spans [around the hole], make the shape of a triangle, its edges three spans long, in the chamber. Place the body in the lotus position in this cell that defies birth. (1915) One's own land; a road; a dyke; the land at a river confluence; a beautiful flower garden; an area in a town; impenetrable forest; steep mountain slopes: these are sites suitable for making chambers. (1916) The good chamber is five feet broad on the four sides, nine feet deep, three feet square [internally?]. The [yogi's] attendants should construct it. (1917) It is made by spreading five metals and nine jewels, pressing them firmly, placing a pedestal over it, spreading *muñja* grass, sprinkling white holy ash and putting golden turmeric powder on it too. (1918) Make four squares in the centre of the chamber and over it place a honeyed flower garland, sandal paste, the perfume of musk, pure sandal [and] civet perfume mixed with rose water, and gladly offer bright light. (1919) Smear glorious white ash over the body as a coat, put it on the pedestal and decorate it with flowers, grass, powder and ash, and spread them over the pedestal. (1920) After spreading these, pave it on all four sides and place on it tender shoots, fried vegetables, cooked rice and succulent coconuts. After having a [last] blessed look [at the yogi] place the ceremonial cloth on the body. (1921) Pour on white ash, scented powder, lots of flowers, *darbha* grass and *bilva* leaves. Bathe the feet with holy water and over the earth build a shrine three feet by three feet square. (1922) Plant one of either a peepul tree or a Śiva *liṅga* over the pedestal and perform sixteen homages, facing north or east.

Glossary

This glossary is a quick reference guide to some of the more common yoga terms. Our definitions here are extremely brief and are intended to give an initial orientation only, rather than convey the full complexity and semantic range of the words. The reader is encouraged to consult the index in order to see how these terms are used in practice within the texts.

ādhāra: A 'support' for meditation, a feature of the yogic body; (Ādhāra) 'the Base', a specific focus for meditation at the bottom of the central channel.

Āgama: A category of text, especially in tantra.

Ājīvaka: A type of Śramaṇa ascetic contemporary with early Buddhists and Jains.

Akula: The transcendental aspect of divinity in Śaiva tantra. See also Kula.

aṅga: 'Limb'; an auxiliary division of a body of knowledge or practice; see *yogāṅga*.

apāna: One of the five principal breaths.

ariṣṭa: A sign of approaching death.

āsana: Seat; posture.

aṣṭāṅgayoga: Yoga of eight auxiliaries, most commonly associated with Patañjali's *Yogaśāstra*.

ātman: The self.

Āyurveda: An Indian system of medicine.

bandha: 'Lock'; in *haṭhayoga* a bodily constriction.

bhāṣya: A commentary to a text.

bindu: 'Drop' or 'point'; a tantric *tattva* and focus for meditation, sometimes located in the body; in *haṭhayoga*, 'semen'.

Brahmā: One of the three chief gods of Hinduism, together with Śiva and Viṣṇu.

Brahman: The absolute, the supreme principle of Vedānta (in Sanskrit, *brahman*); a member of Hinduism's priestly caste (in Sanskrit, *brāhmaṇa*).

Brahmanical: Descriptive of practices, texts, etc., performed or practised by Brahmans.

brahmarandhra: 'The aperture of Brahmā/Brahman'; the fontanelle, through which the vital principle of the yogi exits at death.

cakra: 'Wheel'; a focus for visualization in the yogic body.

citta: The mind, the activity of which is to be suppressed in Patañjali's and other yoga traditions.

dhāraṇā: 'Fixation'; a meditative practice often included among the auxiliaries of yoga.

dharma: Law, justice, religious observance, societal or caste duty.

dhyāna: 'Meditation'.

doṣa: One of three bodily substances (*kapha*, *pitta* and *vāta*), which, according to Āyurveda, need to be kept in balance in order to maintain health.

granthi: 'Knot'; a blockage in the yogic body that must be pierced by means of the breath or Kuṇḍalinī.

guṇa: In the Sāṃkhya system, one of the three qualities that are present in varying proportions in all things (see *rajas*, *tamas* and *sattva*); *guṇa* may also refer to a supernatural power resulting from success in yoga.

haṭhayoga: 'Yoga by force'; a system of yoga that rose to prominence in the second millennium CE (see Introduction).

Iḍā: A subtle channel (*nāḍī*), usually located on the left side of the Suṣumnā.

īśvara: 'The lord/Lord'; God.

Jālandhara: A tantric sacred site in north-west India; (*jālandhara*) a type of yogic lock.

japa: The repetition of mantras.

jīva: The vital principle in each individual.

kaivalya: Lit. 'aloneness'. Liberation from death and rebirth (see *mokṣa*, *nirvāṇa*).

kalā: 'Part'; a tantric *tattva* and focus for meditation, sometimes located in the body; a digit of the moon.

kanda: A 'bulb' located below the navel, which is the source of the *nāḍīs*.

kapha: One of the three *doṣas*, akin to phlegm.

Kaula: A reformist tantric school which includes transgressive practices in its teachings.

Khecarī: Lit. 'she who moves through the sky', a particular type of Yoginī; (*khecarī*) a type of *mudrā* or yogic seal.

Kula: Lit. 'clan' or 'family'; in Śaiva tantra originally indicated families of Yoginīs; later, in the yogi's body as microcosm (see Chapter 5), the highest (non-transcendental) level of divinity, sexual energy and the goddess Śakti.

kumbhaka: Breath-retention; in *haṭhayoga*, specific methods of inhalation and/or exhalation used in conjunction with breath-retention.

Kuṇḍalinī: 'She who is coiled'. The power of the divine feminine, residing within the body of the yogi.

laya: Dissolution (e.g. of the self into the deity in tantric systems).

liṅga: An aniconic representation of Śiva; the penis.

manas: The mind.

maṇḍala: 'Disc' or 'orb'; a focus for meditation; an area in which ritual is performed.

marman: A vital point within the body.

mokṣa: Liberation from the cycle of death and rebirth (see *nirvāṇa*, *kaivalya*).

mudrā: Lit. 'seal'; a gesture used in tantric ritual; a technique for manipulating the vital energies in *haṭhayoga*.

nāda: 'Resonance'; a tantric *tattva* and focus for meditation, sometimes located in the body; in *haṭhayoga*, internal sounds to be meditated upon.

nāḍī: A subtle channel in the body which carries vital energy.

Nāth: An order of householder and ascetic yogis.

nirvāṇa: Lit. 'extinction'. Liberation from death and rebirth, especially in Buddhism. See also *mokṣa*, *kaivalya*.

Pātañjala yoga: Yoga as described in Patañjali's *Yogaśāstra* (the *Pātañjalayogaśāstra*) and its commentaries.

Piṅgalā: A channel (*nāḍī*), usually located on the right side of the Suṣumnā.

pitta: One of the three *doṣas*, akin to bile.

prakṛti: The principle of matter in the Sāṃkhya philosophical system.

prāṇa: Breath, the vital energy that animates all living things; or one of five principal breaths.

prāṇāyāma: Breath-control.

pratyāhāra: Withdrawal of the senses (often included among the auxiliaries of yoga).

Purāṇa: Lit. 'old'. A category of theistic Hindu literature mainly concerned with mythological tales of gods.

puruṣa: Lit. 'person'. The principle of spirit in the Sāṃkhya philosophical system.

rajas: One of the *guṇa*s, characterized by passion and activity; alternatively, female menstrual or generative fluid (which in some yogic systems is also said to exist within men).

sādhana: (Spiritual) practice.

Śaiva: Lit. 'pertaining to Śiva'; a devotee of the god Śiva; descriptive of traditions or texts in which Śiva is the principal deity.

Śākta: Lit. pertaining to Śakti, the goddess; a devotee of the goddess; descriptive of traditions or texts in which Śakti is the principal deity.

śakti: Lit. 'power'; the divine feminine; (Śakti) a/the goddess, usually the consort of the god Śiva.

samādhi: 'Absorption'. The ultimate cognitive state of yoga.

samāna: One of the five principal 'winds' in the body.

Sāṃkhya: An ancient dualist philosophical system, which became one of the orthodox Brahmanical philosophies.

Saṃnyāsī: A renouncer; a particular ascetic order.

saṃsāra: The cycle of death and rebirth, 'cyclic existence'.

saṃyama: (In the *Pātañjalayogaśāstra*) the combined practices of fixation (*dhāraṇā*), meditation (*dhyāna*) and absorption (*samādhi*).

śastra: An instructional treatise.

sattva: One of the *guṇa*s, characterized by light and harmony.

siddha: An adept, a perfected yogi.

siddhi: 'Success' or supernatural power.

smṛti: Lit. 'that which is remembered': the corpus of Brahmanical texts transmitted by human teachers. Orthodox Brahmanical texts other than the Vedas. See *śruti*.

Śramaṇa: A type of renunciant ascetic, first attested in the fifth century BCE in north-east India.

śruti: Lit. 'that which is heard': the corpus of revealed Brahmanical texts, i.e. those that were heard by the Vedic sages. The Vedas, including the Brāhmaṇas and the Upaniṣads. See *smṛti*.

Suṣumnā: The central channel (*nāḍī*) in the body.

tamas: One of the *guṇa*s, characterized by darkness and heaviness.

tantra: A type of text; a body of knowledge, ritual and praxis regarded as distinct from – and more powerful than – Vedic revelation.

tapas: Lit. 'heat'; asceticism, in particular physical austerities.

tattva: 'Reality' or 'truth'; in metaphysics, an element or level of reality.

Terāpanthīs: A modern revivalist sect of Jainism.

udāna: One of the five principal breaths in the body.

Uḍḍiyāna: A tantric sacred site in north-west India; (*uḍḍiyāna*) a type of yogic lock.

utkrānti: Suicide by means of yoga (literally 'upward progression').

Vaiṣṇava: Lit. pertaining to Viṣṇu; a devotee of Viṣṇu; descriptive of traditions or texts in which Viṣṇu is the principal deity.

vajra: 'Thunderbolt'; a mythical weapon; name of a yoga posture.

vāta: One of the three *doṣa*s, akin to wind.

vāyu: Breath (literally 'wind').

Vrātya: A member of a male brotherhood mentioned in the *Atharva Veda*.

vyāna: One of the five principal breaths in the body.

yogāṅga: An auxiliary practice of yoga.

Yoginī: A type of tantric goddess; (*yoginī*) a female practitioner of yoga.

yoni: Female genitals; can also refer to the perineum of male yogis.

Primary Sources

Ācārāṅga Cūrṇi of Jinadāsagaṇi, ed. unknown (Ratnapur (Mālavā): Keśarīmalajī Śvetāmbar Sāhitya Saṃsthā, 1931).

Ācārāṅga Cūrṇi of Jinadāsagaṇi, ed. unknown (Suriyapuri: Śrī Jain-ānanda Mudraṇālaya, 1998).

Ācārāṅga Sūtra, in *Jaina Sūtras*, Part 1, pp. 1–213, trans. Hermann Jacobi, ed. Max Muller, Sacred Books of the East 22 (Delhi: Motilal Banarsidass, 1994 [1884]).

Amanaska, ed. Jason Birch, from 'The *Amanaska*: King of All Yogas. A Critical Edition and Annotated Translation with a Monographic Introduction', DPhil. thesis, University of Oxford, 2013.

Amaraughaprabodha of Gorakṣanātha, ed. K. Mallik, in Mallik 1954.

Amaraughaśāsana of Gorakṣanātha, ed. Pandit Mukund Rām Śāstrī, Kashmir Series of Texts and Studies 20 (Srinagar, 1918).

Amṛtasiddhi, critical edition in preparation by James Mallinson and Péter-Dániel Szántó, based on China Nationalities Library of the Cultural Palace of Nationalities S005125 (21), Maharaja Mansingh Pustak Prakash, Jodhpur, Acc. Nos. 1242 and 1243, and other witnesses.

Aṅguttaranikāya, Parts 1 and 2, ed. R. Morris (London: Pali Text Society, 1885 and 1888).

Anubhavanivedanastotra, ed. and trans. Lilian Silburn, from *Hymnes de Abhinavagupta*, Publications de l'Institut de civilisation indienne, fasc. 31 (Paris: Institut de civilisation indienne with the Centre national de la recherche scientifique, 1970).

Aparokṣānubhūti, Vidyāraṇyakṛtayā Aparokṣadīpikākhyaṭīkayā saṃvalitā, ed. Kamla Devi (Akṣayavaṭa Prakāśana, 1988).

Āpastambadharmasūtra: Based on the edition by G. Bühler, Bombay Sanskrit Series Nos. LIV and L, 3rd ed. 1932, with variant readings taken from the edition by A. Chinnaswami, Kashi Sanskrit Series No. 93, Benares 1932.

Arāīsh-i-maḥfil; or, The Ornament of the Assembly, trans. Henry Court, 2nd edn (Calcutta, 1882).*

Ariyapariyesanā Sutta in *Majjhimanikāya*, vol. 1, pp. 160–75.

Arthaśāstra, ed. R. P. Kangle (Delhi: Motilal Banarsidass, 1992). Reprinted from the second edition (Bombay University, 1969).

Aṣṭa Mudrā, p. 247 in *Gorakhbāṇī*.

Āśvalāyanaśrautasūtra, with the commentary of Gārgya Nārāyaṇa, ed. Rāmanārāyaṇa Vidyāratna, Bibliotheca Indica 49 (Calcutta: Royal Asiatic Society, 1864–74).

Atharvavedasaṃhitā, in the Śaunakīya recension with the commentary (*bhāṣya*) of Sāyaṇācārya, ed. Shankar Pândurang Pandit (Bombay: Government Central Book Depot, 1895).

Baḥr al-ḥayāt, Chapter 4, trans. Carl Ernst. Available at http://www.asia.si.edu/explore/yoga/ocean-of-life.asp.

Baudhāyana-Dharmasūtra with the 'Vivaraṇa' Commentary by Śrī Govinda Svāmī, ed. Umeśa Candra Pāṇḍeya with critical notes by M. M. A. Chinnasvāmī Śāstrī (Varanasi: Chowkhamba Sanskrit Series Office, 1972).

Bhagavadgītā, ed. and trans. J. A. B. van Buitenen in *The Bhagavadgītā in the Mahābhārata: Text and Translation* (Chicago: University of Chicago Press, 1981).

Bhāgavatapurāṇa, ed. Vasudeva Śarman (Bombay: Nirnaya Sagar, 1905).

Bhartṛharinirveda, see Gray 1904.

Bodhasāra: An Eighteenth Century Sanskrit Treasure by Narahari, ed. and trans. Jennifer Cover and Grahame Cover with contributions from Kanchan V. Mande (Charleston: CreateSpace, 2010).

Brahmasiddhi by Ācārya Maṇḍanamiśra with Commentary by Śaṅkhapāṇi, ed. Kuppuswami Sastri. Madras Government Oriental Manuscripts Series 4. (Madras, 1937).

Brahmasūtrabhāṣya, in Vācaspatimiśra, *The Bhāmatī of Vācaspati on Śaṅkara's Brahmasūtrabhāṣya (Catussūtrī)*, ed. and trans. Chittenjoor Kunhan Raja and S. S. Sūryanārāyaṇa Śāstrī (Adyar: Theosophical Publishing House, 1933).

Brahmayāmalatantra or *Picumata*: Chapters 1, 2, 5, 73 and 99, ed. and trans. Shaman Hatley in 'The *Brahmayāmalatantra* and Early Śaiva Cult of Yoginīs', PhD dissertation, University of Pennsylvania, 2007; Chapters 3, 21 and 45, ed. and trans. Csaba Kiss in *The Brahmayāmalatantra or Picumata*, Vol. 2: *The Religious Observances and Sexual Rituals of the Tantric Practitioner* (Pondicherry: Institut français de

* The Urdu text is published as the *Arayish-i maḥfil* of Shir 'Ali Khan Afsus, ed. Kalb 'Alī Khān Fā'iq, Urdū kā Klāsikī Adab 31 (Lahore, 1963).

Pondichéry/Paris: École française d'Extrême-Orient/Hamburg: Asien-Afrika-Institut, Universität Hamburg, 2015).

Bṛhadāraṇyaka Upaniṣad, in Olivelle 1998.

Bṛhadāraṇyakopaniṣat, with the *bhāṣya* attributed to Śaṇkara, ed. S. Subrahmanya Shastri (Varanasi: Mahesh Research Institute, 1986).

Bṛhadyogiyājñavalkyasmṛti, ed. Swami Kuvalayananda and Pandit Raghunathashastri Kokaje (Lonavla: Kaivalyadhāma S. M. Y. M. Samiti, 1976).

Bṛhatkhecarīprakāśa, Scindia Oriental Research Institute Library (Ujjain) manuscript no. 14575.

Buddhacarita of Aśvaghoṣa, see Johnson 1972 [1936].

Candrāvalokana, Government Oriental Manuscripts Library, Madras, manuscript no. D 4345.

Chāndogya Upaniṣad, in Olivelle 1998.

Chos drug gi man ngag zhes bya ba ('The Oral Instruction of the Six Yogas') by Mahasiddha Tilopa, in Mullin, 2006 [1997], pp. 23–30.

Cūḷavedalla Sutta, in *Majjhimanikāya*, vol. 1, pp. 209–305.

Dattātreyayogaśāstra, working edition by James Mallinson, based on *Dattātreyayogaśāstra*, ed. Brahmamitra Avasthī (Delhi: Svāmī Keśavānanda Yoga Saṃsthāna, 1982), and on the following manuscripts: Maharaja Man Singh Pustak Prakash no. 1936, Wai Prajñā Pāṭhaśālā 6/4–399 and 6163, Baroda Oriental Institute 4107, Mysore Government Oriental Manuscripts Library 4369 and Thanjavur Palace Library B6390.

Dharmaputrikā, ed. Anil Kumar Acharya and Nirajan Kafle. Forthcoming.

Dighanikāya, vol. 1, ed. T. W. Rhys Davids and J. Estlin Carpenter (London: Pali Text Society, 1890).

Fawā'id al-fu'ād of Amīr Hasan Dehlavī (Lahore, 1966).

Gheraṇḍasaṃhitā, ed. and trans. James Mallinson (New York: YogaVidya.com, 2004).

Gorakhbāṇī, ed. P. D. Baḍathvāl (Prayāg: Hindī Sāhity Sammelan, 1960).

Gorakṣa Bijaẏ, see Ondračka 2011.

Gorakṣaśata, ed. and trans. Fausta Nowotny (Cologne: K. A. Nowotny, 1976).

Gorakṣaśataka, Government Oriental Manuscripts Library, Madras, manuscript no. R 7874.

Gorakṣavijaya of Vidyāpati, ed. Harimohan Miśra (Paṭnā: Bihār Rāṣṭrabhāṣā Pariṣad, 1984).

Haṃsavilāsa of Haṃsamiṭṭhu, ed. Swami Trivikrama Tirtha and Mahamahopadhyaya Hathibhai Shastri of Jamnagar, Gaekwad's Oriental Series 81 (Baroda: Oriental Institute, 1937).

Haribhaktivilāsa of Gopāla Bhaṭṭa Gosvāmin, with *Digdarśiṇī ṭīkā* of Sanātana Gosvāmin, 2 vols, ed. Haridāsa Śāstri (Vṛndāvana: Śrī Gadādhara Gaurahari Press, 1986).

Haṭhābhyāsapaddhati, manuscript no. 46/440 in the collection of the Bhārat Itihās Saṃśodhak Maṇḍal, Pune. Catalogued as *Āsanayogaḥ*.

Haṭhapradīpikā, Long Recension: *Haṭhapradīpikā Siddhāntamuktāvalī*, manuscript no. 6756 at Maharaja Man Singh Pustak Prakash, Jodhpur.

Haṭhapradīpikā of Svātmārāma, ed. Svāmī Digambarjī and Dr Pītāmbar Jhā (Lonavla: Kaivalyadhāma S. M. Y. M. Samiti, 1970).

Haṭhapradīpikājyotsnā of Brahmānanda, ed. Svāmī Maheśānanda, Dr Bāburām Śarmā, Jñānaśaṃkar Sahāy and Ravindranāth Bodhe (Lonavla: Kaivalyadhāma S. M. Y. M. Samiti, 2002).

Haṭharatnāvalī of Śrīnivāsayogī, ed. M. L. Gharote, P. Devnath and V. K. Jha (Lonavla: Lonavla Yoga Institute, 2002).

Haṭhasaṃketacandrikā, unpublished edition by Jason Birch based on Mysore Government Oriental Library manuscript no. R3239, ff. 165v–166r and Man Singh Pustak Prakash manuscript no. 2255, ff. 83r–83v.

Haṭhatatvakaumudī: A Treatise on Haṭhayoga by Sundaradeva, ed. M. L. Gharote, Parimal Devnath and Vijay Kant Jha (Lonavla: Lonavla Yoga Institute, 2007).

Ḥawż al-ḥayāt, unpublished translation by Carl Ernst, based on a collation of twenty-five manuscripts.

Hevajratantra, ed. David L. Snellgrove, in *The Hevajra Tantra: A Critical Study*, Part 2: *Sanskrit and Tibetan Texts* (London: Oxford University Press, 1959).

Īśvaragītā, in *Kūrmapurāṇa*, ed. A. S. Gupta (Varanasi: All-India Kashiraj Trust, 1967).

Jātaka, ed. V. Faussell, 4 vols (London: Trübner & Co., 1877–87).

Jayadrathayāmala, National Archives, Kathmandu, manuscript no. 1–1468. Nepal–German Manuscript Preservation Project reel no. B 122/4.

Jayākhyasaṃhitā, ed. Embar Krishnamacharya (Baroda: Oriental Institute, 1957).

Jīvanmuktiviveka, ed. and trans. Robert Goodding, in 'The Treatise on Liberation-in-Life: Critical Edition and Annotated Translation of the *Jīvanmuktiviveka* of Vidyāraṇya', PhD thesis, University of Texas, 2002.

(Śrī)-Jñāneśvarī of Jñānadeva, ed. G. S. Naṇadīkar, 5 vols (Mumbai: Prakāś Gopāl Naṇadīkar, 2001).

Jogpradīpakā of Jayatarāma, ed. M. L. Gharote (Jodhpur: Rajasthan Oriental Research Institute, 1999).

Kathāsaritsāgara of Somadevabhaṭṭa, ed. Pandit Durgāprasāda and Kāśīnātha Pāṇḍuraṅga Paraba (Bombay: Nirnaya Sāgara Press, 1889).

Kaṭhopaniṣad, in Olivelle 1998.

Kaulajñānanirṇaya, ed. Prabodh Chandra Bagchi, in *Kaulajñānanirṇaya and Some Minor Texts of the School of Matsyendranātha* (Calcutta: Metropolitan Printing and Publishing House, 1934).

Kevaddha Sutta, in *Dīghanikāya*, vol. 1, pp. 211–23.
Khecarīvidyā: *The Khecarīvidyā of Ādinātha: A Critical Edition and Annotated Translation of an Early Text of Haṭhayoga*, ed. and trans. James Mallinson (London: Routledge, 2007).
Kubjikāmatatantra, Kulālikāmnāya version, ed. T. Goudriaan and J. A. Schoterman (Leiden: E. J. Brill, 1988).
Kumārasambhava with the Commentary of Mallinātha, ed. Narayana Bhatta Parvanikar and Kashinatha Panduranga Parab, 2nd, rev. edn (Bombay: Nirnaya Sagara Press, 1886).
Kumbhakapaddhati of Raghuvīra, ed. M. L. Gharote and Parimal Devnath (Lonavla: Lonavla Yoga Institute, 2005).
Kuṭṭanīmatam of Dāmodaragupta, ed. Csaba Dezső and Dominic Goodall (Groningen: Egbert Forsten, 2012).
Lallā-Vākyāni: or, The Wise Sayings of Lal Ded, A Mystic Poetess of Ancient Kashmir, ed. and trans. George Grierson and Lionel D. Barnett (London: Royal Asiatic Society, 1920).
Liṅgapurāṇa, Gurumandal Series 15 (Calcutta, 1960).
Mahābhārata: *The Mahābhārata: For the First Time Critically Edited*, 19 vols, ed. V. S. Sukthankar (1927–43) and S. K. Belvalkar (from 1943), with the co-operation of Shrimant Balasaheb Pant Pratinidhi, S. K. Belvalkar, R. N. Dandekar, S. K. De, F. Edgerton, A. B. Gajendragadkar, P. V. Kane, R. D. Karmakar, V. G. Paranjpe, V. K. Rajavade, N. B. Utgikar, P. L. Vaidya, V. P. Vaidya, Raghu Vira, M. Winternitz, R. Zimmerman, et al. (Poona: Bhandarkar Oriental Research Institute, 1933–66).*
Mahābhāratam: With the Commentary of Nīlakaṇṭha, ed. R. Kiṃjavaḍekara, 6 vols (Poona: Chitrashala Press, 1929–36).
Mahākālasaṃhitā of Ādinātha, *Guhyakālīkhaṇḍa*, ed. Kiśoranāth Jhā, 3 vols (Allahabad: Gaṅgānāth Jhā Kendrīya Saṃskṛta Vidyāpīṭha, 1976, 1977, 1979).
Mahāsaccaka Sutta, in *Majjhimanikāya*, vol. 1, pp. 237–51.
Majjhimanikāya, vol. 1, ed. V. Trenckner (London: Pali Text Society, 1888).
Majjhimanikāya, vol. 3, ed. R. Chalmers (London: Luzac and Co. (for the Pali Text Society), 1967).
Mālinīvijayottaratantra, *adhikāra*s 1–4, 7 and 11–17, ed. Somdeva Vasudeva, in Vasudeva 2004.
Mālinīvijayottaratantra, ed. Madhusūdan Kaul Śāstrī, Kashmir Series of Texts and Studies 37 (Srinagar, 1922).

* We have used the critical edition (and its numbering), but have occasionally silently emended to the readings used by the sixteenth-century commentator Nīlakaṇṭha (and have occasionally drawn on his commentary in our translations).

Mānavadharmaśāstra: Manusmṛti with the Sanskrit Commentary Manvartha-muktāvalī of Kullūka Bhaṭṭa, ed. N. L.Shastri (Delhi: Motilal Banarsidass, 1983).

Mañjuśriyamūlakalpa: *The Âryamanjusrîmûlakalpa*, 3 vols, ed. T. Gaṇapati Sâstrî, Trivandrum Sanskrit Series 70, 76 and 84 (Trivandrum, 1920, 1922 and 1925).

Mantrarājarahasyam of Śrīsiṃhatilakasūri, ed. Acharya Jina Vijaya Muni (Bombay: Bharatiya Vidya Bhavan, 1980).

Mārkaṇḍeyapurāṇa, ed. K. M. Banerjea (Calcutta: Bishop's College Press, 1862).

Mataṅgapārameśvarāgama, with the commentary (*vṛtti*) of Bhaṭṭa Rāmakaṇṭha: *Mataṅgapārameśvarāgama (Vidyāpāda) avec le commentaire de Bhaṭṭa Rāmakaṇṭha*, ed. N. R. Bhatt, Publications de l'Institut français d'Indologie [IFI] 56 (Pondicherry: IFI, 1977).

Mataṅgapārameśvarāgama, *kriyāpāda*, *caryāpāda* and *yogapāda*, with the commentary (*vṛtti*) of Bhaṭṭa Rāmakaṇṭha up to *kriyāpāda* 11.12b: *Mataṅgapārameśvarāgama (Kriyāpāda, Yogapāda et Caryāpāda) avec le commentaire de Bhaṭṭa Rāmakaṇṭha*, ed. N. R. Bhatt, Publications de l'Institut français d'Indologie [IFI] 65 (Pondicherry: IFI, 1982).

Matsyendrasaṃhitā, ed. and trans. Csaba Kiss, Chapters 1–13 and 55, (thesis, University of Oxford, 2009). See Kiss 2009.

Miragāvatī of Kutubana: Avadhī text with critical notes, ed. D. F. Plukker (thesis, Universiteit van Amsterdam, 1981).

Mokṣopāya/Yogavāsiṣṭha: *Bhāskarakaṇṭha's Mokṣopāya-ṭīkā: A Commentary on the Earliest Available Recension of the Yogavāsiṣṭha. I, Vairāgyaprakaraṇam*, ed. Jürgen Hanneder and Walter Slaje, Geisteskultur Indiens 1, Indologica Halensis (Aachen: Shaker, 2002).

Mṛgendratantra: *Mṛgendrāgama (Kriyāpāda et Caryāpāda) avec le commentaire de Bhaṭṭa-Nārāyaṇakaṇṭha*, ed. N. R. Bhatt, Publications de l'Institut français d'Indologie [IFI] 23 (Pondicherry: IFI, 1962).

Muṇḍaka Upaniṣad, in Olivelle 1998.

Nādabindūpaniṣad, in *Yoga Upaniṣads*.

Netratantra, with the commentary (*uddyota*) by Kṣemarāja, ed. Madhusūdan Kaul Śāstrī, Kashmir Series of Texts and Studies 46 (Srinagar, 1926).

Niśvāsatattvasaṃhitā: *The Earliest Surviving Śaiva Tantra*, vol. 1: *A Critical Edition and Annotated Translation of the Mūlasūtra, Uttarasūtra and Nayasūtra*, ed. Dominic Goodall in collaboration with Alexis Sanderson and Harunaga Isaacson (Pondichéry: Institut français de Pondicherry/Paris: École française d'Extrême-Orient/Hamburg: Asien-Afrika-Institut, Universität Hamburg, 2015).

Padārthadharmasaṃgraha of Praśastapāda, with Śrīdhara's *Nyāyakandalī*, ed. D. Jh. Sarma (Varanasi, 1963).

Pādmasaṃhitā (Part 1), ed. S. Padmanabhan and R. N. Sampath (Madras: Pancaratra Parisodhana Pariṣad, 1974).

Parākhyatantra, ed. and trans. Dominic Goodall (Pondicherry: Publications de l'Institut français d'Indologie 98, 2004).

Paramokṣanirāsakārikāvṛtti, ed. Alex Watson, Dominic Goodall and S. L. P. Anjaneya Sarma (Pondicherry: Publications de l'Institut français d'Indologie 122, 2013).

Pāśupatasūtra (= *Pañcārtha*), with the commentary (*Pañcārthabhāṣya*) of Bhagavat Kauṇḍinya, ed. R. Anantakrishna Sastri, Trivandrum Sanskrit Series 143 (Trivandrum: University of Travancore, 1940).

Pātañjalayogaśāstra, ed. Kāśinātha Śāstrī Āgāśe: *Vācaspatimiśraviracitaṭīkāsaṃvalitavyāsabhāṣyasametāni Pātañjalayogasūtrāṇi, tathā bhojadevaviracitarājamārtaṇḍābhidhavṛttisametāni pātañjalayogasūtrāṇi. sūtrapāṭhasūtravarṇānukramasūcībhyāṃ ca sanāthīkṛtāni* [. . .], (Pune: Ānandāśramamudraṇālaye, 47, 1904).

Pātañjalayogaśāstravivaraṇa: *Pātañjala-Yogasūtra-Bhāṣya-Vivaraṇa of Śaṅkara-Bhagavatpāda*, critically edited with introduction by Polakam Sri Rama Sastri and S. R Krishnamurthi Sastri. (Madras: Government Oriental Manuscript Library, 94, 1952) See also Harimoto 2014.

Pātravidhi, ed. and trans. Diwakar Acharya, in 'The Pātravidhi: A Lakulīśa Pāśupata Manual on Purification and Use of the Initiate's Vessel', in *Saṃskṛta-sādhutā, Goodness of Sanskrit: Studies in Honour of Professor Ashok N. Aklujkar*, ed. C. Watanabe, M. Desmarais and Y. Honda (New Delhi: D. K. Printworld, 2011), pp. 1–28.

Rājayogāmṛta, part of the *Rājayogasiddhāntarahasya* in an unnumbered manuscript in the collection of the Wai Prajñāpāṭhaśālā.

Rāmāyaṇa: *The Vālmīki-Rāmāyaṇa: Critically Edited for the First Time*, 7 vols, ed. G. H. Bhatt, P. L. Vaidya, P. C. Divanji, D. R. Mankad, G. C. Jhala, Umakant Premanand Shah (Baroda: Oriental Institute, 1960–75).

The Reḥla of Ibn Baṭṭūṭa, ed. and trans. Mahdi Husain (Baroda: Oriental Institute, 1953).

Rtsa rlung gsang ba'i lde mig ('The Secret Key to the Channels and Winds'), a chapter from Pema Lingpa's 'Compendium of Enlightened Spontaneity' (*Rdzogs chen kun bzang dgongs 'dus*), translated in Baker 2012.

Rudrayāmalatantra, ed. Sudhakar Malaviya. Published on the website of the Muktabodha Indological Research Institute: www.muktabodha.org (20 September 2011).

Saccavibhaṅga Sutta, in *Majjhimanikāya*, vol. 3, pp. 248–53.

Saddharmasmṛtyupasthānasūtra, ed. Daniel M. Stuart, in *A Less Traveled Path: Saddharmasmṛtyupasthānasūtra, Chapter 2. Critically Edited with a Study on Its Structure and Significance for the Development of Buddhist Meditation*, 2 vols (Beijing: China Tibetology Publishing House/Vienna: Austrian Academy of Sciences Press, 2015).

Sāmbapañcāśikā, with the commentary of Kṣemarāja, ed. Paṇḍit Kedārnātha and Wāsudeva Laxmaṇ Shāstrī Paṇashīkar, Kāvyamālā 13 (Bombay, 1910).

Sanatkumārasaṃhitā, ed. V. Krishnamacharya and Venkatarama Raghavan (Madras: Adyar Library, 1969).

Saṅgītaratnākara of Śārṅgadeva, with the *Kalānidhi* of Kallinātha and the *Saṃgītasudhākara* of Siṃhabhūpāla, ed. S. Subrahmanya Sastri, 2nd edn ed. V. Krishnamacharya (Madras: Adyar Library and Research Centre, 1976 [1959]).

Śaṅkaradigvijaya of Śrīvidyāraṇya, Ānandāśrama Sanskrit Series 22 (Poona: Ānandāśramamudraṇālaye, 1891).

Śāradātilakam of Lakṣmaṇadeśikendra, *paṭala* 25, ed. G. Bühnemann. See Bühnemann 2011.

Śārṅgadharapaddhati, ed. Peter Peterson (Bombay: Government Central Book Depot, 1888).

Sarvajñānottara Yogapāda, ed. K. Ramachandra Sarma and revised by R. Thangaswami Sarma, *Adyar Library Bulletin* 62, pp. 181–231 (1998, appeared 1999).

Sarvāṅgayogapradīpikā, in *Sundar-granthāvalī*, ed. Purohit Hari N. Śarmā (Calcutta, 1936).

Satipaṭṭhāna Sutta, in *Majjhimanikāya*, vol. 1, pp. 55–63.

Ṣaṭkarmasaṃgraha, ed. and trans R. G. Harshe (Lonavla: Kaivalyadhāma, 1970).

Sekha Sutta, in *Majjhimanikāya* vol. 1, pp. 353–59.

Siddhānt Paṭal bhāṣā ṭīkā sahit (Ṭhākur Prasād eṇḍ sans bukselar [i.e. 'and sons bookseller'], Rājā Darvāzā, Vārāṇasī, n.d.).

Siddhasiddhāntapaddhati of Gorakṣanātha, ed. M. L. Gharote and G. K. Pai (Lonavla: Lonavla Yoga Institute, 2005).

Siddhayogeśvarīmata, ed. Judit Törzsök, DPhil thesis, University of Oxford, 1999.

Śivasaṃhitā, ed. and trans. J. Mallinson (New York: YogaVidya.com, 2007).

Śivasvarodaya, in *Svar Yog* by Svāmī Satyānand Sarasvatī (Muṅger: Bihār Yog Vidyālay Yoga Publications Trust, 2006).

Śivayoga(pra)dīpikā of Sadāśivayogin, ed. the paṇḍits of the Ānandāśrama and Hari Nārāyaṇa Āpṭe (Madras: Ānandāśrama, 1907).*

Skandapurāṇa, ed. Kṛṣṇaprasāda Bhaṭṭarāī (*Skandapurāṇasya Ambikākhaṇḍaḥ*) (Kathmandu: Mahendrasaṃskṛtaviśvavidyālayaḥ, 1988).

Spandakārikā, with the commentary (*vivṛti*) of Rāmakaṇṭha, ed. J. C. Chatterji, Kashmir Series of Texts and Studies 6 (Srinagar, 1913).

Spandasaṃdoha of Kṣemarāja, Kashmir Series of Texts and Studies 16 (Srinagar, 1917).

Śrītattvanidhi, see Sjoman 1996.

Sthānāṅgasūtra, ed. Muni Jambūvijaya, Jaina Āgama Series 3 (Bombay: Mahāvīra Jaina Vidyālaya, 1985).

Svacchandatantra, ed. M. Kaul Shāstrī, *The Svacchanda Tantram, with Commentary by Kshemarāja*, 6 vols, Kashmir Series of Texts and Studies 31, 38, 44, 48, 51 (vol. 5a), 51 (vol. 5b), 56 (Bombay: The Research Department of Jammu and Kashmir State, 1921–35).

Śvetāśvatara Upaniṣad, in Olivelle 1998.

Taittirīya Āraṇyaka, ed. Subramania Sarma, Chennai 2004, based on Grantha manuscripts and on *The Taittiriya Aranyaka*, 3 vols in one, ed. A. Mahadeva Sastri et al. (Delhi: Motilal Banarsidass, 1985). www.sanskritweb.net/yajurveda/#TA.

Tantravārttika of Kumārila Bhaṭṭa, in *Śrīmajjaiminipraṇīte Mīmāṃsādarśane*, 2 vols, ed. K. V. Abhayaṅkara and G. Jośī (Pune: Ānandāśrama, 1970).

Tashrīh al-Aqvāṃ, British Library APAC Add. 27255.

Tirumandiram, ed. T. N. Ganapathy, 7 vols, Yoga Siddha Research Center Publication Series (Quebec: Babaji's Kriya Yoga and Publications, 2010).

Vaikhānasadharmasūtra, ed. K. Rangachari, Ramanujachari Oriental Institute Publication 3 (Madras: Diocesan Press, 1930).

Vairocanābhisaṃbodhi Sūtra, see Giebel 2005.

Vaiśeṣikasūtra, with the commentary of Praśastapāda, see Wezler 1982 and Isaacson 1993.

Vajrāvalī of Abhayākaragupta, ed. Masahide Mori, 2 vols, Buddhica Britannica Series Continua XI (Tring, UK: The Institute of Buddhist Studies, 2009).

Vajravārāhī Sādhana, ed. Elizabeth English, in English 2002, pp. 225–314.

* This edition of the text calls it the *Śivayogadīpikā*, but all its manuscript witnesses and citations call it the *Śivayogapradīpikā*, so we refer to it as such. We thank Seth Powell for alerting us to the discrepancy (personal communication, 12 October 2016.)

Vasiṣṭhasaṃhitā (Yogakāṇḍa), ed. Swami Digambarji, Pitambar Jha, Gyan Shankar Sahay (first edition); Swami Maheshananda, B. R. Sharma, G. S. Sahay, R. K. Bodhe (revised edition) (Lonavla: Kaivalyadhāma Śrīmanmādhav Yogamandir Samiti, 2005).

Vāyavīyasaṃhitā of the *Śivapurāṇa*, unpublished edition by Christèle Barois.

Vāyupurāṇa (Revākhaṇḍa), ed. (as *Śrīskandamahāpurāṇam*) Kṣemrāj Śrīkṛṣṇadās (Bombay: Veṅkateśvara Steam Press, 1910).

Vāyupurāṇa, see Grönbold 1996, p. 4.

Vijñānabhairava, ed. and trans. J. Singh (Delhi: Motilal Banarsidass, 1979).

Vimalaprabhā: Śrīmañjuśrīyaśoviracitasya Paramādibuddhoddhṛtasya Śrīlaghukālacakratantrarājasya Kalkinā Śrīpuṇḍarīkeṇa viracitā ṭikā, ed. Samdhong Rinpoche et al., Rare Buddhist Texts Series 13, vol. 3, 1994.

Vimānārcanākalpa, ed. Raghunāthacakravārtin and Setu Mādhavācārya (Madras: Venkateshwar Press, 1926).

Vīṇāśikhatantra, ed. T. Goudriaan, in *Vīṇāśikhatantra: A Śaiva Tantra of the Left Current. Edited with an Introducation and Translation* (Delhi: Motilal Banarsidass, 1985).

Viṣṇupurāṇa: *The Critical Edition of the Viṣṇupurāṇam*, 2 vols, ed. M. M. Pathak (Vadodara: Oriental Institute, 1997 and 1999).

Viṣṇusaṃhitā, ed. Gaṇapati Śāstrī (Trivandrum: Trivandrum Sanskrit Series, 1925).

Visuddhimagga of Buddhaghosa, see Warren and Kosambi 1989 [1950].

Vivekamārtaṇḍa of Gorakṣadeva, Oriental Institute of Baroda Library, Acc. no. 4110.

Yogabīja, ed. Rām Lāl Śrīvāstav (Gorakhpur: Śrī Gorakhnāth Mandir, 1982).*

Yogacintāmaṇi of Godāvaramiśra, see Gode 1954.

Yogacintāmaṇi of Śivānanda Sarasvatī, manuscript no. 9784, Kaivalyadhāma Yoga Institute Library, Lonavla.

Yogamārgaprakāśikā of Yugaladāsa, ed. Giridhara Śāstrī (Bombay: Venkateshvar Steam Press, 1904).

Yogasārasaṃgraha of Vijñānabhikṣu, edited and translated by Gaṅgānātha Jhā (Bombay: Tattva-Vivechaka Press, 1894).

Yogaśāstra of Hemacandra, ed. and trans. Olle Qvarnström, Harvard Oriental Series 60 (Cambridge, MA: Harvard University Press, 2002).

Yogaśāstra and *Svopajñavṛtti* of Hemacandra, ed. Muni Jambūvijaya, 3 vols (Bombay: Jain Sāhitya Vikāsa Maṇḍala, 1971, 1981 and 1986).

* We have also used readings from Nepal–German Manuscript Preservation Project manuscript A-0939-19.

Yogaśataka of Haribhadrasūri, with auto-commentary along with his *Brahmasiddhāntasamuccaya*, ed. Munirāja Śrī Puṇyavijayajī, Lalbhai Dalpatbhai Series 4, Bhāratīya Saṃskṛti Vidyāmandira (Ahmedabad: Bhāratīya Saṃskṛti Vidyāmandira, 1965).

Yogaśikhā Upaniṣad, see *Yoga Upaniṣads*.

Yogatārāvalī, working edition by Jason Birch based on multiple editions and manuscripts.

Yoga Upaniṣads, with the commentary of Śrī Upaniṣadbrahmayogin, ed. Pandit A. Mahadeva Sastri (Madras: Adyar Library and Research Centre, 1968).

Yogavāsiṣṭha, see *Mokṣopāya*.

Yogayājñavalkya, ed. P. C. Divanji (Bombay: Royal Asiatic Society, 1954).

Secondary Literature

Acharya, Diwakar. 2008. Major Points of Vācaspati's Disagreement with Maṇḍana. *Logic and Belief in Indian Philosophy.* Warsaw Indological Studies 3: 421–33.

————. 2013. 'NÉTI NÉTI: Meaning and Function of an Enigmatic Phrase in the Gārgya-Ajātaśatru Dialogue of *Bṛhadāraṇyaka Upaniṣad* II.1 and II.3. *Indo-Iranian Journal* 56: 3–39.

Alter, Joseph S. 2004. *Yoga in Modern India: The Body between Science and Philosophy.* Princeton: Princeton University Press.

Angot, Michel. 2012 [2008]. *Le* Yoga-Sūtra *de Patañjali et le* Yoga-Bhāṣya *de Vyāsa: La parole sur le silence.* Paris: Les Belles Lettres. 2nd, corrected and expanded edition.

Ashby, Muata. 2005. *Egyptian Yoga: Postures of the Gods and Goddesses. The Ancient Egyptian System of Physical Postures for Health, Meditation and Spiritual Enlightenment and the Ancient Egyptian Origins of Hatha Yoga.* Miami: Sema Institute.

Aurobindo, Sri. 1914–20 [1998]. *The Secret of the Veda.* In *The Complete Works of Sri Aurobindo*, Vol. 15. Pondicherry: Sri Aurobindo Ashram.

Avalon, Arthur [Sir John Woodroffe] (ed. and trans). 1919. *The Serpent Power: Being the Shaṯ-chakra-nirûpaṉa and Pâdukâ-panchaka. Two Works on Tantrik Yoga.* London: Luzac & Co.

Baker, Ian A. 2012. Embodying Enlightenment: Physical Culture in Dzogchen as Revealed in Tibet's Lukhang Murals. *Asian Medicine* 7: 225–64.

————. 2015. Tibetan Yoga: Somatic Practice in Vajrayāna Buddhism and Dzogchen. Draft of a chapter to be published in Philipp A. Maas and Karin Preisendanz (eds.), *Yoga in Transformation: Historical and Contemporary Perspectives on a Global Phenomenon.* Vienna: V&R Unipress (in the series 'Wiener Forum für Theologie und Religionswissenschaft').

Bansat-Boudon, Lyne. 2013. The Contribution of Nondual Śaivism of Kashmir to the Debate on *Jīvanmukti*: A Thematic Perspective on the

Question of Periodization. In Eli Franco (ed.), *Periodization and Historiography of Indian Philosophy*. Publications of the De Nobili Research Library 37. Vienna: Sammlung de Nobili, Institut für Südasien-, Tibet- und Buddhismuskunde der Universität Wien, pp. 53–90.

Barois, Christèle. 2012. Texte révisé de la *Vāyavīyasaṃhitā* à partir des éditions de Calcutta (1890) et de Bénarès (1963, 1998) du *Śivapurāṇa*. Vol. 3 of the thesis dissertation 'La *Vāyavīyasaṃhitā*: Doctrine et rituels śivaïtes en contexte *purāṇique*', Université Paris-III–Sorbonne nouvelle, Paris.

———. Unpublished paper. On a list of sixty-four *guṇa*s in Purāṇic literature.

Bedekar, V. M. 1959. The *Mokṣadharma* Studies: The Place and Functions of the Psychical Organism. *Annals of the Bhandarkar Oriental Research Institute* 40: 262–88.

———. 1962a. The *Dhyānayoga* in the *Mahābhārata* (XII 188). *Bhāratīya Vidyā* 20–21 (1960–61): 116–25.

———. 1962b. *Dhāraṇā* and *Codanā* in the *Mokṣadharmaparvan* of the *Mahābhārata* in Their Relation with the *Yogasūtras*. *Bhāratīya Vidyā* 22: 25–32.

———. 1963. The place of *Japa* in the *Mokṣadharmaparvan* (Mbh 12.189–93) and the *Yoga Sūtras*: A Comparative Study. *Annals of the Bhandarkar Oriental Research Institute* 44: 63–74.

———. 1968. Yoga in the *Mokṣadharmaparvan* of the *Mahābhārata*. In *Beiträge zur Geistesgeschichte Indiens. Festschrift für Erich Frauwallner. Wiener Zeitschrift für die Kunde Süd- und Ostasiens und Archiv für indische Philosophie* 12–13 (1968–9), pp. 43–52.

Bigger, Andreas, Rita Krajnc, Annemarie Mertens, Markus Schüpbach and Heinz Werner Wessler (eds.). 2010. *Release from Life – Release in Life: Indian Perspectives on Individual Liberation*. Bern and New York: Peter Lang.

Birch, Jason. 2013. The *Amanaska*: King of All Yogas. A Critical Edition and Annotated Translation with a Monographic Introduction. DPhil thesis, Balliol College, University of Oxford.

———. Forthcoming. Did Āyurveda Influence Medieval Yoga Traditions? Preliminary Remarks on their Shared Terminology, Theory and Praxis.

Birch, Jason and Jacqueline Hargreaves. 2014. Yoganidrā: An Understanding of the History and Context. http://theluminescent.blogspot.co.uk/2015/01/yoganidra.html.

Bloomfield, Maurice. 1917. On the Art of Entering Another's Body: A Hindu Fiction Motif. *Proceedings of the American Philosophical Society*, 56 (1): 1–43.

Bouillier, Véronique. 2008. *Itinérance et vie monastique: Les ascètes Nāth Yogīs en Inde contemporaine*. Paris: Éditions de la Maison des sciences de l'homme.

Bouy, Christian. 1994. *Les Nātha-yogin et les Upaniṣads: Étude d'histoire de la littérature hindoue*. Paris: de Boccard.

Braid, James. 1850. *Observations on Trance: or, Human Hybernation*. London: John Churchill.

Briggs, G. W. 1989 [1938]. *Gorakhnāth and the Kānphaṭa Yogīs*. Delhi: Motilal Banarsidass.

Brockington, John. 2003. Yoga in the *Mahābhārata*. In Ian Whicher and David Carpenter (eds.), *Yoga: The Indian Tradition*. London and New York: RoutledgeCurzon, pp. 13–24.

Bronkhorst, Johannes. 1981. Yoga and Seśvara Sāṃkhya. *Journal of Indian Philosophy* 9: 309–20.

————. 1985. Patañjali and the Yoga Sūtras. *Studien zur Indologie und Iranistik* 10: 191–212.

————. 1993. *The Two Traditions of Meditation in Ancient India*. Delhi: Motilal Banarsidass.

————. 2007. *Greater Magadha: Studies in the Culture of Early India*. Handbook of Oriental Studies, Section Two, India, Vol. 19. Leiden: Brill.

————. 2011a. The Brāhmaṇical Contribution to Yoga. In 'Contextualizing the History of Yoga in Geoffrey Samuel's *The Origins of Yoga and Tantra*: A Review Symposium'. *International Journal of Hindu Studies* 15 (3): 303–57, at 318–22.

————. 2011b. *Buddhism in the Shadow of Brahmanism*. Leiden: Brill.

Brunner, Hélène. 1994. The Place of Yoga in the Śaivāgamas. In P.-S. Filliozat, S. P. Narang and C. P. Bhatta (eds.), *Pandit N. R. Bhatt: Felicitation Volume*. Delhi: Motilal Banarsidass, pp. 425–61.

Brunner-Lachaux, Hélène (ed. and trans.). 1977. *Somaśambhupaddhati: Troisième partie*. Pondicherry: Institut français d'Indologie.

Bühnemann, Gudrun. 2011. The *Śāradātilakatantra* on Yoga: A New Edition and Translation of Chapter 25. *Bulletin of SOAS* 74 (2): 205–35.

Burchett, Patton. 2012. My Miracle Trumps Your Magic: Encounters with *Yogīs* in Sufi and *Bhakti* Hagiographical Literature. In Knut A. Jacobsen (ed.), *Yoga Powers*. Leiden: Brill, pp. 345–80.

Campbell, Joseph. 1953 [1949]. *The Hero with a Thousand Faces*. New York: Pantheon Books.

Chandik, Bissessur Nath. 1898. *The Second or the Last Elements of the Yoga*. Madras: Hoe & Co.

Chaoul, M. A. 2006. Magical Movements (*'phrul 'khor*): Ancient Yogic Practices in the Bön Religion and Contemporary Medical Perspectives. Rice University, Houston, dissertation.

———. 2007. Magical Movement (*'phrul 'khor*): Ancient Tibetan Yogic Practices from the Bön Religion and their Migration into Contemporary Medical Settings. *Asian Medicine: Tradition and Modernity* 3 (1): 130–55.

Colas, Gérard. 1988. Le yoga de l'officiant Vaikhanasa. *Journal Asiatique* 276 (3–4): 245–83.

Coward, Harold. 1982. Review of *Theravada Meditation: The Buddhist Transformation of Yoga* by Winston L. King. *Philosophy East and West* 32 (4): 463–5.

Davidson, Ronald M. 2002. *Indian Esoteric Buddhism: A Social History of the Tantric Movement*. New York: Columbia University Press.

de la Vallée Poussin, Louis. 1937a. Le Bouddhisme et le Yoga de Patañjali. *Mélanges chinois et bouddhiques* 5: 223–42.

———. 1937b. Musīla et Nārada. *Mélanges chinois et bouddhiques* 5: 189–222.

De Michelis, Elizabeth. 2004. *A History of Modern Yoga: Patañjali and Western Esotericism*. London: Continuum.

———. 2008. Modern Yoga: History and Forms. In Mark Singleton and Jean Byrne (eds.), *Yoga in the Modern World: Contemporary Perspectives*. London: Routledge, pp. 17–35.

Deleanu, Florin. 2009. Sedi, Vidi, Vici: A Brief Introduction to Meditation in Indian Buddhism. Unpublished paper. Enlarged version of presentation at the symposium 'Imag(in)ing the Buddhist Brain', Leiden Institute for Brain and Cognition, 20 March 2009.

Dhaky, M.A. 1995. Umāsvāti in Epigraphical and Literary Tradition. In *Śri Nāgābhinandanam: Dr M. S. Nagaraja Rao Festschrift Essays on Art, Culture, History, Archaeology, Epigraphy and Conservation of Cultural Property of India and Neighbouring Countries*, Vol. 2, ed. L. K. Srinivasan and S. Nagaraju. Bangalore: Dr M. S. Nagaraja Rao Felicitation Committee, pp. 505–22.

Diamond, Debra. 2013. *Yoga: The Art of Transformation*. Washington, DC: Arthur M. Sackler Gallery, Smithsonian Institution.

Digby, Simon. 1970. Encounters with Jogīs in Indian Sufi Hagiography. Unpublished paper presented at a seminar on 'Aspects of Religion in South Asia' at the School of Oriental and African Studies (SOAS), University of London.

———. 2000. *Wonder-tales of South Asia*. Jersey: Orient Monographs.

Dundas, Paul. 1998. Becoming Gautama: Mantra and History in Śvetāmbara Jainism. In John E. Cort (ed.), *Open Boundaries: Jain Communities and Cultures in Indian History*. Albany, NY: State University of New York Press, pp. 31–52.

Dyczkowski, Mark S. G. 1995–6. Kubjikā the Erotic Goddess: Sexual Potency, Transformation and Reversal in the Heterodox Theophanies of the Kubjikā Tantras. *Indologica Taurinensia* 21–22: 123–40 (available at http://www.indologica.com/volumes/vol21-22/vol21-22_art08_DYCZKOWSKI.pdf).

Einoo, Shingo. 2004. The Signs of Death and Their Contexts. In Shoun Hino and Toshihiro Wada (eds.), *Three Mountains and Seven Rivers*. Delhi: Motilal Banarsidass, pp. 871–86.

Eliade, Mircea. 1973 [1954]. *Yoga: Immortality and Freedom*. Princeton: Princeton University Press.

English, Elizabeth. 2002. *Vajrayoginī: Her Visualizations, Rituals and Forms. A Study of the Cult of Vajrayoginī in India*. Boston: Wisdom Publications.

Ernst, Carl W. 2007. Accounts of Yogis in Arabic and Persian Historical and Travel Texts. *Jerusalem Studies in Arabic and Islam* 33: 409–26.

Falconer, W. (trans.). 1857. *The Geography of Strabo*, Vol. 3. London: Henry G. Bohn.

Feuerstein, Georg, Subhash Kak and David Frawley. 1995. *In Search of the Cradle of Civilization: New Light on Ancient India*. Wheaton, IL: Quest Books.

Fitzgerald, James L. 2011. A Prescription for *Yoga* and Power in the *Mahābhārata*. In David Gordon White (ed.), *Yoga in Practice*. Princeton: Princeton University Press, pp. 43–57.

———. 2012. The Sāṃkhya-Yoga 'Manifesto' at *MBh* 12.289–290. In John Brockington (ed.), *Battle, Bards and Brāhmins*. Delhi: Motilal Banarsidass, pp. 259–300.

Flagg, William J. 1898. *Yoga: or, Transformation: A Comparative Statement of the Various Religious Dogmas Concerning the Soul and Its Destiny, and of Akkadian, Hindu, Taoist, Egyptian, Hebrew, Greek, Christian, Mohammedan, Japanese and Other Magic*. New York: J. W. Bouton/London: George Redway.

Flood, Gavin. 2006. *The Tantric Body: The Secret Tradition of Hindu Religion*. London: I. B. Tauris.

Fort, Andrew O. 1998. *Jīvanmukti in Transformation: Embodied Liberation in Advaita and Neo-Vedanta*. Albany, NY: State University of New York Press.

Fort, Andrew O. and Patricia Y. Mumme (eds.). 1996. *Living Liberation in Hindu Thought*. Albany, NY: State University of New York Press.

Franco, Eli (ed.), in collaboration with Dagmar Eigner. 2009. *Yogic perception, Meditation and Altered States of Consciousness*. Vienna: Verlag der Österreichischen Akademie der Wissenschaften.

Frawley, David. 1991. *Gods, Sages and Kings: Vedic Secrets of Ancient Civilization*. Delhi : Motilal Banarsidass.

———. 2001. *The Rig Veda and the History of India (Rig Veda Bharata Itihasa)*. New Delhi: Aditya Prakashan.

Fujii, Masato. 1989. Three Notes on the *Jaiminīya-Upaniṣad-Brāhmaṇa* 3, 1–5. *Journal of Indian and Buddhist Studies* 37 (2): 1002–994 (23–31).

Gerety, Finnian McKean Moore. 2015. This Whole World is OM: Song, Soteriology, and the Emergence of the Sacred Syllable. Doctoral dissertation, Harvard University.

Gethin, Rupert. 2004. On the Practice of Buddhist Meditation according to the Pali Nikāyas and Exegetical Sources. *Buddhismus in Geschichte und Gegenwart* 9: 201–21.

———. 2015. How Only Buddhists Can Stop Thinking and Get Away with It: A Theory of 'the Attainment of Cessation' (*nirodha-samāpatti*) in Early Buddhist Literature. Lecture at the School of Oriental and African Studies (SOAS), London, 12 March.

Gharote, Manmath L. 1989. Āsana: A Historical and Definitional Analysis. *Yoga-Mīmāṃsā* 28 (2): 29–43.

Gharote, M. L. (ed.-in-chief), V. K. Jha, Parimal Devnath and S. B. Sakhalkar (eds.). 2006. *Encyclopaedia of Traditional Asanas*. Lonavla: Lonavla Yoga Institute.

Giebel, Rolf W. (ed. and trans.). 2005. *The Vairocanābhisaṃbodhi Sūtra. Translated from the Chinese* (Taishō Volume 18, Number 848). BDK English Tripiṭaka Series. Berkeley: Numata Center for Buddhist Translation and Research.

Gode, P. K. 1954. *Studies in Indian Literary History*, Vol. 2. Bombay: Singhi Jain Śāstra Śikshāpīth Bhāratīya Vidyā Bhavan.

Gold, Daniel. 1999. Nāth Yogis as Established Alternatives: Householders and Ascetics Today. *Journal of Asian and African Studies* 34 (1): 68–88.

Gonda, Jan 1963. *The Vision of the Vedic Poets*. The Hague: Mouton & Co.

Goodall, Dominic (ed. and trans.). 2004. *The Parākhyatantra: A Scripture of the Śaiva Siddhānta. A Critical Edition and Annotated Translation*. Pondicherry: Institut français de Pondichéry.

———. 2011. The Throne of Worship: An 'Archaeological Tell' of Religious Rivalries. *Studies in History* 27 (2): 221–50.

Goodall, Dominic and Harunaga Isaacson. 2011. Tantric Traditions. In Jessica Frazier (ed.), *The Continuum Companion to Hindu Studies*.

London and New York: Continuum, pp. 122–37, 189–91 (notes), 361–400 (bibliography, joint for the whole volume).

Goodall, Dominic (ed and trans.) in collaboration with Alexis Sanderson and Harunaga Isaacson. 2015. *Niśvāsatattvasaṃhitā: The Earliest Surviving Śaiva Tantra*, Vol.: *A Critical Edition and Annotated Translation of the Mūlasūtra, Uttarasūtra and Nayasūtra*. Pondicherry: Institut français de Pondichéry/Paris: École française d'Extrême-Orient/Hamburg: Asien-Afrika-Institut, Universität Hamburg.

Granoff, Phyllis. 1996. The Ambiguity of Miracles: Buddhist Understandings of Supernatural Power. *East and West* 46: 79–96.

Gray, Louis H. 1904. The *Bhartṛharinirveda* of Harihara, Now First Translated from the Sanskrit and Prākrit. *Journal of the American Oriental Society* 25: 197–230.

Green, Nile. 2004. Oral Competition Narratives of Muslim and Hindu Saints in the Deccan. *Asian Folklore Studies* 63 (2): 221–42.

———. 2008. Breathing in India, *c.* 1890. *Modern Asian Studies* 42 (2–3): 283–315.

Greene, Eric M. 2014. Healing Breaths and Rotting Bones: On the Relationship between Buddhist and Chinese Meditation Practices during the Eastern Han and Three Kingdoms Period. *Journal of Chinese Religions* 42 (2): 145–84.

Grönbold, Günter. 1996. *The Yoga of Six Limbs: An Introduction to the History of Ṣaḍaṅgayoga*. Trans. Robert L. Hütwohl. Santa Fe, NM: Spirit of the Sun Publications.

Guggenbühl, Claudia. 2008. Mircea Eliade and Surendranath Dasgupta: The History of Their Encounter; Dasgupta's Life, His Philosophy and His Works on Yoga; A Comparative Analysis of Eliade's Chapter on Patañjali's *Yogasūtra* and Dasgupta's *Yoga as Philosophy and Religion*. Unpublished paper written as part of the project 'Yoga between Switzerland and India: The History and Hermeneutics of an Encounter', sponsored by the Swiss National Fund for Scientific Research and guided by Prof. Maya Burger (University of Lausanne) and Prof. Peter Schreiner (University of Zurich).

Halbfass, Wilhelm. 1988. *India and Europe: An Essay in Understanding*. Albany, NY: State University of New York Press.

Hanegraaff, Wouter J. 1998. *New Age Religion and Western Culture*. Albany, NY: State University of New York Press.

Hara, Minoru. 1966. Materials for the Study of Pāśupata Śaivism. PhD thesis, Harvard University.

———. 1999. Pāśupata and Yoga: *Pāśupata-sūtra* 2.12 and *Yogasūtra* 3.37. *Asiatische Studien* 53 (3): 593–608.

Hardy, Friedhelm. 1983. *Viraha-bhakti: The Early History of Kṛṣṇa Devotion in South India*. Delhi: Oxford University Press.

Harimoto, Kengo (ed. and trans.). 2014. *God, Reason and Yoga: A Critical Edition and Translation of the Commentary Ascribed to Śaṅkara on Pātañjalayogaśastra 1.23–28*. Hamburg: Department of Indian and Tibetan Studies, Universität Hamburg.

Hatley, Shaman. 2010. Tantric Śaivism in Early Medieval India: Recent Research and Future Directions. *Religion Compass* 4 (10): 615–28.

———. 2013. 'Nābhi' and 'Nābhikanda'. In Dominic Goodall and Marion Rastelli (eds.), *Tāntrikābhidhānakośa: Dictionnaire des termes techniques de la littérature hindoue tantrique*, Vol. 3. Vienna: Verlag der Österreichischen Akademie der Wissenschaften, pp. 284–86.

———. 2015. Representations of Women in the *Brahmayāmala*. Paper given at a symposium on 'Tantric Communities in Context: Sacred Secrets and Public Rituals' at the University of Vienna, February.

———. 2016. Kuṇḍalinī. In Arvind Sharma (ed.), *Encyclopedia of Indian Religions*, Vol.3 Netherlands: Springer.

Heelas, Paul. 1996. *The New Age Movement: The Celebration of the Self and the Sacralization of Modernity*. Oxford: Blackwell.

Heesterman, J. C. 1962. Vrātya and Sacrifice. *Indo-Iranian Journal* 6 (1): 1–37.

———. 1985. Brahmin, Ritual and Renouncer. In J. C. Heesterman, *The Inner Conflict of Tradition*. Chicago: University of Chicago Press, pp. 26–44.

Heiligjers-Seelen, D. 1994. *The System of Five Cakras in Kubjikāmatatantra 14–16*. Groningen: Egbert Forsten.

Hidas, Gergely. 2015. Dhāraṇī Sūtras. In Jonathan, A. Silk (ed.-in-chief), Oskar von Hinüber and Vincent Eltschinger (consulting eds.), *Brill's Encyclopedia of Buddhism*, Vol. 1. Leiden: Brill.

Hopkins, E. Washburn. 1901. Yoga-technique in the Great Epic. *Journal of the American Oriental Society* 22: 333–79.

Husain, Mahdi (ed. and trans.). 1953. *The Reḥla of Ibn Baṯṭūṭa*. Baroda: Oriental Institute.

Huxley, Aldous. 1946 [1945]. *The Perennial Philosophy*. London: Chatto & Windus.

Isaacson, Harunaga. 1993. Yogic Perception (*yogipratyakṣa*) in Early Vaiśeṣika. *Studien zur Indologie und Iranistik* 18: 139–60.

Isaacson, Harunaga and Dominic Goodall. 2016. On the Shared 'Ritual Syntax' of the Early Tantric Traditions. In Harunaga Isaacson and Dominic Goodall (eds.), *Tantric Studies: Fruits of a Franco-German*

Project on Early Tantra. Pondicherry: Institut français de Pondichéry / Paris: École française d'Extrême/Orient/Hamburg: Asien-Afrika-Institut, Universität Hamburg, pp. 1–76.

Iyengar, B. K. S. 2008. *Light on Life: The Journey to Wholeness, Inner Peace and Ultimate Freedom*. London: Rodale.

———. 2012.ṭ *Aṣṭadaḷa Yogamālā: The Collected Works of B. K. S. Iyengar*, 8 vols. New Delhi: Allied Publishers Pvt. Ltd.

Jackson, Roger R. (ed. and trans.). 2004. *Tantric Treasures: Three Collections of Mystical Verse from Buddhist India*. Oxford: Oxford University Press.

Jacobi, Hermann (trans.). 1964 [1884]. *Jaina Sutras, Part 1: Ācārāṅga Sūtra. Kalpa Sūtra*. Delhi: Motilal Banarsidass.

Jacobsen, Knut A. (ed.). 2005. *Theory and Practice of Yoga: Essays in Honour of Gerald James Larson*. Leiden: Brill.

——— (ed.). 2012. *Yoga Powers*. Leiden: Brill.

Johnson, E. H. (ed. and trans.). 1972 [1936]. *The Buddhacarita: or, Acts of the Buddha. Part 1: Sanskrit Text. Part 2: Cantos I to XIV translated from the Original Sanskrit Supplemented by the Tibetan Version, together with an Introduction and Notes*. New Delhi: Oriental Books Reprint Corporation. [Reprint of the Lahore 1936 edn.]

Jung, C. G. 1996. *The Psychology of Kundalini Yoga: Notes of the Seminar Given in 1932 by C. G. Jung*, ed. Sonu Shamdasani. London: Routledge.

Kane, Pandurang Vaman. 1941. *History of Dharmaśāstra*, Vol. 2, Part 1. Poona: Bhandarkar Oriental Research Institute.

Kieffer-Pülz, Petra. 1992. *Die Sīmā: Vorschriften zur Regelung der buddhistischen Gemeindegrenze in älteren buddhistischen Texten*. Monographien zur indischen Archäologie, Kunst und Philologie 8. Berlin: Reimer.

Kiehnle, Catharina. 2000. Love and Bhakti in the Early Nāth Tradition of Mahārāṣṭra: The Lotus of the Heart. In M. K. Gautam and G. H. Schokker (eds.), *Bhakti Literature in South Asia*. Leiden: Kern Institute, pp. 255–76.

———. 2005. The Secret of the Nāths: The Ascent of Kuṇḍalinī according to *Jñāneśvarī* 6.151–328. *Bulletin des études indiennes* 22–3: 447–94.

———. 2006. The Signs of Death according to the Jñāndev Gāthā. In Monika Horstmann (ed.), *Bhakti in Current Research, 2001–2003. Proceedings of the Ninth International Conference on Early Devotional Literature in New Indo-Aryan Languages, Heidelberg, 23–26 July 2003*. New Delhi: Manohar, pp. 179–200.

Killingley, Dermot. 2013. Manufacturing Yogis: Swami Vivekananda as a Yoga Teacher. In Mark Singleton and Ellen Goldberg (eds.), *Gurus of Modern Yoga*. New York: Oxford University Press.

Kiss, Csaba. 2009. Matsyendranātha's Compendium (*Matsyendrasaṃhitā*), a Critical Edition and annotated translation of *Matsyendrasaṃhitā* 1–13 and 55 with analysis. DPhil thesis, Balliol College, University of Oxford.

———. 2011. The *Matsyendrasaṃhitā*: A Yoginī-centered Thirteenth-century Text of the South Indian Śāmbhava Cult. In David N. Lorenzen and Adrián Muñoz (eds.), *Yogi Heroes and Poets: Histories and Legends of the Nāths*. Albany, NY: State University of New York Press, pp. 143–62.

Kragh, Ulrich Timme (ed.). 2013. *The Foundation for Yoga Practitioners: The Buddhist Yogācārabhūmi Treatise and Its Adaptation in India, East Asia and Tibet*. Cambridge, MA: Harvard University Press.

Larson, Gerald James. 1979. *Classical Sāṃkhya: An Interpretation of Its History and Meaning*, 2nd, rev. edn. Delhi: Motilal Banarsidass.

———. 1989. An Old Problem Revisited: The Relation between Sāṃkhya, Yoga and Buddhism. *Studien zur Indologie und Iranistik* 15: 129–46.

Larson, Gerald James, and Bhattacharya, Ram Shankar (eds.). 2008. *Yoga: India's Philosophy of Meditation*. Delhi: Motilal Banarsidass.

Leadbeater, C. W. 1927. *The Chakras*. Adyar: Theosophical Publishing House.

Lidke, Jeffrey S. 2005. Interpreting Across Mystical Boundaries: An Analysis of Samādhi in the Trika-Kaula Tradition. In Knut A. Jacobsen (ed.), *Theory and Practice of Yoga: Essays in Honour of Gerald James Larson*. Leiden: Brill, pp. 143–79.

Lindquist, Sigurd. 1935. *Siddhi und Abhiññā. Eine Studie über die klassischen Wunder des Yoga*. Uppsala Universitets Årsskrift 1935:2. Uppsala: A.-B. Lundequistska Bokhandeln.

Maas, Philipp. 2008. Valid Knowledge and Belief in Classical Sāṁkhya-Yoga. *Logic and Belief in Indian Philosophy*. Warsaw Indological Studies, Vol. 3: 371–80.

———. 2009. The So-called Yoga of Suppression in the *Pātañjala Yogaśāstra*. In Eli Franco (ed.) in collaboration with Dagmar Eigner, *Yogic Perception, Meditation and Altered States of Consciousness*. Vienna: Verlag der Österreichischen Akademie der Wissenschaften, pp. 263–82.

———. 2013. A Concise Historiography of Classical Yoga Philosophy. In Eli Franco (ed.), *Periodization and Historiography of Indian Philosophy*. Publications of the De Nobili Research Library 37.

Vienna: Sammlung de Nobili, Institut für Südasien-, Tibet- und Buddhismuskunde de Universität Wien, pp. 53–90.
———. Forthcoming. *Reader on Yoga: A Historical Sourcebook in the Classical Dualist Philosophy of Spiritual Liberation* [provisional title]. In the series Historical Sourcebooks of Classical Indian Thought, ed. Sheldon Pollock. New York: Columbia University Press.
McEvilley, Thomas. 1981. An Archaeology of Yoga. *Res* 1: 44–77.
Malinar, Angelika. 2012. Yoga Powers in the *Mahābhārata*. In Knut A. Jacobsen (ed.), *Yoga Powers*. Leiden: Brill, pp. 33–60.
Mallinson, James. 2005. Rāmānandī Tyāgīs and Haṭha Yoga. *Journal of Vaishnava Studies* 14 (1): 107–21.
——— (ed. and trans.). 2007a. *The Khecarīvidyā of Ādinātha: A Critical Edition and Annotated Translation of an Early Text of Haṭhayoga*. London: Routledge.
——— (ed. and trans.). 2007b. *The Shiva Samhita: A Critical Edition and an English Translation*. New York: YogaVidya.com.
———. 2011a. The Original *Gorakṣaśataka*. In David Gordon White (ed.), *Yoga in Practice*. Princeton: Princeton University Press, pp. 257–72.
———. 2011b. Nāth Saṃpradāya. In Knut A. Jacobsen (ed.-in-chief), Helene Basu, Angelika Malinar and Vasudha Narayanan (eds.), *Brill's Encyclopedia of Hinduism*, Vol. 3, pp. 407–28.
———. 2011c. Haṭha Yoga. In Knut A. Jacobsen et al. (eds.), *Brill's Encyclopedia of Hinduism*, Vol. 3, pp. 770–81.
———. 2012. *Siddhi* and *Mahāsiddhi* in Early *Haṭhayoga*. In Knut A. Jacobsen (ed.), *Yoga Powers*. Brill: Leiden, pp. 327–44.
———. 2014. The Yogīs' Latest Trick. *Journal of the Royal Asiatic Society* 24(1): 165–80.
———. 2015. Śāktism and *Haṭhayoga*. In Bjarne Wernicke Olesen (ed.), *Goddess Traditions in Tantric Hinduism: History, Practice and Doctrine*. London: Routledge, pp. 109–40.
———. Forthcoming (a). Yoga and Sex: What is the Purpose of *Vajrolīmudrā*? In *Yoga in Transformation: Historical and Contemporary Perspectives on a Global Phenomenon*. Vienna: V&R Unipress (in the series 'Wiener Forum für Theologie und Religionswissenschaft').
———. Forthcoming (b). The *Amṛtasiddhi*: *Haṭhayoga*'s Tantric Buddhist Source Text. In *Śaivism and the Tantric Traditions: A Festschrift for Alexis Sanderson*. Leiden: Brill.
Meulenbeld, G. J. 1974. *The Mādhavanidāna and Its Chief Commentary, Chapters 1–10: Introduction, Translation and Notes*. Leiden: E. J. Brill.
Monier-Williams, Monier. 1960 [1872]. *A Sanskrit-English Dictionary, Etymologically and Philologically Arranged, with Special Reference to Cognate Indo-European Languages*. Oxford: Clarendon Press.

Mullin, Glenn H. (ed. and trans.). 2006. *The Practice of the Six Yogas of Naropa*. Ithaca, NY: Snowlion.

Mumme, Patricia Y. 1996. Conclusion: Living Liberation in Comparative Perspective. In Andrew O. Fort and Patricia Y. Mumme (eds.), *Living Liberation in Hindu Thought*. Albany, NY: State University of New York Press, pp. 247–70.

Mundy, Peter. 1914. *The Travels of Peter Mundy, in Europe and Asia, 1608–1667*, ed. Richard Carnac Temple Vol. 2: *Travels in Asia, 1628–1634*. London: Hakluyt Society.

Nelson, Lance E. 1986. *Bhakti* in Advaita Vedânta: A Translation and Study of Madhusûdana Sarasvatî's *Bhaktirasâyana*. McMaster University, Open Access Dissertations and Theses, Paper 3453.

———. 1996. Living Liberation in Śaṅkara and Classical Advaita: Sharing the Holy Waiting of God. In Andrew O. Fort and Patricia Y. Mumme (eds.), *Living Liberation in Hindu Thought*. Albany, NY: State University of New York Press, pp. 17–62.

Newcombe, Suzanne. 2009. The Development of Modern Yoga: A Survey of the Field. *Religious Compass* 3 (6): 986–1002.

Nicholson, Andrew J. 2010. *Unifying Hinduism: Philosophy and Identity in Indian Intellectual History*. New York: Columbia University Press.

———. 2013. Is Yoga Hindu? On the Fuzziness of Religious Boundaries. *Common Knowledge* 19 (3): 490–505.

Oberhammer, Gerhard. 1977. *Strukturen yogischer Meditation. Untersuchungen zue Spiritualität des Yoga*. Vienna: Verlag der Österreichischen Akademie der Wissenschaften.

Oertel, Hanns. 1896. The Jāiminīya or Talavakāra Upaniṣad Brāhmaṇa: Text, Translation and Notes. *Journal of the American Oriental Society* 16: 79–260.

Ohira, Suzuko. 1982. *A Study of Tattvārthasūtra with Bhāṣya: With Special Reference to Authorship and Date*. Ahmedabad: L. D. Institute of Indology.

Olivelle, Patrick. 1984. Renouncer and Renunciation in the Dharmaśāstras. In Richard W. Lariviere (ed.), *Studies in Dharmaśāstra*. Calcutta: Firma KLM, pp. 81–152.

——— (ed. and trans.). 1998. *The Early Upaniṣads: Annotated Text and Translation*. New York and Oxford: Oxford University Press.

Ondračka, Lubomír. 2011. What Should Mīnanāth Do to Save His Life? In David N. Lorenzen and Adrián Muñoz (eds.), *Yogi Heroes and Poets: Histories and Legends of the Nāths*. Albany, NY: State University of New York Press, pp. 129–41.

Padoux, André. 1992. *Vāc: The Concept of the Word in Selected Hindu Tantras*. Delhi: Sri Satguru Publications.

———. 2002. Corps et cosmos: L'image du corps du yogin tantrique. In Véronique Boullier and Gilles Tarabout (eds.), *Images du corps dans le monde hindou*. Paris: CNRS Éditions, pp. 163–87.

Pratibhāprajñā, Samaṇī. 2015a. Tantric Elements in Prekṣā Meditation. Paper presented at the 17th Jaina Studies Workshop, SOAS, University of London, 20 March.

———. 2015b. Prekṣā Meditation History and Methods. Unpublished PhD thesis, SOAS, University of London.

Prothero, Stephen. 2010. *God is Not One: The Eight Rival Religions that Run the World – and Why Their Differences Matter*. New York: HarperOne.

Puri, Purāṇ (1792). His account of his travels, published as 'Oriental Observations, No. X – The Travels of Prán Puri, a Hindoo, Who Travelled over India, Persia, and Part of Russia', *The European Magazine and London Review*, vol. 57, pp. 261–71, 341–52.

Quarnström, Olle and Jason Birch. 2011. Universalist and Missionary Jainism: Jain Yoga of the Terāpanthī Tradition. In David Gordon White (ed.), *Yoga in Practice*. Princeton: Princeton University Press, pp. 365–82.

Rastogi, Navjivan. 1992. The Yogic Disciplines in the Monistic Śaiva Tantric Traditions of Kashmir: Threefold, Fourfold, and Six-limbed. In Teun Goudriaan (ed.), *Ritual and Speculation in Early Tantrism: Studies in Honor* of *André Padoux*. Albany, NY: State University of New York Press, pp. 247–80.

Reigle, David. 2012. The *Kālacakra Tantra* on the *Sādhana* and *Maṇḍala*: A Review Article. *Journal of the Royal Asiatic Society*, Series 3, 22 (2): 439–63.

Rizvi, Saiyid Athar Abbas. 1970. Sufis and Natha Yogis in Mediaeval Northern India (XII–XVI Centuries). *Journal of the Oriental Society of Australia* 7: 119–33.

Rukmani, T. S. 2005. Revisiting the Jīvanmukti Question in Sāṃkhya in the Context of the *Sāṃkhyasūtra*. In Knut A. Jacobsen (ed.), *Theory and Practice of Yoga: Essays in Honour of Gerald James Larson*. Leiden: Brill, pp. 61–74.

Rüping, Klaus. 1977. Zur Askese in indischen Religionen. *Zeitschrift für Missionswissenschaft und Religionswissenschaft* 61 (2): 81–98.

Sakaki, Kazuyo. 2005. Yogico-tantric Traditions in the *Ḥawḍ al-Ḥayāt*. *Journal of the Japanese Association for South Asian Studies* 17: 135–56.

Samuel, Geoffrey. 2008. *The Origins of Yoga and Tantra: Indic Religions to the Thirteenth Century*. Cambridge: Cambridge University Press.

Sanderson, Alexis. 1986. Comments in discussion at end of 'Kubjikā's

Samayamantra and Its Manipulation in the *Kubjikāmata*', by Teun Goudriaan, in *Mantras et diagrammes rituelles dans l'hindouisme*, ed. André Padoux. Équipe no. 249, L'hindouisme: textes, doctrines, pratiques. Paris: Éditions du centre national de la recherche scientifique, pp. 141–67.

———. 1988. Śaivism and the Tantric Traditions. In Stewart Sutherland et al. (eds.), *The World's Religions*. London: Routledge, pp. 660–704.

———. 1990. The Visualisation of the Deities of the Trika. In André Padoux (ed.), *L'Image divine: Culte et méditation dans l'hindouisme*. Paris: Éditions du CNRS, pp. 31–88.

———. 1999. Yoga in Śaivism: The Yoga Section of the *Mṛgendratantra*: An Annotated Translation with the Commentary of Bhaṭṭa Nārāyaṇakaṇṭha. Unpublished paper.

———. 2007a. Śaivism, Society and the State. Unpublished paper.

———. 2007b. Atharvavedins in Tantric Territory: The *Āṅgirasakalpa* Texts of the Oriya Paippalādins and Their Connection with the Trika and the Kālīkula. With Critical Editions of the *Parājapavidhi*, the *Parāmantravidhi* and the *Bhadrakālīmantravidhiprakaraṇa*. In Arlo Griffiths and Annette Schmiedchen (eds.), *The Atharvaveda and Its Paippalāda Śākhā: Historical and Philological Papers on a Vedic Tradition*. Geisteskultur Indiens: Text und Studien 11, Indologica Halensis. Aachen: Shaker Verlag, pp. 195–311.

———. 2009. The Śaiva Age: The Rise and Dominance of Śaivism during the Early Medieval Period. In Shingo Einoo (ed.), *Genesis and Development of Tantrism*. Institute of Oriental Culture Special Series 23. Tokyo: Institute of Oriental Culture, University of Tokyo, pp. 41–350.

———. 2013. The Śaiva Literature. *Journal of Indological Studies* 24–5: 1–113.

Saraogi, Olga Serbaeva. 2010. Liberation in Life and After Death in Early Śaiva Mantramārgic Texts: The Problem of *Jīvanmukti*. In Andreas Bigger, Rita Krajnc, Annemarie Mertens, Markus Schüpbach and Heinz Werner Wessler (eds.), *Release from Life – Release in Life: Indian Perspectives on Individual Liberation*. Bern and New York: Peter Lang, pp. 211–34.

Śāstrin, Govindaśaraṇa. 1972. Śrīnimbārkācārya se Paravartī Vedāntācārya. In Vrajavallabhaśaraṇa (ed.), *Śrī Nimbārkācārya aura unakā Sampradāya*. Salemābāda: Śrīnimbārkācārya Pīṭha, pp. 20–65.

Satapathy, B. and G. S. Sahay. 2014. A Brief Introduction of 'Yogāsana-Jaina': An Unpublished Yoga Manuscript. *Yoga-Mīmāṃsā* 46: 43–55.

Schmithausen, Lambert. 1981. On Some Aspects of Descriptions or Theories of 'Liberating Insight' and 'Enlightenment' in Early Buddhism. In

Klaus Bruhn and Albrecht Wezler (eds.), *Studien zum Jainismus und Buddhismus: Gedenkschrift für Ludwig Alsdorf*. Wiesbaden: Franz Steiner, pp. 199–250.

Schneider, Johannes. 2010. *Vāgīśvarakīrtis* Mṛtyuvañcanopadeśa*: Eine buddhistische Lehrschrift zur Abwehr des Todes*. Vienna: Verlag der Österreichischen Akademie der Wissenschaften.

Schreiner, Peter. 2010. How to Come Out of Samādhi? In Andreas Bigger, Rita Krajnc, Annemarie Mertens, Markus Schüpbach and Heinz Werner Wessler (eds.), *Release from Life – Release in Life: Indian Perspectives on Individual Liberation*. Bern and New York: Peter Lang, pp. 197–210.

Sferra, Francesco (ed. and trans.). 2000. *The Ṣaḍaṅgayoga by Anupamarakṣita, with Raviśrījñāna's Guṇabharaṇīnāmaṣaḍaṅgayogaṭippaṇī*. Serie orientale Roma 85. Rome: Istituto Italiano per L'Africa e l'Oriente.

———. 2005. Constructing the Wheel of Time: Strategies for Establishing a Tradition. In Federico Squarcini (ed.), *Boundaries, Dynamics and Construction of Traditions in South Asia*. Florence: Firenze University Press/New Delhi: Munshiram Manoharlal, pp. 253–85.

Shee, Monika. 1986. *Tapas und Tapasvin in den erzählenden Partien des Mahābhārata*. Reinbek: Dr Inge Wezler Verlag für Orientalische Fachpublikationen.

Sheridan, Daniel P. 1996. Direct Knowledge of God and Living Liberation in the Religious Thought of Madhva. In Andrew O. Fort and Patricia Y. Mumme (eds.), *Living Liberation in Hindu Thought*. Albany, NY: State University of New York Press, pp. 91–110.

Siegel, Lee. 1991. *Net of Magic: Wonders and Deceptions in India*. Chicago and London: University of Chicago Press.

Silk, Jonathan A. 1997. Further Remarks on the *Yogācāra Bhikṣu*. In Bhikkhu Tampalawela Dhammaratana and Bhikkhu Pāsādika (eds.), *Dharmadūta: Mélanges offerts au Vénérable Thích Huyên-Vi à l'occasion de son soixante-dixième anniversaire*. Paris: Éditions You Feng, pp. 233–50.

———. 2000. The *Yogācāra Bhikṣu*. In Jonathan A. Silk (ed.), *Wisdom, Compassion, and the Search for Understanding: The Buddhist Studies Legacy of Gadjin M. Nagao*. Honolulu: University of Hawai'i Press, pp. 265–314.

Singleton, Mark. 2010. *Yoga Body: The Origins of Modern Posture Practice*. New York: Oxford University Press.

Singleton, Mark and Jean Byrne (eds.). 2008. *Yoga in the Modern World: Contemporary Perspectives*. London: Routledge.

Sivananda, Swami. 2000 [1939]. *Easy Steps to Yoga*. World Wide Web edition, http://www.dlshq.org/download/easysteps.htm. Shivanandanagar, Uttar Pradesh: The Divine Life Society.

———. n.d. The Unity that Underlies All Religions. Available at http://www.dlshq.org/religions/unirel.htm.

Sjoman, N. E. 1996. *The Yoga Tradition of the Mysore Palace*. New Delhi: Abhinav.

Skoog, Kim. 1996. Is the *Jīvanmukti* State Possible? Rāmānuja's Perspective'. In Andrew O. Fort and Patricia Y. Mumme (eds.), *Living Liberation in Hindu Thought*. Albany, NY: State University of New York Press, pp. 63–90.

Slaje, Walter. 2000. Liberation from Intentionality and Involvement: On the Concept of *Jīvanmukti* according to the Mokṣopāya. *Journal of Indian Philosophy* 28: 171–94.

Smith, Frederick M. 2006. *The Self Possessed: Deity and Spirit Possession in South Asian Literature and Civilization*. New York: Columbia University Press.

———. 2011. *Yogasūtras* II.25 and the Conundrum of *Kaivalya*. In Jonathan Duquette and Pratap Penumala (eds.), *Classical and Contemporary Issues in South Asian Studies: In Felicitation of Prof. T. S. Rukmani*. New Delhi: D. K. Printworld (P) Ltd, pp. 66–78.

Smith, Huston. 1991. *The World's Religions: Our Great Wisdom Traditions*. San Francisco: HarperSanFrancisco.

Snellgrove, David. 1959. *The Hevajra Tantra: A Critical Study*. London: Oxford University Press.

Sprockhoff, Joachim Friedrich. 1976. *Saṃnyāsa: Quellenstudien zur Askese im Hinduismus*. Vol. 1 of 2: *Untersuchungen über die Saṃnyāsa-Upaniṣads*. Wiesbaden: Franz Steiner.

Staal, Frits. 1989. Vedic Mantras. In Harvey P. Alper (ed.), *Understanding Mantras*. Albany, NY: State University of New York Press, pp. 48–95.

Strauss, Sarah. 2005. *Positioning Yoga: Balancing Acts across Cultures*. Oxford: Berg.

Stuart, Daniel M. 2015. See *Saddharmasmṛtyupasthānasūtra*.

Szántó, Péter-Dániel. 2012. Selected Chapters from the *Catuṣpīṭhatantra* (1/2: Introductory Study with the Annotated Translation of Selected Chapters. DPhil thesis, Balliol College), University of Oxford.

Taylor, Kathleen. 2001. *Sir John Woodroffe, Tantra and Bengal: 'An Indian Soul in a European Body'?* Richmond: Routledge Curzon.

Törzsök, Judit. 2014. Women in Early Śākta Tantras: *Dūtī*, *Yoginī* and *Sādhakī*. *Cracow Indological Studies* 16: 339–67.

Vasudeva, Somdeva (ed. and trans.). 2004. *The Yoga of the Mālinīvijayottaratantra: Chapters 1–4, 7, 11–17. Critical Edition, Translation and*

Notes. Pondicherry: Institut français de Pondichéry/École française d'Extrême-Orient.

———. 2011. Haṃsamiṭṭhu: 'Pātañjalayoga is Nonsense'. *Journal of Indian Philosophy* 39 (2): 123–45.

———. 2012. Powers and Identities: Yoga Powers and the Tantric Śaiva Traditions. In Knut A. Jacobsen (ed.), *Yoga Powers*. Leiden: Brill, pp. 265–302.

Vidyāratna, Tārānātha (ed.). 1913. *Shatchakranirūpana and Pādukāpanchaka*. Vol. 2 of the series 'Tantrik Texts' edited by Arthur Avalon [Sir John Woodroffe]. Calcutta: Sanskrit Press Depository/London: Luzac & Co.

Walter, Michael. 2000. Cheating Death. In David Gordon White (ed.), *Tantra in Practice*. Princeton: Princeton University Press, pp. 605–23.

Warren, Henry Clarke and Dharmananda Kosambi. 1989 [1950]. *Visuddhimagga of Buddhaghosâcariya*. Delhi: Motilal Banarsidass. [Reprint of the Harvard 1950 edn.]

Watson, Alex, Dominic Goodall and S. L. P. Anjaneya Sarma (eds. and trans.). 2013. *An Enquiry into the Nature of Liberation: Bhaṭṭa Rāmakaṇṭha's* Paramokṣanirāsakārikāvṛtti. *A Commentary on Sadyojyotiḥ's Refutation of Twenty Conceptions of the Liberated State (mokṣa). For the First Time Critically Edited, Translated into English and Annotated*. Pondicherry: Institut français de Pondichéry/École française d'Extrême-Orient.

Werner, Karel. 1994 [1977]. The Longhaired Sage of RV 10, 136: A Shaman, a Mystic or a Yogi? In Karel Werner (ed.), *The Yogi and the Mystic: Studies in Indian and Comparative Mysticism*. Durham Indological Series 1. London: Curzon Press [1st edn 1989], pp. 33–53. [Original version of essay published as: Yoga and the Ṛg *Veda*: An Interpretation of the *Keśin* Hymn (RV 10, 136). *Religious Studies* 13 (3) (1977): 289–302.]

Wezler, Albrecht. 1982. Remarks on the Definition of 'Yoga' in the *Vaiśeṣikasūtra*. In L. A. Hercus et al. (eds.), *Indological and Buddhist Studies: Volume in Honour of Professor J. W. de Jong on His Sixtieth Birthday*. Bibliotheca Indo-Buddhica 27. Canberra: Australian National University, Faculty of Asian Studies, pp. 643–86.

White, David Gordon. 1996. *The Alchemical Body*. Chicago: University of Chicago Press.

——— (ed.). 2000. *Tantra in Practice*. Princeton: Princeton University Press.

———. 2003. *Kiss of the Yoginī: 'Tantric Sex' in its South Asian Contexts*. Chicago: University of Chicago Press.

———. 2009. *Sinister Yogis*. Chicago: University of Chicago Press.

———. 2014. *The Yoga Sutra of Patanjali: A Biography*. Princeton and Oxford: Princeton University Press.

Wujastyk, Dominik. 1998. *The Roots of Āyurveda: Selections from Sanskrit Medical Writings*. New Delhi and London: Penguin.

———. 2002. Interpréter l'image du corps humain dans l'Inde pré-moderne. In Véronique Boullier and Gilles Tarabout (eds.), *Images du corps dans le monde hindou*. Paris: CNRS Éditions, pp. 71–99.

———. 2009. Interpreting the Image of the Human Body in Premodern India. *International Journal of Hindu Studies* 13(2): 189–228.

———. 2011. The Path to Liberation through Yogic Mindfulness in Early Āyurveda. In David Gordon White (ed.), *Yoga in Practice*. Princeton: Princeton University Press, pp. 31–42.

———. Forthcoming. Some Problematic Yoga Sutras and Their Buddhist Background. In Philipp A. Maas and Karin Preisendanz (eds.), *Yoga in Transformation: Historical and Contemporary Perspectives on a Global Phenomenon*. Vienna: V&R Unipress (in the series 'Wiener Forum für Theologie und Religionswissenschaft').

Wynne, Alexander. 2003. The Origins of Buddhist Meditation. DPhil thesis, University of Oxford.

———. 2007. *The Origin of Buddhist Meditation*. London and New York: Routledge.

Yadav, K. C. (ed.). 2003 [1976]. *The Autobiography of Dayanand Saraswati*. Gurgaon: Hope.

Zin, Monika. 2006. *Mitleid und Wunderkraft: Schwierige Bekehrungen und ihre Ikonographie im indischen Buddhismus*. Wiesbaden: Harrassowitz.

Notes

ONE

Yoga

1. The meaning 'magic' or 'trick' is particularly common in first-millennium literary and śāstric texts. See, for example, *Kāmasūtra* 1.3.7: 'A princess or daughter of a minister who knows yoga can control her husband even if he has a thousand women in his harem.'
2. A particularly idiosyncratic understanding of yoga, which perhaps fits our heuristic definition, is in the *Yājñavalkyasmṛti* (3.110–16), which identifies yoga with singing the Vedas and other songs, and playing the veena and the drum, adding that if one does not reach the supreme level through those methods, one should become a follower of Rudra and sport with him.
3. See Pratibhāprajñā 2015b: 17-18. Yoga in the restricted sense is also present in later non-canonical Jain texts. See, for example, Hemacandra's *Yogaśāstra* 1.5–7 and 15.
4. But not with Śiva himself: the *Parākhyatantra* claims that would be impossible on account of Śiva being all-pervading (14.97).
5. '*patañjalimuner uktiḥ kāpy apūrvā jayaty asau | puṃprakṛtyor viyogo 'pi yoga ity*' (*Yogasūtrarājamārtaṇḍa* 1.1). Bhojarāja further says that in this context the verbal root √*yuj*, from which *yoga* is derived, means the act of concentration or *samādhi* (1.1 '*yogo yuktiḥ-samādhānam | yuja samādhau*'), implicitly rejecting etymologies of *yoga* in which √*yuj* is taken to have the alternative meaning of union (*yujir yoge*), such as that of Nārāyaṇakaṇṭha at *Mṛgendra Yogapāda* 2ab (see 1.1.17).
6. See Nicholson 2010: 121.
7. Contrary to widespread popular and even scholarly belief, the *Bhagavadgītā* does not teach a triad of *karmayoga*, *jñānayoga* and *bhaktiyoga*. While there are five instances in the text of

karmayoga, the compound word *jnānayoga* appears only twice, and *bhaktiyoga* only once. Moreover, the three never appear together. Many other kinds of – or means to – yoga are also named in the text, as our selections show. Killingley suggests that the notion of the *Bhagavadgītā*'s triad of yogas, which was popularized in the modern period by Swami Vivekananda, may originate with the sixteenth-century commentator Madhusūdana Sarasvatī, who divides the text into six chapters on *karma*, six on *bhakti* and six on *jñāna* (Killingley 2013: 37, n.22).

8. The yoga of touch is associated with breath-control. The yoga of being is beyond the yogas of mantra and touch, and purifies the mind. The yogas of non-being and the great yoga are described in the section from the *Īśvaragītā* included in this chapter (1.2.4); the former is the absence of mental activity, held as the goal of yoga in the *Pātañjalayogaśāstra* and in the latter the yogi meditates on the true nature of Śiva.
9. See Birch 2011.
10. See Mallinson forthcoming (a).
11. According to Sanderson (1999:31–2) this sense of *aṅga* derives from the terminology of the Mīmāṃsā school of philosophy and indicates a subsidiary factor which leads to the accomplishment of a goal. For an extensive discussion of the term *aṅga* as used in texts of yoga see Vasudeva 2004: 367–82.
12. '*Ṣaḍaṅgayoga* is set forth as a subsidiary to the principal conquest of realities (this is also the relationship between the *aṅga*s and the *tattvajaya* seen in most Saiddhāntika scriptures). It is to be understood as a collection of helpful or even indispensable yogic techniques which enable the prospective yogi to achieve the required "coalescence" or "identification" (*tanmayatā* , lit. the "consisting-of-that-ness") with the object of contemplation' (Vasudeva 2004: 369). Note that the earliest known tantra, the *Niśvāsatattvasaṃhitā* (*Nayasūtra* 4.24) speaks of an 'unsupported' (*nirālamba*) yoga that goes beyond six-limbed yoga, so although it does not teach a six-limbed yoga, it clearly knew of one.
13. See Sferra 2000: 14. As Sferra remarks, however, the majority of Pāñcarātra Saṃhitās teach a yoga of eight auxiliaries.
14. Grönbold (1996: 35–47) makes the case for an unbroken lineage of sixfold yoga within the Buddhist Vajrayāna tradition. See Sferra 2000: 11–16 for a detailed treatment of *ṣaḍaṅga* systems.
15. 'While the majority of surviving Śaiva scriptures generally agree on which these six auxiliaries are, there is no consensus as to their order, their definition, or even their subdivisions. Such disagreement

reflects doctrinal divergences in the various Śaiva Tantras and also indicates deliberate shifts of emphasis [. . .] these systems are not simply indiscriminately reshuffled versions of an original "correct" order' (Vasudeva 2004: 286–7). See Goodall 2004: 353, fn.736 for further discussion of this matter.

16. Wujastyk (2011: 31) notes that in later Sanskrit medical literature the term *aṣṭāṅga* becomes so standard as to become a synonym for medicine.
17. Although in some Śaiva teachings (e.g. *Śivayogapradipīkā* 2.6), the positions of meditation and fixation are reversed. *Pace* Sferra (2000: 14, n.12), the *Pādmasaṃhitā* (*Yogapāda* 1.4) does not substitute *niyama* with *tapas* (*tapas* is the first of the *niyama*s at 1.9) and the *Jayākhyasaṃhitā* (Chapter 33) does not say that it teaches an eightfold yoga, nor does it list the *aṅga*s of its yoga. The elements of the classic eightfold scheme of the *Pātañjalayogaśāstra* are given new interpretations in the *Netratantra* (on which, see Rastogi 1992: 259–60).
18. Kṣemarāja, in his *Uddyota* commentary on *Svacchandatantra* 1.17, quotes the *Śrīpūrvaśāstra* as saying that *tarka* is the best of yoga's *aṅga*s. Where other Śaiva works have *tarka* in their sixfold yogas, the *Śivadharmottarapurāṇa* (10.115) has *japa*. Vajrayāna Buddhist texts have *anusmṛti* ('recollection') in the place of the Śaiva *tarka* in their sixfold systems (see Sferra 2000: 16).
19. The notion that the absence of *yama*s and *niyama*s in tantric texts is because of the presence of transgressive practices which would make the observance of such ethical instructions difficult or impossible seems flawed. For one thing, tantric works usually contain plenty of ethical instruction and rules in passages other than their teachings on yoga (on this point, see Brunner 1994: 440). Furthermore, if they were practised at all, such transgressive practices were likely to have been restricted to a very small number of initiates into highly esoteric cults.
20. For a succinct presentation of the place of Īśvara in the *Pātañjalayogaśāstra* (PYŚ), see Jacobsen 2005: 5–17.
21. Cf. Vasudeva 2004: 373.
22. Birch 2011: 541, n.105.
23. Mallinson 2007: 172, n.47.
24. Birch 2013.
25. Vasudeva 2011: 139.
26. On *khecarīmudrā*, see Chapter 6.
27. See Nicholson 2013.
28. As edited in Wezler 1982. Wezler (ibid: 665) suggests that this passage is an addition to the earliest layer of the text.
29. We have translated the text as edited in Barois 2012.

30. Translation by Dominic Goodall.
31. Translation by Kengo Harimoto (2014: 189–91).
32. Translation by Somdeva Vasudeva (2004: 241).
33. Translation by Alexis Sanderson (1999: 4–5).
34. Translation by Dominic Goodall (Goodall et al. 2015: 385).
35. Here we have emended *parameśvaraḥ*, as found in all witnesses of the text, to *pārameśvaraḥ*.
36. Translation by Glenn H. Mullin (2006: 27–9).
37. On the Suṣumnā, see Chapter 5, p. 172
38. i.e. a man's semen does not flow during sexual intercourse.
39. Translation by Alexis Sanderson (1999: 5).
40. In this passage Sanderson translates *prāṇāyāma* as 'breath-extension', following the analysis of the commentator Nārāyaṇakaṇṭha (Sanderson 1999: 2, n.4).
41. On this passage, and sections 1.5.2–4, see Nicholson 2013.
42. The term *kula* here signifies the highest (non-transcendental) divine state of Śiva. On the multiple meanings of this term see *Tāntrikābhidhānakośa* (s.v. Kula), and the Glossary.
43. On *prāṇa* and *apāna* see Chapter 5, p. 173. On mantra, see Chapter 7.
44. i.e. *ṣaṇmukhīmudrā*, whose technique is taught as part of *yonimudrā* in the *Gheraṇḍasaṃhitā* (6.2.13).
45. The wearing of conch-shell earrings is given as one of the symbols of the yogi at *Siddhasiddhāntapaddhati* 5.13. It is not clear that this is what is referred to in this verse and the referents of the other instances of *dhāraṇa* in it are equally obscure. The Sanskrit word used is the neuter *dhāraṇam*, not the feminine *dhāraṇā*, which is the sixth of the *aṅgas* of Patañjali's eightfold yoga.
46. This practice is obscure. It may involve the nose or nasal fluids, since at *Siddhasiddhāntapaddhati* 2.23 the bodily station (*ādhāra*) called *kapāṭa* is said to be at the base of the nose.
47. This practice is obscure. It may involve fluid from the eyes since *kharpara* is a type of eye application.

TWO
Preliminaries

1. See Brunner 1994: 450 on the relationship between initiation and yoga (and the part yoga plays within initiation rituals) in Āgamic texts.
2. In contrast with the *Pātañjalayogaśāstra*, the *Amṛtasiddhi*'s grades correspond to the aptitude of the aspirant, rather than the intensity of his method, hence the alternative translations of the different grades.

3. In the tantric context, Brunner (1994: 451) translates *ṣaṭkarma* as 'the six magical acts'. *Kuṭṭanīmatam* 249 gives an early (ninth-century) instance of a pun on the Brahmanical and tantric meanings of this term.
4. As well as an additional 'dry *basti*' technique and three versions of *kapālabhāti*.
5. Philipp Maas notes the following: 'The five obligations (*yama*s) that a yogi has to commit himself to throughout his spiritual career are very similar in name and content to the five vows that Jain monks permanently have to keep. See the discussion of the commitments (*yama*s) in *Pātañjalayogaśāstra* 2.30–31, which is largely parallel to the vows of Jain monks as they are outlined in *Tattvārthasūtra* 7.8–12. The exposition of the Jain vows in the *Tattvārthasūtra*, which according to Dhaky (1995: 519) is probably roughly contemporary with the *Pātañjalayogaśāstra*, is based on the much older canonical *Ācārāṅgasūtra*' (personal communication, February 2016).
6. See Jacobi 1964 [1884].
7. Other tenfold lists occur, for example, in the *Śivayogapradīpikā*, and in three Pāñcarātra/Vaikhānasa texts: the *Pādmasaṃhitā*, the *Vimānārcanākalpa* and the *Ahirbudhnyasaṃhitā*.
8. As Nicholson points out, although *āstikya* is most commonly taken to indicate belief in the authority of the Vedas, it is a contested term which is also used by Jains (such as Haribhadra) and Buddhists (such as Asaṅga) to refer to themselves (Nicholson 2013: 172–6).
9. However, see Kiss (2011: 153): 'The absence of *yama-niyama* rules in a yogic text that is modelled on Pātañjala yoga is significant and can be accounted for by the fact that many of the practices included in the MaSam [*Matsyendrasaṃhitā*] (e.g. the practices with human skulls in *paṭala* 33 or sexual practices of *paṭala* 40) would be difficult to harmonize with rules such as *brahmacarya* ("continence") and *śauca* ("purity") (*Yogasūtra* 2.30, 32).' On this see also Chapter 1, note 19.
10. See Gold 1999 for a discussion of householder Nāths and their varying social positions. The Nāths are an order of Śaiva renunciate ascetics and householders often associated with *haṭhayoga* (see Mallinson 2011b).
11. See Brunner 1994.
12. e.g. the Maithili *Gorakṣavijaya* and the Sanskrit *Bhartṛharinirveda*.
13. See Bouillier 2008: 68, n.15.
14. e.g. *Amaraughaprabodha* 44cd, *Śivasaṃhitā* (5.4–5), *Haṭhapradīpikā* 1.61ab and *Gheraṇḍasaṃhitā* (**2.2.8**), statements which appear to derive from the *Amṛtasiddhi* (see **2.1.2**).

15. However, see also *Haṭhapradīpikā* 1.62, which (citing Gorakṣa) recommends against 'the use of fire, women and travelling', but does not specify that this refers only to the beginning stages of practice. The same is true of the *Śivasaṃhitā* – although, in apparent contradiction to this injunction, the text later states that through mastering *vajrolīmudrā* the yogi's semen is not wasted, even if he has sex with 100 women (4.103cd). Similar claims are made in other descriptions of *vajrolī*; these, however, do not imply that the women with whom the yogi has sex were practitioners of yoga.
16. See *Dattātreyayogaśāstra* 155–6 (**6.2.2**); *Haṭhapradīpikā* 3.84, 3.95–8; *Haṭharatnāvalī* 2.109.
17. A *yoginī* is either a female human practitioner of yoga or a type of goddess.
18. See also Olivelle 1984: 114–15.
19. See Birch 2013: 122 and Gode 1954: 9–14.
20. See Sanderson 2007a: 70–72.
21. See Sanderson 2013: 312.
22. *Brahmayāmala*, Chapter 45 (Hatley 2015: 7; see also Törszök 2014).
23. See Kiehnle 2000: 265.
24. Cf. *Śārṅgadharapaddhati* 4383–4.
25. i.e. Kṛṣṇa.
26. Andrew Nicholson has suggested to us that, given that Cārvākas are defined specifically by their *lack* of faith (in an afterlife, in reincarnation and, ergo, in the liberation from cyclic existence afforded by yoga), it is possible that there is some intended irony here – a reading which disrupts a simple interpretation of this passage as a statement that yoga is a secular practice open to all.
27. Unpublished translation by Bruce Wannell, with input on the content by James Mallinson.
28. Literally 'four fingers' wide and 'fifteen *hastas*' long, with one *hasta* being measured from the elbow to the tip of the outstretched middle finger (approximately forty-five centimetres).
29. *Kapālabhāti* literally means 'skull-shine'.
30. On this practice, see **6.2.13**.
31. There are several alternative names for this practice, which is most commonly known as *kapālabhāti* (and is taught as such in the *Haṭhapradīpikā* (**2.5.1**)): in the manuscripts of the *Haṭharatnāvalī* alone it is variously called *mastakabhrānti*, *kapālabhāti*, *kapālabhrānti*, *kapālabhastrī* and *kapālabhastrikā*.
32. *Vajrolī* is not among the eight cleansing techniques, but is one of the *mudrās* (see Chapter 6).

33. *Kāṣṭhamauna* literally means 'silence like [a piece of] wood'. In the *Tattvavaiśāradī*, Vācaspatimiśra's commentary on the *Pātañjalayogaśāstra*, *kāṣṭhamauna* is explained as not even using any gestures to make known what one means, and *ākāramauna* is simply not speaking (*kāṣṭhamaunam iṅgitenāpi svābhiprāyāprakāśanam | avacanamātram ākāramaunam*).

THREE

Posture

1. In other types of text *āsana* most commonly means a 'seat'. The earliest known usage of *āsana* to refer to a physical posture is found in Aśvaghoṣa's *c.* 50 CE *Buddhacarita* (v. 12.120; Gharote 1989).
2. Kauṇḍinya's *c.* 400–550 CE commentary on the *Pāśupatasūtra*, which is roughly contemporaneous with the *Pātañjalayogaśāstra*, lists the following as the postures which may be adopted for *prāṇāyāma* (*ad* 1.17): '*padmaka*, *svastika*, *upasthāñjalika*, *ardhacandra*, *pīṭhaka*, *daṇḍāyata*, *sarvatobhadra*, etc.'
3. In Śaṅkara's commentary on *Brahmasūtrabhāṣya* 4.1.10 he advocates the use of specific postures such as the lotus posture, as taught in 'the yoga *śāstra*'.
4. The Pali word used to denote this cross-legged posture is *pallaṅka* (Sanskrit *paryaṅka*), which means 'couch'. It is not explained in the Pali canon, but in the Sanskrit *Buddhacarita* (12.120) the future Buddha is said to assume a *paryaṅka* position which is 'unshakeable' (*akampyam*) and 'compact like the coils of a sleeping snake' (*suptoragabhogapiṇḍitam*), and in the *c.* 400 CE Pali *Visuddhimagga*, Buddhaghosa explains *pallaṅka* with *samantato ūrubaddhāsanam* (223.26), which most probably means a posture in which the feet are pressed tightly against the thighs, i.e. the lotus posture.
5. No Vedic texts (the early Upaniṣads included) mention postures for meditation, although modes of sitting for ritual are taught in the *Ṛg Veda* and subsequent works (see Gharote 1989 for references).
6. Vasudeva 2004: 399 and n.81. Cf. *Bhāgavatapurāṇa* 11.28.39, which says that disturbances that arise in the course of yoga practice may be overcome by *āsana*s (as well as fixation (*dhāraṇā*), asceticism, mantra and herbs).
7. A small number of practices involving bodily postures other than simple seated positions are taught in tantric texts (but not as *āsana*s, nor indeed as specifically yogic methods). The *Pāśupatasūtra* prescribes dancing as part of the worship of Paśupati (1.8, 2.3.1). The

Niśvāsatattvasaṃhitā's *Nayasūtra* (1.29ff.) teaches the practitioner how to reproduce the shapes of the letters of the alphabet with his body. Some letters are already present in the body and do not require the adoption of particular postures (e.g. 1.34–35a), while others involve holding parts of the body in particular attitudes (e.g. 1.43). *Jayadrathayāmala* 4.2.612–22 (**6.1.2**) teaches a seal (*mudrā*) which requires the practitioner to adopt a seated position in which one leg is extended. Among the various means for sublimating consciousness taught in the *Vijñānabhairava* is a practice in which one sits on one buttock and extends an arm and leg (v. 78, **9.2.4**). The *Bhūmiparigrahavidhi* of the tantric Buddhist *Vajrāvalī* prescribes seated yogic *āsana*s together with various more dynamic movements, including threatening gestures and dancing, as a method of driving away beings from a *maṇḍala* before practising rituals inside it. Circumambulation while performing *aṣṭāṅga praṇāma*s or *namaskāra*s, i.e. prostrations in which eight parts of the body touch the ground, is often taught in tantric works as a method of purifying a *maṇḍala* or worshipping the guru (**2.4.2**).

8. The approximately contemporaneous *Tattvavaiśāradī*, a commentary on the *Pātañjalayogaśāstra*, gives a description of the hero's pose (*vīrāsana*) which may perhaps be understood as instructing the yogi to stand on one foot with the other folded back and placed on the thigh.
9. Falconer 1857: 111–13.
10. The Buddha himself is never said to have undertaken any of the postural austerities, but one Buddhist text, the fifth-century CE *Visuddhimagga*, includes among various ascetic methods the 'sitting-man's practice' in which the ascetic never lies down (2.13).
11. e.g. *Jātaka* 1, 493 (*Naṅguṭṭhajātaka*), *Jātaka* 3, 232–7 (*Setaketu Jātaka*), *Kassapasīhanāda Sutta* (*Dīghanikāya* 1) 166–7, *Aṅguttaranikāya* 1.295–6.
12. e.g. *Mahābhārata* 1.81.9–16, 1.201.1–20, 3.13.1–15.
13. See, for example, *Skandapurāṇa* 34.70, *Mārkaṇḍeyapurāṇa* 31.24, *Kūrmapurāṇa* 2.27.29–30, *Matysapurāṇa* 35.17, *Vāyupurāṇa* (*Revākaṇḍa*) 54.50, *Bhāgavatapurāṇa* 7.3.2 and *Liṅgapurāṇa* 1.69.76. Cf. *Kathāsaritsāgara* 6.4.11.
14. Hemacandra is likely to have based this statement on statements in early Jain sources such as the *Ācārāṅga Sutta* (1.9.4.14), *Ācārāṅga Cūrṇi* (15.38) and *Ācārāṅga Cūlā* (15.38). We are grateful to Samaṇī Pratibhāprajñā for providing us with these references.
15. In Madhva's *Mahābhāratatātparyanirṇaya*, when Duryodhana is fighting Bhīma at the very end of the great battle, he tries to trick

Bhīma by putting his head on the ground and his legs upwards, but Bhīma then smashes both his thighs. Bhīma thus not only fulfils his promise to break Duryodhana's thighs because Duryodhana asked Draupadī to sit on them, but also avoids flouting a rule of *gadā-yuddha*, the type of fight they are engaged in, which says that one must not hit 'below the belt'. This detail is not found in the *Mahābhārata* itself, where Bhīma's breaking of Duryodhana's thighs sees him accused of violating *dharma* (*Śalya parvan* 32). We thank Vishal Sharma for pointing out to us this convincing explanation of the name *duryodhanāsana*.

16. The modern usages of *sarvāṅgāsana* to denote the shoulderstand and *śīrṣāsana* to denote the headstand are not found in pre-modern Sanskrit texts.
17. A key difference between modern postural yoga and pre-modern yoga practice is the absence in the latter of standing postures other than the simple upright *kāyotsargāsana* and *vṛkṣāsana* (e.g. *Gheraṇḍasaṃhitā* 2.36).
18. Satapathy and Sahay 2014.
19. *Āsana*s are identified with *tapas* in texts of the Jain tradition, in particular the specific external *tapas* called *kāyakleśa* ('bodily suffering'). For examples, see Muni Jambuvijaya's commentary to Hemacandra's *Yogaśāstra* 4.125.
20. Similarly, difficult yogic postures in *c.* eighteenth-century depictions on temple walls in South India are identified in accompanying inscriptions as *tapas* (Anna Seastrand, personal communication, 2 April 2014).
21. Some ascetic yogis in India today do perform a variety of postures as part of their yoga practice – for example, those Rāmānandī *sādhu*s who practise *āsana*s at the end of their ritual fire penance – but such practice is subsidiary to remaining for longer periods in single postures, whether for meditation, mantra-repetition or *tapas*.
22. Mundy 1914: 254.
23. e.g. Chaoul 2006.
24. The closest parallel between the techniques of *'khrul 'khor* and those of *haṭhayoga* is found in the twentieth of the twenty-three techniques taught in 'The Secret Key to the Channels and Winds' (3.9), which corresponds closely to the *mahāvedha* technique as taught in the *Dattātreyayogaśāstra* and subsequent *haṭha* texts (on which see Chapter 6). In those texts, however, the yogi is to sit with his heel under the perineum, before raising himself with his arms and dropping himself on to it, while in the *'khrul 'khor* technique

he sits in the lotus posture. Furthermore, the *mahāvedha* is to be done gently, whereas the Tibetan practice is more forceful.

25. Baker 2015: 6, n.17; 12.
26. A small number of textual descriptions of *āsana*s are predicated on descriptions of *āsana*s given earlier in the same text, e.g. Hemacandra's *Yogaśāstra* 4.127 (3.5), in which the description of *vajrāsana* proceeds from the *vīrāsana* posture that has already been taught; or the *Haṭhābhyāsapaddhati*, which at 25–31 (3.14) gives a description of *gajāsana*, which is followed by six postures which are variations thereof (and there are other similar sequences elsewhere in that text). Nowhere, however, do we find complex and well-defined posture sequences like those central to the teachings on *āsana* propagated in the twentieth century by T. Krishnamacharya and some of his students. Furthermore, the Sanskrit word *vinyāsa* used (with considerable variation of meaning) by Krishnamacharya and his students to denote a stage in one of these linked sequences is not found with this meaning in pre-modern texts on yoga. Related verbal forms (*vinyāsa* is a nominal formation from from the verbal root √*ās* prefixed by *vi-* and *ni-*), such as the absolutive *vinyasya*, are found in a handful of posture descriptions with the meaning 'having placed [*x* on *y*]', e.g. *Vasiṣṭhasaṃhitā* 1.72 (3.6) ('Hav[ing] placed one foot on one thigh, and the other foot under the other thigh'). *Vinyāsa* and related words are more common in tantric texts, where they usually refer to the installation of mantras on the body. The compound *vinyāsakrama*, which has been used by Krishamacharya and his students to denote a particular sequence of linking poses, is not found in pre-modern yoga texts. We have found five instances of it in tantric works. In four it refers to a sequential installation of mantras; in the fifth, Kṣemarāja's commentary on verse 9 of the *Sāmbapañcāśikā*, it is used to refer to the sequence of strides across the three worlds taken by Viṣṇu in his Vāmana incarnation. The modern usage of *vinyāsa* is thus a reassignment of the meaning of a common Sanskrit word; the usage in modern yoga parlance of the word *viniyoga* (which in Sanskrit means 'appointment', 'employment' or 'application') to mean tailoring yoga to individual needs is a similar reassignment, albeit closer to its pre-modern usage (in contexts other than yoga), while the word *pratikriyāsana*, used in the Krishnamacharya tradition to mean a 'counter pose', is a modern coinage not found in any pre-modern Sanskrit texts.
27. In the nineteenth century the sun salutation (*sūryanamaskāra*) was yet to be associated with yoga; this is its only known textual

mention prior to the twentieth century and here it is identified as a strenuous physical exercise detrimental to yoga practice if practised to excess. In earlier texts, procedures for performing acts of homage known as *namaskāra*s and *praṇāma*s, some of which involve repeated full-body prostrations, are common (see *Haribhaktivilāsa* 8.357–392 for passages from a variety of texts which describe such procedures), but they are not taught as techniques of yoga nor are any directed at the sun.

28. The translations of the names *bhadrāsana* and *svastikāsana* are those of Dominik Wujastyk and Philipp Maas (unpublished paper, 2015).
29. Cf. Hemacandra on *bhadrāsana* at 3.5.
30. Manu 2.72: *saṃhatya hastāv adhyeyaṃ sa hi brahmāñjaliḥ smṛtaḥ* |
31. Translated by Dominic Goodall (Goodall et al. 2015: 466 and 483–4).
32. There is an addition in brackets here in the text which is corrupt but appears to say 'one should place the ankles so that the left is on the right side, the left is at the right thigh. That is the cow's mouth posture.'
33. 'With mouth closed' for the lion pose seems odd, but we don't see any other way of taking *saṃvṛtāsya*.
34. At the beginning of this description there is *brāhmaṃ jānvantaradvayamagnam aṅguṣṭhaṃ nigūhya bhrūmadhyekṣaṇaṃ*, which appears to be a corruption derived from the description of *brahmāsana*.
35. The compound is ambiguous as to whether one or both feet are on the ground. If one, then this hero's pose could be like that of the *Tattvavaiśāradī* mentioned later in this section.
36. At the suggestion of Samaṇī Pratibhāprajñā, we are taking *lagaṇḍa* to be equivalent to *laguḍa*.
37. *Haṭhapradīpikā* 1.36 calls this *siddhāsana*, the 'adept's pose'.
38. From an unpublished translation by Carl Ernst.
39. Ernst: 'Evidently this means that yoga is at first hard, like the extreme seasons, but later becomes easier, like the temperate seasons. One Persian translation (Per2B) treats the seasons as corresponding to four progressive degrees of discipline, while another (Per2A) merely says, "striving in the beginning is winter, and in the end is spring". While these expressions appear metaphorical, the Persian translation of Muhammad Ghawth (Per1) treats the seasons concretely: 'The season for austerity is when it is winter, especially towards the end, and when it is the rainy season (*barashkal*) and spring.'
40. Translation by Ian Baker (Baker 2015: 245–57).
41. Translation by Carl Ernst (http://www.asia.si.edu/explore/yoga/ocean-of-life.asp).

42. The name *kāṇṭhava* is obscure and there is no corresponding description in the body of the text.
43. A mythical animal said to inhabit the Himalayas.
44. See Puri 1810.
45. The English in this extract (which is a translation of Purāṇ Puri's Hindi statement) has been left unchanged, but the Hindi words and place names have been adapted according to current methods of transcription (e.g. Jumna has been changed to Yamuna).
46. *Cāraṇā* is a noun derived from the causative of the root √*car*, 'to move'.
47. A *hasta* is usually the distance from the elbow to the tip of the hand, but this meaning would leave the yogi too far from the wall to lean his chest on it.
48. The name of this posture is not found in the manuscript and has been taken from the *Śrītattvanidhi* (v. 65).
49. We have used 'centipede' to differentiate the name from that in the next verse ('caterpillar'), but we are not sure of the exact referents of either Sanskrit name.

FOUR
Breath-control

1. See also *Mahābhārata* 12.304.9.
2. *Amaraughaprabodha* 4c: *yas tu prabhañjanapidhānarato haṭhaḥ saḥ* | (°*pidhāna*° em. Sanderson, °*vidhāna*° Ed.).
3. Cf. *Dharmaputrikā* 1.23–5, *Īśvaragītā* 11.42, *Mārkaṇḍeyapurāṇa* 36.35c–36d, *Matsyendrasaṃhitā* 6.1 and 7.77, *Vivekamārtaṇḍa* 94–5, *Jogpradīpikā* 433–6, etc.
4. *Tantrāloka* 4.91a.
5. *Pratyabhijñāhṛdaya* 21.
6. *Yogaśāstra* 6.2ab.
7. Elsewhere, however, Hemacandra does say that control of the breath will lead to liberation (5.3).
8. *Mṛgendratantravṛtti ad Yogapāda* 1.2cd. Cf. the fourth-century CE Chinese *Chu yao jing*, which says that Buddhist breathing meditation (*ānāpāna*) 'through a disturbance of the internal winds, can lead to death if performed improperly' (Greene 2014: 148, n.9).
9. Exceptions to this understanding of the word *āyāma* in this compound can be found in the *Parākhyatantra* (4.10) and Nārāyaṇakaṇṭha's commentary on the *Mṛgendratantra*, in which it is taken to mean 'extension' (4.11, see also Sanderson 1999: 2, n.4). The

Mṛgendratantra itself defines *prāṇāyāma* as 'exhausting' or 'exercising' the breath. Kauṇḍinya, in his commentary on the *Pāśupatasūtra* (4.7), and the *Mataṅgapārameśvara* (4.12) both understand *āyāma* to mean 'suppression', i.e. holding of the breath. For more definitions of *prāṇāyāma* in tantric texts, see Vasudeva 2004: 388.

10. e.g. *Aitareya Brāhmaṇa*, *passim*.
11. See, for example, *Āpastambadharmasūtra* 1.9.26.14 in which a penance includes reciting the Sāvitrī 1,000 times either with or without *prāṇāyāma*. Cf. *Āpastambadharmasūtra* 2.5.12.15.
12. See e.g *Amṛtasiddhi* 6.11.
13. See e.g. *Baudhāyanadharmasūtra* 4.1.1–10, *Vasiṣṭhadharmasūtra* 26.1–4.
14. In the Pāśupata tradition, *prāṇāyāma* may also be used to purify objects external to the yogi (*Pātravidhi* 1).
15. See Kane 1941: 317.
16. *Āśvalāyanaśrautasūtra* 2.7, *Āpastambhadharmasūtra* 2.5.12.15. Cf. *Śvetāśvatara Upaniṣad* 2.9 (2.2.3).
17. See Vasudeva 2004: 388–9.
18. e.g. *Svacchandatantra* 2.33ab.
19. Kṣemarāja, in his *Uddyota* commentary to *Svacchandatantra* 7.294cd–295ab explains that the purification of the channels means pacifying the winds therein (*marutapraśamana*).
20. Analysis of the movement of the breath is one of the ways in which a yogi can tell whether death is close at hand. If it is he may use various methods to avoid it. See Chapter 11 for more details. The flow of the breath is also used to predict the future and to determine auspicious times to undertake specific actions. These prognostications, whose method is known as *svarodaya*, are taught in several texts. See e.g. Nārāyaṇakaṇṭha's *vṛtti* on *Mṛgendratantra Yogapāda* 20c–27b (4.11), Hemacandra's *Yogaśāstra* 5.225–47 and, for a text devoted to this subject, the *Śivasvarodaya*. Persian and Arabic texts written in India also display a keen interest in *svarodaya* (see Sakaki 2005: 139–40).
21. Like the vast majority of yoga texts, the *Dattātreyayogaśāstra* uses the words *pūraka*, *kumbhaka* and *recaka* for 'inhalation', 'retention' and 'exhalation'. These are not found in the *Pātañjalayogaśāstra* and appear to be innovations of the tantric tradition: Kauṇḍinya's *Pañcārthabhāṣya* mentions *pūraṇa* and *recaka* (4.7); the *Niśvāsatattvasaṃhitā* is the first to teach the triad of *pūraka*, *kumbhaka* and *recaka*, to which it adds a quiescent state of breath-control, *supraśānta* (4.9); see Goodall et al. 2015: 488–90.

22. e.g. *Pātañjalayogaśāstra* 2.50, *Mālinīvijayottaratantra* 17.6–7.
23. For a detailed discussion of different systems of 'number' (*saṃkhyā*) and 'time' (*kāla*) in teachings on *prāṇāyāma*, see Vasudeva 2004: 403–8.
24. See also Vasudeva 2004: 403–8.
25. The haṭhayogic *kumbhaka*s all have feminine names, which is curious since the word *kumbhaka* itself is neuter. Furthermore, *kumbhaka* means 'breath-retention', so to use it as a name for practices whose distinguishing features are their methods of inhalation and exhalation is also odd. The most likely explanation is that the names arose in a different context, but we have been unable to find any references to them in texts prior to the *Gorakṣaśataka*. There are, however, a small number of references to practices similar to the haṭhayogic *sahita kumbhaka*s, but which do not bear their names. For example, one of the eight *sahita kumbhaka*s is *mūrcchā*, a method of inducing fainting, and it is perhaps significant that *Niśvāsatattvasaṃhitā Nayasūtra* 4.138 mentions fainting as a result of *prāṇāyāma*; *Mālinīvijayottaratantra* 17.5 names the upper palate as one of the possible locations of inhalation, which is redolent of the haṭhayogic *ujjāyī kumbhaka*; and *Vivekamārtaṇḍa* 119 teaches an unnamed practice that is very similar to the *Gorakṣaśataka*'s *śītalī kumbhaka* (but the *Vivekamārtaṇḍa* may be contemporaneous with the *Gorakṣaśataka*).
26. See e.g. *Mataṅgapārameśvara Yogapāda* 7.1–6b and *Sārdhatriśatikālottaravṛtti* p. 30, ll. 19–p. 31, l. 3.
27. On *udghāta* see *Tāntrikābhidhānakośa* II p. 302 s.v. *udghāta* and Vasudeva 2004: 402–9. *Pace* Wynne (2003: 95, n.367), the *codanā*s described in connection with *prāṇāyāma* in the *Mahābhārata* (e.g. 12.294.11, 12.304.11 and 12.307.9–10; see also Bedekar 1962b) appear to us to be forerunners of *udghāta*.
28. Translation by Alexis Sanderson (1999: 12, n.37).
29. Vasudeva 2004: 409.
30. The *Svacchandatantra* also describes an internal upwards expulsion of breath called *ūrdhvarecaka* (see *Tāntrikābhidhānakośa* III, pp. 585–6), which is similar to *udghāta*, but associated with the *uccāraṇa* of a mantra (on which see Chapter 7).
31. *Bhagavadgītā* 6.34 is also suggestive of this notion: it says that restraining the fickle mind is as difficult as restraining the wind (Vidyāraṇya in his *Jīvanmuktiviveka* understands this as referring to *haṭhayoga*; see 1.5.7). At the end of his teachings on *prāṇāyāma*, Patañjali says that it makes the mind capable of performing the fixations (2.53; cf. 1.34, which says that mental steadiness may result from the exhalation and retention of the breath). Some tantric texts

identify the breath as the seat of consciousness, e.g. *Parākhyatantra* 4.117cd and *Mataṅgapārameśvara Yogapāda* 2.10–15b.

32. e.g. *Svacchandatantroddyota* 7.294–5.
33. *Mālinīvijayottaratantra* 18.8c–10b.
34. See also Vasudeva 2004: 410–19.
35. On *utkrānti*, see Mallinson 2007a: 238, n.448.
36. On *parakāyapraveśa*, see Chapter 11 and Mallinson 2007a: 237, n.439.
37. The *Gheraṇḍasaṃhitā* (4.21) uses the terms *sabīja* ('with a seed-syllable') and *nirbīja* ('without a seed-syllable').
38. Ernst 2007: 411; see also ibid., 415.
39. We are aware of one exception to this: the *Kumbhakapaddhati*, which teaches fifty-seven *kumbhakas*.
40. Translated by Dominic Goodall (Goodall et al., 2015: 486–91). *Niśvāsatattvasaṃhitā Nayasūtra* 4.119a–144b describes the benefits of the yogi moving the breath to various bodily locations (see 5.1.8).
41. Translation by Dominic Goodall (2004: 354).
42. Translation by Alexis Sanderson (1999: 5–21).
43. In this passage Sanderson translates *prāṇāyāma* as 'breath-extension', following the analysis of the commentator Nārāyaṇakaṇṭha (Sanderson 1999: 2, n.4).
44. Cf. *Baudhāyanadharmasūtra* 4.1.28 (see 4.4).
45. From an unpublished translation by Carl Ernst. Ernst notes that the manuscripts give several variant readings for these seed-syllables.
46. *Haṃsa*, the union of the out- (*haṃ*) and in- (*saḥ*) breaths, literally means 'goose'.
47. i.e. at four o'clock in the morning, at noon and at eight o'clock in the evening.
48. When instructing the yogi to inhale, the text uses the verbs *ucār* and *bhākh*, which mean 'to say' – i.e. the yogi's inhalation should make a noise.

FIVE

The Yogic Body

1. On the empirical and bio-medical body of modern yoga see Alter 2004.
2. See (Dominik) Wujastyk 2002 and 2009 on 'the many bodies of pre-modern India'. The relationship between Āyurveda and yoga is the topic of a five-year research project (2015–2020) at the University of Vienna headed by Dagmar Wujastyk and funded by the

European Research Council, entitled 'Entangled Histories of Yoga, Ayurveda and Alchemy in South Asia' (see the project website www.ayuryog.org). As an observation preliminary to the project's findings, we note here that until the sixteenth-century CE āyurvedic terminology is infrequent in yogic texts, even those of the *haṭhayoga* tradition, but becomes more prevalent from the sixteenth to eighteenth century (see e.g. the *Yuktabhavadeva*). See also Birch forthcoming. Dominik Wujastyk's *The Roots of Āyurveda* (1998) is a key resource for textual sources on Āyurveda and was an important model in the conception phase of this book.

3. Wujastyk 2009; Flood 2006.
4. For some examples of contradictory interpretations of the yogic body and the practices associated with it, see the section '*Bindu*' in this chapter.
5. The figure of 72,000 for the total number of channels subsequently became widely accepted, but it may have arisen through confusion with the numbering of the verses in the *Śatapathabrāhmaṇa* and originally been a more vague 'thousands' (Acharya 2013: 15, n.21).
6. The *Bṛhadyogiyājñavalkyasmṛti* also teaches a *nāḍī* system in which Iḍā and Suṣumnā are lateral channels (9.96–8), but it adds a central channel, called Amā.
7. The central channel is known by a variety of names other than Suṣumnā. For a comprehensive list, see *Haṭhapradīpikā* 3.4.
8. Goodall et al. (in the introduction to their edition of the *Niśvāsatattvasaṃhitā*, pp. 33–5) argue that early upaniṣadic notions of subtle channels must be understood as distinct from later instantiations of the yogic body (such as that of the *Niśvāsatattvasaṃhitā*) insofar as the former are blood vessels and the latter conduits for the breaths (which may in turn push fluids about the body) and that the familiar upaniṣadic tally of 72,000 blood vessels was only mapped on to the model of wind tubes some time after the composition of the *Niśvāsatattvasaṃhitā*'s *Uttarasūtra*. However, although this distinction is useful for highlighting two distinctive discourses of the yogic body, it may not be quite so hard and fast: for example, in some tantric texts such as the *Sārdhatriśatikālottara*, *prāṇa* flows along the subtle channels *along with* the blood (see Flood 2006: 159), much as it appears to in upaniṣadic models.
9. On which see Wynne 2003: 78. Wynne notes that, although 'the yogic method is not described' in this passage, it is exceptional with regard to other passages in the *Mokṣadharma* section of the

Mahābhārata, which are almost all 'variations, or extrapolations, of the ideas found in the yogic passages of the early Upaniṣads'.

10. On the Sahasrāra *cakra* which is sometimes added to this schema, see below, pp. 177–8.
11. See, for example, the Theosophist C. W. Leadbeater's Western esoteric rendering of tantric physiology in his *The Chakras* (1927), and C. G. Jung's psychological interpretations of Kuṇḍalinī from 1932, both of which greatly influenced conceptions of the 'yogic body' in modern, global contexts.
12. On the subtle body in the Śaivāgamas (i.e. Saiddhāntika Āgamas) see Brunner 1994: 435–9. Brunner points out that there is agreement on *nāḍīs* and *vāyus*, but wide differences of opinion across texts on *ādhāras* and *granthis*. In the Saiddhāntika Āgamas there are many lists of *granthis*, which usually number five, and which 'obviously play the same role as the *cakras* of the Śakta tradition; but the latter word is almost never used in this connection' (437).
13. According to Alexis Sanderson, this is likely to be the case in some less detailed and more schematic texts like the *Mṛgendra*, but not so much in other works where the treatments are more detailed (e.g. the *Mataṅga* and *Mālinīvijayottara*). Furthermore, 'Yoga as seen in the texts that seem more au fait with the subject seems not to have been the object of lively interest on the parts of the exegetes' such as Bhaṭṭa Rāmakaṇṭha and Abhinavagupta. Personal communication on 21 November 2014.
14. Snellgrove 1959: 14 dates the *Hevajratantra* to the late eighth century. However, the text postdates the *Laghuśaṃvara*, which itself is probably post-900 CE (Sanderson 2009: 163–4). Comparable descriptions of the yogic body within Buddhism, albeit couched in more mystical language, can be found in Kāṇha's *Treasure of Couplets* (esp. vv. 4–5, 13–16, 25–7; see Jackson 2004: 117–28).
15. Older teachings on physical locations as focuses for fixation (*dhāraṇā*) are found in the *Mahābhārata* and *Pātañjalayogaśāstra* (8.2.3, 8.2.4).
16. Later chapters of the *Kubjikāmatatantra* list five *cakras* only, not linked to Kuṇḍalinī but associated with the elements (see Padoux 2002 and Heiligjers-Seelen 1994).
17. 'Kaulism developed into four main systems. These were known as the Four Transmissions (*āmnāya*) or as the Transmissions of the Four Lodges (*gharāmnāya*) (eastern, western, northern and southern). Each has its own distinctive set of deities, *mantras*, *maṇḍalas*, mythical saints, myths of origin and the like' (Sanderson 1988: 680).

18. The *Saṃgītaratnākara* passage is followed by a section describing how mastery of particular aspects of playing music and singing may arise through locating the self in particular petals of particular *cakras*.
19. i.e. which brings the cosmos, or reality, into existence.
20. The earliest mention of Kuṇḍalinī in Jain texts is in the thirteenth-century *Mantrarājarahasya* (Pratibhāprajñā 2015a).
21. See Desikachar, *Religiousness in Yoga*, pp. 243–5; Desikachar perhaps derives this notion from the *Yogayājñavalkya* (4.21–4), whose teachings on Kuṇḍalinī are taken from the *Pādmasaṃhitā*.
22. The female equivalent of this, occasionally mentioned in our texts, is *rajas*, uterine fluid.
23. Secondary literature on yoga practice often states that semen is refined as it moves upwards towards the head (e.g. White 1996: 40–41). This notion, which may result from confusion with descriptions of Kuṇḍalinī's rarefication during her ascent, is not found in textual sources.
24. Cf. the *Padmamālāvidhi* of the fourth chapter of the *Brahmayāmala*, which teaches a system of nine knots (*granthis*) and instructs the yogi to visualise lotuses at their locations. Here it seems that the knots are real entities while the lotuses are to be imagined. We thank Shaman Hatley for this observation.
25. The ontological clash between features of the yogic body as imaginatively generated focuses for meditation and as physical realities takes a new turn from the mid-nineteenth century onwards, when *cakras*, Kuṇḍalinī, etc. begin to be reinterpreted in the context of modern scientific rationalism as corresponding to physical features of the biological body. The cognitive dissonance which this sometimes generates is nicely illustrated by a (perhaps apocryphal) story of Ārya Samāj founder Dayānanda Sarasvatī, who dissects a corpse in order to ascertain for himself the truth of the *cakras*: when he fails to find them, he throws his yoga texts into the river in disgust (Yadav 2003 [1976]: 41; see Singleton 2010: 49–53 for a discussion of scientific rationalism and the yogic body).
26. On fasting according to the phases of the moon and heating austerities, see also *Pātañjalayogaśāstra* 2.32 (2.6.2). The *Jīvanmuktiviveka* (3.10.18) draws a distinction between ascetic practices and yoga, declaring the latter to be superior because it is a means of attaining the highest realm (see 1.2.12).
27. *Prāṇāyāma* is associated with *tapas* from its earliest textual mentions and it is likely to be through this association that Kuṇḍalinī is said to dry the body.

28. For example, the *kośa*s are an important part of B. K. S. Iyengar's theorization of the yogic body. Those interested in tracing his interpretation of the concept might begin by consulting the eight volumes of his collected works, *Astadala Yogamala* (2012; the index on p. 331 of vol. 8 shows forty references to the *kośa*s across vols. 1–8). Thanks to Louie Ettling for this reference. The *kośa*s are also prominent within the popular teachings of the early twentieth-century guru Swami Sivananda, although perhaps with less integration into praxis than with Iyengar. See, for example, Sivananda 2000 [1939]: 86, where a part of 'the process of yoga' is characterized as 'the stilling of the discordant vibratory tempo of the lower Kosas'.
29. Translation by Dominic Goodall (Goodall et al. 2015: 395).
30. Translation by Dominic Goodall (2004: 364–70).
31. Reigle (2012: 442) shows that the word *karṇikā*, which is usually translated with 'pericarp', is more accurately translated as 'central receptacle'.
32. This passage is paraphrased, in verse, in Chapter 7 of the *Yogayājñavalkya*, which is cited by Nīlakaṇṭha *ad Mahābhārata* 12.307 (cf. Hopkins 1901: 345). The raising of the breath through the vital points is here equated with sense withdrawal (*pratyāhāra*), on which see Chapter 8.
33. The only other instance of the word *citi* that we have found is in the *Gheraṇḍasaṃhitā* (2.14), where it appears to mean 'the shin'.
34. We know of no other instances of *kaṇṭhakūbara*; perhaps it is a corruption of *kaṇṭhakūpa*, which is used in several yoga texts to refer to the Adam's apple.
35. Translation Dominic Goodall (Goodall et al. 2015: 491–5).
36. In this context, these represent the first and last letters of the Sanskrit syllabary: thus Kuṇḍalinī encompasses all speech.
37. At dawn, noon and dusk.
38. On this term, see Mallinson 2007a: 216, n.305.
39. A pun is being made here: *guṇa* can mean 'thread'.
40. Translation by Dominic Goodall (2004: 371–2).
41. Various texts give different locations for this esoteric centre.
42. The aperture of Brahman is the fontanelle.
43. On the location of *bindu* in the forehead, see Mallinson 2007a: 219, n.325.
44. i.e. the seven openings in the head.
45. Unpublished translation by Shaman Hatley for his edition for the Nepal-German Manuscript Preservation Project (A48) 1, p. xxii.
46. The meaning of *Saṃvara* here may be either 'bliss' or the god Hevajra himself.

47. The locations of these *cakra*s are not given in the *Hevajratantra* itself, but are found in its Tibetan translations and commentaries (see Snellgrove 1959: 49).
48. A *daṇḍa* is a unit of time whose length in this context is unclear.
49. It may be that *nāḍī* here means a unit of time equal to the more common *ghaṭikā*, i.e. twenty-four minutes (see Birch 2013: 264, n.44), but in light of the earlier reference to thirty-two *nāḍī*s as channels, we have understood it to refer to channels here.
50. A *prahara* is a unit of time lasting three hours (see Birch 2013: 264, n.45).
51. We have drawn on the commentaries of Kallinātha and Siṃhabhūpāla in our translation of the root text.
52. Bandhūka (*Pentapetes phoenicea* Linn.) flowers are bright red.
53. The bee cave is on the thousand-petalled lotus in the head (*Jogpradīpakā* 932 (9.3.9); cf. *Śārṅgadharapaddhati* 4366, *Gorakhbāṇī*, *pad*s 28.2, 30.4).
54. The five elements, together with the mind, intellect and ego. Cf. *Bhagavadgītā* 7.4.
55. On *śakticālana*, see Chapter 6, p. 231.
56. On this practice, see Chapter 6, pp. 230–31.
57. i.e. The fluid that flows from elephants' temples when they are in rut.
58. A sequence of four blisses experienced in the course of sexual ritual is a common feature of tantric Buddhism.
59. Translation by Catharina Kiehnle (2005: 477–80).
60. Translation by Lubomír Ondračka (Ondračka 2011).
61. Translation by Catharina Kiehnle (2005: 473–6).
62. See also *Yogabīja* 34–5 on raw and cooked bodies (1.2.7).

SIX

Yogic Seals

1. Some texts (e.g. *Haṭhapradīpikājyotsnā* 3.91) identify *rajas*, which is variously interpreted as menstrual or generative uterine fluid, as the equivalent of *bindu* in female bodies. On *bindu* see Chapter 5.
2. The exact meaning of *vajrolīmudrā* is unclear; it perhaps derives from tantric Buddhist traditions and means 'the Vajra lineage *mudrā*' (Mallinson forthcoming (a)).
3. The *Amṛtasiddhi*'s *vedha* or 'piercing' involves a slightly different technique from that taught in all subsequent texts.

4. For an overview of the use of *mudrās* in early tantra see Isaacson and Goodall 2016: 49–51.
5. Some *mudrās* taught in tantric texts do involve manipulation of the vital energies, in particular the breath. See e.g. the thirty-second *āhnika* of the *Tantrāloka*. In addition, a number of tantric texts teach yogic methods called *karaṇas*, which share some features with the haṭhayogic *mudrās*. For examples of parallels with the haṭhayogic *khecarīmudrā*, see Mallinson 2007a: 20–26.
6. Mallinson 2007a: 25–6.
7. At three places in the *Bhāgavatapurāṇa* (which is not a tantric work) the yogi is instructed to press his anus with his heel in the manner of the haṭhayogic *mahāmudrā* and (in some descriptions) *mūlabandha* (2.2.19, 11.15.24 and 4.23.14). Kṣemarāja, an eleventh-century Kashmiri exegete of Śaiva tantric works, does prescribe squeezing and relaxing the anus in order to make Śakti, the goddess, enter the central channel (commentary on *Netratantra* 7.30), but we are not aware of clear-cut forerunners of the haṭhayogic *mudrās* in earlier tantric texts.
8. See Mallinson 2007a: 17–19.
9. Most textual descriptions of the Inverter do not specify how it is to be performed beyond saying that the body is to be inverted. Chandik (1898: 35) says that it may be done either by standing on one's head or hanging from a tree.
10. The *Amaraughaśāsana* (8.2) associates a squatting position (*utkaṭāsana*) with the raising of Kuṇḍalinī, the main aim of *mudrā* practice in later haṭhayogic texts.
11. See Sanderson 2007b: 250, n.119 and Birch 2013: 70–78. See also Kṣemarāja's *Spandasaṃdoha* commentary on *Spandakārikā* 1.11 (9.1.9), which describes a version of *bhairavīmudrā* as a method of *samādhi*.
12. On the Kaula tantric appropriation of the techniques of *haṭhayoga* see Mallinson 2015.
13. On *vajrolīmudrā* and the problems with this understanding of its purpose, see Mallinson forthcoming (a).
14. In the *Amṛtasiddhi* (13.1), *yonimudrā* is found as a variant name for *mahāmudrā*, a different practice from the *Śivasaṃhitā*'s *yonimudrā*. *Śivasaṃhitā* 4.66 says that *yonimudrā* is perfected by *mūlabandha*; it is probably as a variant of *mūlabandha* that the *Vivekamārtaṇḍa* (v. 53, which is also found at *Haṭhapradīpikā* 3.42 and *Śivasaṃhitā* 4.82, cf. *Śivasaṃhitā* 4.97) prescribes *yonimudrā* as a means of preventing ejaculation.

15. On the connection between *yonimudrā* and mantra practices made by the commentator Rāghavabhaṭṭa in the context of *Śāradātilaka* 2.111, see Sanderson 2007b: 249, n.118.
16. Translation by Dominic Goodall (Goodall et al. 2015: 372–4).
17. On *bindu*, see Chapter 5.
18. In *Amṛtasiddhi* 2.5 and 13.8, goddesses are said to dwell at the base of the central channel and gods along it and at the top.
19. On the breaths, see Chapter 4 (on breath-control) and 5 (on the yogic body).
20. On the piercing of the knots, see Chapter 5.
21. Translation by Catharina Kiehnle (Kiehnle 2005: 467–9).
22. Translation by Carl Ernst (http://www.asia.si.edu/explore/yoga/ocean-of-life.asp).
23. Lit. 'she who has horses'.
24. As noted in the introduction to this chapter, the *Gheraṇḍasaṃhitā*'s identification of these practices of fixation as *mudrā*s is anomalous. Several comparable element fixations are included in section 2 of Chapter 8.

SEVEN
Mantra

1. The use of mantras in yoga is distinct from the practice of *nāda*, listening to the internal sound, taught in tantric and haṭhayogic texts as a means of accomplishing *samādhi*.
2. As pointed out to us by Finnian Moore Gerety (personal communication, 3 October 2015), a significant exception to this is found in the Sāmavedic songs called *gāna*s, many of which include meaningless syllables and distorted phrases called *stobha*s. See Staal 1989 on the parallels between Sāmavedic *stobha*s and tantric *bīja*s.
3. But see *Bhagavadgītā* 8.12–13 (discussed in the next section of this introduction).
4. Patañjali makes no place for the use of Vedic mantras other than *oṃ*: in the commentary to *sūtra* 2.32, *svādhyāya*, which in a Vedic context would mean the recitation of Vedic hymns, is defined as 'the study of texts on liberation or the repetition of *oṃ*'.
5. For an overview of the use of mantra in early tantra, see Isaacson and Goodall 2016. On mantra in Saiddhāntika tantric traditions, see Brunner 1994.
6. Brunner 1994: 440, 452–9.

7. The *Khecarīvidyā*'s *khecarīmantra* remains impossible to extract with certainty. One of the most likely candidates is *hskhphrīṃ* (Mallinson 2007a: 199, n.225).
8. Cf. *Jaiminīya Upaniṣad Brāhmaṇa* 3.5.4–5.
9. An exception is the Pāśupata tradition, whose earliest text, the *Pāśupatasūtra*, enjoins the recitation of Vedic mantras (1.17).
10. On mantra in early Jainism, see Dundas 1998. On the early (first century CE onwards) Buddhist mantra-type spells called *dhāraṇīs* see Hidas 2015.
11. Mallinson 2015.
12. For further Śaiva references to the Haṃsa mantra and analysis of it see Goodall 2004: 375, n.821 and Padoux 1992: 139–42. See also *Vijñānabhairava* 154–6.
13. The *Śāradātilaka*, which is contemporaneous with the *Vivekamārtaṇḍa*, also calls the involuntary repetition of Haṃsa Ajapā. We know of no earlier instances of this name.
14. Here we follow Finnian Moore Gerety's translation of this passage (Gerety 2015: 255), which is in turn drawn from that of Fujii (Fujii 1989: 996–7).
15. Translation by Alexis Sanderson (1999: 8).
16. From an unpublished translation by Carl Ernst.
17. [Ernst's footnote:] Here the translator compares the yogic mantras with the Greatest Name (*al-ism al-a'zam*) of God, which according to Islamic (as well as Jewish and Christian) tradition is the key to all knowledge. The Persian text goes further with its comparison: 'Most of the "friends of God" (*awliya'-i khuda*, Sufi saints) have comprehended and explained these influences from unveiling (*kashf*), and the monks (*rahiban*) of India, who are the yogis, have unveiling that is in agreement with the mystical state of those who have realized the truth. Although the language differs, the explanation is the same.' That is, Muhammad Ghawth equates the mystical experience of the yogis and the Sufi saints.
18. See 2.5.2.
19. The seed mantra of the wind is said to be *ya* at *Gheraṇḍasaṃhitā* 3.62. The lunar channel is the left nostril, the solar channel is the right.
20. This is a reference to the building of a causeway to Laṅkā in the *Rāmāyaṇa*.

EIGHT

Withdrawal, Fixation and Meditation

1. See De Michelis 2004: 8: 'in common English usage (i.e. in Modern Yoga), "yoga" is "postural yoga", and "meditation" is "sitting meditation" [. . .] [T]he first linguistic association that speakers of Indian languages make upon hearing the word "yoga" is with *dhyāna*, "meditation".' De Michelis makes a working typological distinction between 'Modern Postural Yoga' and 'Modern Meditational Yoga' (along with 'Modern Psychosomatic Yoga' and 'Modern Denominational Yoga') (2004: 188). Some Hindi-speaking ascetics distinguish their practice of *yog* (the Hindi pronunciation of Sanskrit *yoga*) from the posture-based *yogā* practised in Indian metropolises and abroad.
2. The *Pātañjalayogaśāstra*'s assertion that when the senses withdraw from sense objects they take on the resemblance of the mind itself is echoed in the *Dattātreyayogaśāstra*'s repeated injunctions to the yogi to cause sense objects to exist in his self (8.1.6) and the *Vivekamārtaṇḍa*'s comparable (and repeated) advice to recognize sense objects as the self (8.1.7).
3. There are exceptions to this order. For example, the *Mālinīvijayottara* is unusual for apparently placing sense-withdrawal (*pratyāhāra*) after *samādhi* as the final and highest auxiliary (although the text does not in fact provide a single, hierarchical list of *aṅgas*). The *Vāyupurāṇa* places withdrawal after breath-control and meditation, and before fixation and recollection (*smaraṇa*) in its fivefold schema of Pāśupata yoga (1.4.5).
4. Compare this with *Parākhyatantra* 14.11a–12b (8.1.3), in which the mind is withdrawn into the heart.
5. Vasudeva 2004: 396.
6. Loc. cit.
7. In the context of the Śaivasiddhānta, Brunner (1994: 441) notes, '*dhāraṇā*'s definition is very much the same as it is in classical yoga, but the form it takes and the use one makes of it are perfectly original. First, our texts do not leave the practitioner every liberty as to the object he must fix his mind on: a limited choice is generally offered [. . .]' But see *Mṛgendratantra* 32c–33b: since one meditates on the divine form within the elements (and not just on material *tattvas*), one may ultimately take anything as an object of meditation (Sanderson 1999: 16). On tantric *Tāntrikābhidhānakośa*, see also *Tāntrikābhidhānakośa* I, s.v. *āgneyī dhāraṇā*, III, s.v. *dhāraṇā*, and Isaacson and Goodall 2016: 7.

8. Goodall et al. (2015: 75) note that 'outside the context of *bhūtaśuddhi* [purification of the elements], early Pāñcarātra sources speak not of five *dhāraṇās* focusing on the five elements, but of only two, namely *dahana* and *plāvana*; other early Saiddhāntika sources speak of four, only the first two of which are clearly associated with elements, namely the *āgneyī* and the *vāruṇī* or *saumyā dhāraṇās*'. See also Brunner (1994: 442), who notes that as well as the five-element *dhāraṇā* practices prevalent in 'orthodox texts' of the Śaivasiddhānta, there is another tradition represented by the *Kiraṇa*, *Raurava* and *Mataṅgapārameśvara*, in which four different *dhāraṇās* are recognized, called *āgneyī* (or *pāvakā*), *saumyā* (or *vāruṇī*), *aiśānī* and *amṛtā*, with places of fixation in the navel, ear, head and no particular spot (respectively). For a further summary of tantric *dhāraṇā* practices in historical context, see Goodall 2004: 360, n.761.
9. Brunner 1994: 441.
10. On this point, see Goodall et al. 2015: 74.
11. See Jacobsen 2005: 15.
12. Gethin 2004: 201.
13. For instance, the *Muṇḍaka Upaniṣad* declares that the self, invisible to the senses, can be perceived by one who meditates and thus has become pure through the light of knowledge (8.3.1). On possible Vedic precedents for yogic practice, see e.g. Gonda 1963 and Werner 1994 [1977].
14. As noted in the main introduction, a helpful, selective summary of de la Vallée Poussin's 1936 list (de la Vallée Poussin 1937a) of the parallels between Patañjali and Buddhism is provided by Franco (2009: 8): 'the four types of concentration (*samādhi*), which correspond to the four levels of *dhyāna* (see YS 1.17); the definition of God (*īśvara*) in YS 1.25 as the one in which the seed of omniscience reaches the highest degree (*niratiśayaṃ sarvajñabījam*), a definition that can only be understood in light of Buddhist Mahāyāna teachings (of Yogācāra and Tathāgatagarbha); the four *brahmavihāras* in YS 1.33; the threefold division of knowledge/wisdom (*prajñā*) into knowledge that "holds the truth" in contradistinction to knowledge which arises from study (*śruta*) or reasoning (*anumāna*) in YS 1.48–49; the interpretation of the doctrine of *karma* (YS 2.12–13,31,34,4.7); the division of suffering into three kinds in YS 2.15 (*pariṇāma-tāpa-saṃskāra-duḥkha*), which is clearly of Buddhist origin; the theory of the existence of three times (past, present and future) in YS 3.13 and 4.12, which is a reflection of the corresponding Sarvāstivāda theory; the doctrine of knowledge of other minds

(*paracittajñāna*) as knowing only whether the cognition of another person is good or bad, but without knowing the object of the cognition (YS 3.20–21); the four perfections of the body (*kāyasampad* YS 3.46); and, of course, the five types of *siddhi* (YS 4.1), which are either innate, produced by the use of herbs, by uttering magical syllables (*mantra*), from the practice of austerities (*tapas*), or through the practice of meditation/concentration (*samādhi*).'

15. Ohira 1982: 90.
16. Bedekar 1962a; Wynne 2007: 26, 45. Although as Wynne (2007: 26) points out, in practice such borrowing probably worked both ways: 'The correspondences allow us to suppose that there was meaningful contact between the two traditions in early times. The similar versions of the chariot metaphor in both the early Buddhist and Brahminic literatures even suggest that early Buddhism was influenced by the meditative ideas of early Brahminism.'
17. Bronkhorst (1993: 45) suggests that the omission of all but the first *dhyāna* is because the later *dhyāna*s 'were an embarrassment for the author of this section because they go beyond his aim in discarding such desirable (see v. 21–22) states as joy (*prīti*) and bliss (*sukha*). The immediate aim in this section of the *Mahābhārata* – as elsewhere in the Epic – is control of the mind and the senses.'
18. Gethin 2015. Namely, the truth of suffering (*duḥkha*), the truth of the origin of suffering, the truth of the cessation of suffering, and the truth of the Eightfold Path leading to the cessation of suffering.
19. Bronkhorst 1993: 85.
20. Bronkhorst 1993: 85; Schmithausen 1981: 216–17; de la Vallée Poussin 1937b: 220.
21. For summaries of the many, varied schemes of meditation in early Buddhism, see Bronkhorst 1993: 55–70 and Deleanu 2009: 8–10.
22. There are three further mentions of meditation in the *Pātañjalayogaśāstra*: as a method to escape the activities of the afflictions (*kleśa*s; see 2.1.1); 'meditation as desired' (1.39) as one among many methods of practice (*abhyāsa*) which overcome distractions and obstacles (1.30); and as an activity which produces no karmic residues (4.6).
23. Oberhammer 1977: 135–61; see also Maas 2009: 264–76.
24. Oberhammer 1977: 162–77; see also Maas: 2009: 276–80.
25. Oberhammer 1977: 177–209.
26. Oberhammer 1977: 209–30.
27. For a detailed examination of the visualization of the deities of Trika Śavism, see Sanderson 1990.
28. Kiss 2011: 159.

29. Goodall 2011.
30. See Sanderson 1999. Similarly, Buddhist tantric yogas commonly begin with a visualization of emptiness (*śūnyatā*) prior to the detailed eidetic meditation on the deity (see Szántó 2012: 33).
31. Translation by Alexis Sanderson (1999: 6–7).
32. This passage is paraphrased, in verse, in Chapter 7 of the *Yogayājñavalkya*, which is cited by Nīlakaṇṭha *ad Mahābhārata* 12.307 (cf. Hopkins 1901: 345).
33. The syntax in these descriptions is defective.
34. For the remainder of this passage, see section 5.1.6.
35. Translation by Rolf Giebel (2005: 156–7).
36. Translation by Alexis Sanderson (1999: 17–19).
37. Translation by Dan Stuart (2015: 491–3).
38. Translation by Dominic Goodall (Goodall et al. 2015: 385–93).
39. These divisions of time are esoteric references to the flow of the breath.
40. Translation by Alexis Sanderson (1999: 7).
41. Translation by Alexis Sanderson (1999: 16–17).
42. Translation by Alexis Sanderson (1990: 51).
43. Vāsudeva, Nārāyaṇa and Acyuta are names of the god Viṣṇu.
44. Adapted from the translation by Csaba Kiss (2009: 262–4).
45. A verse is missing here in the manuscript which we are using as the basis of our edition of the *Vivekamārtaṇḍa*.

NINE

Samādhi

1. As Lidke (2005: 144) states with reference to *samādhi*: 'while many spiritual traditions within India have utilized yogic practices for the attainment of their higher aspirations, there is no consensus as to what such experiences have validated.'
2. 'Egoism' (*asmitā*) is glossed in the commentary as *ekātmikā saṃvid*, 'unitary consciousness'.
3. However, as we saw in Chapter 1, Vijñānabhikṣu, for example, argues that the goals of Sāṃkhyayoga and Vedānta are identical.
4. On this point, see Vasudeva 2000: 286–7 and the section '*Yogāṅgas*: Auxiliaries of Yoga', in Chapter 1 of this book.
5. See Nicholson 2013: 494.
6. Brunner 1994: 429.
7. Kiss 2011: 158.
8. On *bhairavīmudrā*, see Lidke 2005 and 6.2.7.

9. But see also *Mahābhārata* 12.294.14–18 on becoming as still as a stone during meditation.
10. For example *Amanaska* 2.64, *Yogatarāvalī* 24–26, *Haṭhatattvakaumudī* 51.29. See also Birch and Hargreaves 2014.
11. On the interchangeability of *samādhi* and sleep in a purāṇic context see Schreiner 2010: 203–4.
12. Methods of revival from *samādhi* trance similar to that used to bring round Hari Dās are described in *Bṛhatkhecarīprakāśa ad Khecarīvidyā* 3.27–30 (9.1.23) and *Haṭhatattvakaumudī* 51.80. For an overview of accounts of *samādhi* burials, and the use of *khecarīmudrā* therein, see Mallinson 2007a: 234, n.425. For a fictional, filmic representation of the revival of a yogi in *samādhi*, see the opening two scenes of the 1921 film, scripted by Fritz Lang, *The Indian Tomb*. Note that the omniscient yogi Ramagani's tongue appears to be in *khecarīmudrā* and his eyes in *śāmbhavīmudrā*.
13. The term *samādhi* is still commonly used in India to indicate the tomb of a deceased yogi or saint who is considered to have reached *samādhi* at the moment of death.
14. See Mallinson 2007a: 234, n.425, and Siegel 1991: 168–70. Pilot Bābā's *samādhi* includes a daily breakfast *in situ* (Matthew Clarke, personal communication), which puts it at some remove from the 'months without food and drink' of the yogis described by Ibn Baṭṭūṭa. At one point in the 1998 film *Kings with Straw Mats – Yogis and Sadhus of the Kumbh Mela Festival* (a documentary film on the 1986 Kumbh Melā in Haridwar) the director Ira Cohen meets 'the *samādhi* wallah', who is preparing to bury himself for a week.
15. Slaje 2000: 178.
16. As Slaje (2000: 179) puts it, 'A Pātañjala-Yogin, irrespective of his favourite (*nirodha* or *saṃyama*) practice of *samādhi*, can certainly not be expected to walk around or to engage in everyday activities while striving for, or being actually in, the highest stage of concentration (*samādhi*).'
17. The first four of these are said to arise from the practice of *śāmbhavī*, *bhrāmarī*, *khecarī* and *yoni mudrā*s (see Chapter 6).
18. Birch 2013: 48.
19. It is also described as the joining of the mind and self (162) and the identity of the individual self (*jīvātman*) and the supreme self (*paramātman*) in which all conceptions are destroyed (164).
20. Further to this, the text instructs the yogi to drench the body in nectar (*amṛta*) – a procedure which, as we have seen, is characteristic of tantric traditions – and then to focus on the supreme state, making the mind its own object of observation.

21. See Chapter 8 on the dissolution of the elements in the context of fixation, and Chapter 5 for discussion and examples of raising the breath and Kuṇḍalinī up the central channel.
22. For a helpful tabulation of the effects and accomplishments associated with the temporal duration of *laya* in the *Amanaska*, see Birch 2013: 54 and 56.
23. The *Vijñānabhairava* teaches subitist techniques (i.e. leading to direct, immediate realization) which transcend the ritual teachings of the Trika (see Sanderson 1990: 74), including methods such as contemplating the blissful sensations of sex or of a full stomach (**9.2.4**).
24. Vasudeva 2004: 339–42.
25. See Birch 2013: 51.
26. e.g. *Dīrghanikāya* 3.225.
27. Translation by Alexis Sanderson (1999: 7–8).
28. Our translation is based on that of Dominic Goodall (2004: 356).
29. We have adopted the translation 'empathetic imagination' used by Kiss (2011) for the technical term *bhāva*. See introduction to Chapter 8.
30. On *bhairavīmudrā* (as *śāmbhavīmudrā*) see **6.2.7**.
31. On these see **4.16**.
32. i.e. after death: *samādhi* here has the meaning of the permanent *samādhi* that a yogi enters after physical death.
33. Translation by Mahdi Husain (1953: 164).
34. Unpublished translation by Bruce Wannell, with input on the content by James Mallinson.
35. Braid 1850: 11–14.
36. 'Goad' here refers to an *aṅkuśa*, a hook used by elephant drivers to control elephants.
37. We have conjecturally emended *dhyāyen* to *dhyātaṃ* in 1.6a.
38. Translation by T. N. Ganapathy.
39. Translation by Carl Ernst (http://www.asia.edu/explore/yoga/ocean-of-life.asp).

TEN

Yogic Powers

1. These powers are referred to by several names in our texts, for example *siddhi*, *guṇa*, *aiśvarya*, *vibhūti*, *bala*, *vīrya* and *prabhāva* as well as the specifically Buddhist terms *ṛddhi*, *abhijñā*, *adhiṣṭhāna*, *prātihārya* and *vikurvaṇa*. In the *Mahābhārata*, the word *yoga* itself can mean 'yogic power' (see Malinar 2012: 38 for references).

2. Because almost any yogic practice may produce them, supernatural powers are described in several other passages in this book. The abilities of entering another's body (*parakāyapraveśa*) and casting off one's own (*utkrānti*), for example, are included in some lists of yogic powers (e.g. the *Pātañjalayogaśāstra*, selection 10.4 in this chapter) but they are also a corollary of achieving *mukti*, liberation, and we have discussed them in detail in Chapter 11.
3. See the edited volume *Yoga Powers* (Jacobsen 2012) for an overview of this subject (Jacobsen's introduction) and a range of detailed treatments of yogic powers in a wide variety of Indian traditions.
4. See the introduction to Franco 2009 for an overview of the concept of yogic perception, and the first part of the same volume for analyses of how it was understood in a variety of Indian schools of thought.
5. It is not clear how East India Company officials would have reacted to the description of yogis in this text, but the story of the underground *samādhi* of the yogi Hari Dās (9.1.22) shows that some colonial officers were convinced that Indian yogis could perform superhuman feats.
6. See Hara 1999: 603 for references. For further reading on supernatural powers in Buddhist traditions, see e.g. Lindquist 1935 and Granoff 1996.
7. Malinar 2012: 37. Elsewhere in the *Mahābhārata* it is clearly said that such powers must be rejected in order to achieve liberation (e.g. 12.228.37).
8. On *utkrānti*, see Chapter 11.
9. See Vasudeva 2012: 288–9.
10. See e.g. *Niśvāsatattvasaṃhitā Guhyasūtra* 3, *Jayākhyasaṃhitā* 33.1ab.
11. Brunner 1994: 435.
12. *Mahābhārata* 10.7.41, 12.326.51, 13.18.24.
13. For a discussion of different definitions of the members of this group of eight powers in Śaiva tantric texts, see Brunner-Lachaux 1977: 506–8 and Goodall 2004: 379, n.831.
14. e.g. Nārāyaṇakaṇṭha's commentary on *Mṛgendratantra Yogapāda* 65 and *Liṅgapurāṇa* 86 and 88.
15. We thank Dr Christèle Barois for providing us with her unpublished edition and analysis of this passage.
16. Davidson 2002: 200.
17. On this threefold classification, see Vasudeva 2012.
18. We note one exception: in *Yogaśāstra* 8.31, the twelfth-century Jain polymath Hemacandra teaches how visualization of the syllable *oṃ* in different colours will bring about the six malefic acts.

19. On such contests, see Digby 1970 and 2000, Rizvi 1970, Ernst 2007, Green 2004 and Burchett 2012.
20. The powers listed in section (4) are repeated here.
21. Only selections from the commentary have been included here. In some places the commentary has informed our translation of a *sūtra* without itself being translated.
22. On portents (*ariṣṭa*s), see pp. 401–3 and 11.3.
23. On 'yogic suicide', see pp. 401–2 and 11.3.
24. As edited by Harunaga Isaacson (1993: 146).
25. Exceptionally, we have translated *ākāśa* as 'ether' not 'space', because *ākāśa* is followed here by *dik*, for which 'space' is the most appropriate translation.
26. We have used the text as edited by Goodall, Isaacson and Sanderson (*Niśvāsatattvasaṃhitā* introduction pp. 79–80) and followed their translation.
27. Translation by Dominic Goodall (2004: 381–2).
28. We are grateful to Csaba Kiss for his help with the difficult syntax and vocabulary of this passage.
29. A stone-like secretion with purported medicinal qualities found in the stomachs of ruminants (derived from a Persian word meaning 'antidote').
30. Several types of magical movement, such as travelling great distances in one leap, walking on water and using fruits, flowers and leaves etc. as vehicles, are detailed in the commentary to this verse.
31. Translated by Simon Digby in Digby 2000: 229–30.
32. We have used the text as edited by Birch but have made some emendations and adopted some alternative readings.
33. Translated by Court but slightly modified by Carl Ernst according to the Urdu text (see Ernst 2007: 420).

ELEVEN

Liberation

1. Watson et al. 2013: 17.
2. For a concise tabulation of the various views refuted in the *Paramokṣanirāsakārikāvṛtti*, with a partly speculative reconstruction of the groups to which they belong, see Watson et al. 2013: 16.
3. Aldous Huxley's 1945 comparative study of religious mysticism, *The Perennial Philosophy*, and Joseph Campbell's 1949 *The Hero with a Thousand Faces* are key works of popular twentieth-century perennial philosophy. For a critical summary of perennialism in

Western and Indian thought, see Prothero 2010. On the term New Age, see Hanegraaff 1998 and Heelas 1996.

4. The most prominent academic theorist of the perennialist view is Huston Smith: 'It is possible to climb life's mountain from any side, but when the top is reached the trails converge. At base, in the foothills of theology, ritual, and organizational structure, the religions are distinct. Differences in culture, history, geography, and collective temperament all make for diverse starting points . . . . But beyond these differences, the same goal beckons' (Smith 1991: 73). One of the best-known proponents of similar views in modern yoga is Swami Sivananda (see for example his short piece 'The Unity that Underlies All Religions': 'At the present moment all religions contain a mixture of truth, which is divine, and error which is human. The fundamentals or essentials of all religions are the same. There is difference only in the non-essentials' (Sivananda, n.d.)).
5. See Goodall et al. 2015: 73.
6. On liberation and death, see White 2009, chapter 3.
7. Bansat-Boudon remarks that 'one has the sense that Kashmir Śaivism is one of the first systems to seek to *justify* doctrinally the notion of *jīvanmukti*' (2013: 309). However, see the claim made by Saraogi (2010) that the doctrine of *jīvanmukti* only becomes important in Śaivism as a result of the reinterpretations of earlier texts by Kashmiri exegetes such as Abhinavagupta (tenth century) – a process which sometimes, as in the case of the *Svacchandatantra*, led to the actual rewriting of the texts to include the new doctrine.
8. Mumme 1996: 247.
9. On living liberation in Advaita Vedānta, see Nelson 1986 and (especially) Fort 1998. Something similar holds true in the non-dual metaphysics of the Śaiva Trika tradition, where on the absolute level there is in fact no liberation, bondage being merely an empirical, relative phenomenon. In this view, the *jīvanmukta* is one who realizes that he is always already liberated, rather than one who 'attains' the post-emancipatory state of liberation (Bansat-Boudon 2013).
10. On criticisms of *jīvanmukti* from within the dualist (*dvaita*) school of Mādhava, see Sheridan 1996; on Rāmānuja's criticisms from the point of view of qualified non-dual (*viśiṣṭādvaita*) Vedānta, see Skoog 1996.
11. A comparable position (affirming the reality of *jīvanmukti*, but as a state inferior to full liberation) is apparent in the Nimbārka tradition: see Śāstrin 1972: 34–5.

12. Acharya 2008: 424–6.
13. 'Yoga [i.e. the *Pātañjalayogaśāstra*] does not allow the persistence of a trace of *avidyā* after attainment of *ṛtambharā-prajñā*, the highest stage of *saṃprajñāta-samādhi*. In Yoga, the modifications have to be totally abolished before *prajñā* comes into being. Therefore, the belief in the existence of the body of a *jīvanmukta* presents a challenge to the commentators' (Rukmani 2005: 71). In short, a Pātañjala yogi cannot walk around or engage in everyday activities while striving for, or being in, the highest states of *samādhi* (see Slaje 2000: 179, and Chapter 9, n.16).
14. Goodall et al. 2015: 69.
15. Bansat-Boudon 2013: 309.
16. Mumme 1996: 263. The term used by the *Sāṃkhyasūtra* (3.81) to indicate this contradiction is *andhaparamparā*, 'the lineage of the blind' (see Rukmini 2005: 70–71). Mumme further notes that Śaṅkara himself, commenting on *Chāndogya Upaniṣad* 6.14.2, states that one of the reasons *jīvanmukti* must be affirmed is 'the need for authoritative gurus and teachers' (1995: 263).
17. Cheating death (*kāla-* or *mṛtyu-vañcana/ā*) is a key concern in many yoga texts, especially (but not only) tantric texts. On cheating death in the context of tantric Buddhism, see Walter 2000.
18. On the portents of death in yogic and non-yogic contexts, see Einoo 2004; Meulenbeld 1974: 442; and Kiehnle 2006.
19. Bansat-Boudon 2013: 316.
20. We should also note that in some haṭhayogic texts certain postures (*āsanas*) are said to lead to liberation (for example, the adept's posture (*siddhāsana*) at *Haṭhapradīpikā* 1.35, and the lotus posture (*padmāsana*) at *Haṭhapradīpikā* 1.49).
21. See Smith 2006: 286–9.
22. On which see Bloomfield 1917 and the first chapter of White 2009.
23. Smith 2006: 289. Smith further notes: 'Hemacandra is not speaking as a lone voice in Jainism. Cf. Merutuṅga's *Prabandhacintāmaṇi*, p. 12: *parapurapraveśa*; also *Pārśvanāthacaritra* 1.576, 3.119' (ibid., p. 312, n. 15).
24. *Bhāṣya* commentary to 4.33 omitted here.
25. Translation by Alex Watson et al. (2013: 455–64).
26. Translation by Alex Sanderson (1996: 27–8).
27. Translation by Catharina Kiehnle (2005: 484–7).
28. Kiehnle (2005: 487) identifies the *tanmātra* as the subtle element of sound and the half-*mātrā* as the half-syllable situated above the *ṃ* of *oṃ* in the Ājñā *cakra*.
29. Translation by Dominic Goodall (2004: 383–4).

30. On the practice of *khecarīmudrā*, the prerequisite to the practices described here, see Chapter 6.
31. The Varuṇa breath is said in the text to be white and cool and to flow fast downwards to a distance of twelve finger-breadths (5.49).
32. From an unpublished translation by Carl Ernst.
33. [Ernst's note:] The Arabic text is especially incoherent in this paragraph. The Persian version reads with much greater clarity, probably better reflecting the earlier Arabic recension: 'If he wishes to enter a dead body, he can, and that dead body will come alive, while his body dies. When he wishes, he can come back at once into his own body. At a time when he enters the body of another, he protects his body, and tells someone to watch over his body, so that no corruption occurs in it, nor does any demon descend into it. If it is not done in this manner, he cannot come back; even if he wishes [to enter] his body, he cannot imagine [how to do it]. Without his body, he does not die, for it cannot be that a single soul exists between two bodies. If he becomes weakened internally from the living body, he is not overcome, but if he is strong, he overcomes it. When the body is internally strong, he cannot go into it, except when it is unaware. This subject is well known and famous among the masters of this science, and many stories are told and wonders related on this subject. This is not easy except by giving up sexual intercourse and socializing or quarrelling with women.'
34. [Ernst's note:] The Persian version translates thus: 'At the time of meditating on these words, he recites them in the heart, not by the tongue, in the very manner that has been described. In this way, the effect of the magical imagination and the speaking of the words reaches a point so that with a single magical imagination and glance, he gazes at all the figures, and recites all the words in the heart. This is done in such a fashion that one would say that at the moment of imagining those words, he goes out of himself and reaches heaven. When he reaches this station, he attains interior senses other than these senses; by these senses he witnesses the hidden world. Then at this time he becomes unconscious, but then comes back to himself. Life and death appear the same, and sleeping and waking are one. He becomes pure spirit, God willing.'
35. Translation by T. N. Ganapathy.

Acknowledgements

A book of this scope necessarily depends on the work of others. We are particularly grateful to those scholars who have so graciously agreed to allow us to use their translations: Ian Baker (the Tibetan *Rtsa rlung gsang ba'i lde mig*), Carl Ernst (the Arabic *Ḥawż al-ḥayāt* and Persian *Baḥr al-ḥayāt*), Rolf Giebel (the Chinese *Vairocanābhisaṃbodhi Sūtra*), Dominic Goodall (*Parākhyatantra, Niśvāsatattvasaṃhitā, Kiraṇatantra*), Kengo Harimoto (*Pātañjalayogaśāstravivaraṇa*), Harunaga Isaacson (*Niśvāsatattvasaṃhitā*), Shaman Hatley (*Kaulajñānanirṇaya*), Sonam Kachru (the Kashmiri *Lallāvākyāni*), Catharina Kiehnle (the Marathi *Jñāneśvarī*), Glenn H. Mullin (the Tibetan *Chos drug gi man ngag zhes bya ba*), Lubomír Ondračka (the Old Bengali *Gorakṣavijaý*), Alexis Sanderson (the *Yogapāda* of the *Mṛgendratantra* with Bhaṭṭa Nārāyaṇa's commentary, *Niśvāsatattvasaṃhitā, Siddhayogeśvarīmata*), Dan Stuart (*Saddharmasmṛtyupasthānasūtra*), Somdeva Vasudeva (*Yogaśataka*), T. V. Venkataraman (the Tamil *Tirumandiram*), Bruce Wannell (the Persian *Tashrīh al-Aqvāṃ*), Alex Watson (*Paramokṣanirāsakārikā*).

We thank the following scholars for reading and commenting on drafts of each chapter: Frederick M. Smith (Introduction and Chapter 1); Andrew Nicholson (Chapter 2); Jason Birch (Chapters 3 and 5); Somdeva Vasudeva (Chapter 4); Shaman Hatley (Chapter 6); Csaba Kiss (Chapter 7); Dominic Goodall (Chapter 8); Matthew Clark (Chapter 9); Knut Axel Jacobsen (Chapter 10); Alex Watson (Chapter 11). Especial thanks to Graham Burns for offering detailed feedback on a draft of the whole book, and Seth Powell for proof-reading one of its final incarnations. Thanks also to Richard Rosen, Ellen Goldberg and Tara Fraser for their comments.

Many of those mentioned above have helped us in other ways, for which we thank them further. We have also benefited from the help of the following scholars, yogis and friends (categories which are of course not mutually exclusive): Simon Atkinson, Imre Bangha, Christèle Barois, Hartmut Buescher, Whitney Cox, William Dalrymple, Yogirāj Jagannāth Dās, Śrīmahant Raghuvar Dās ('Yogirāj'), Śrī Rām Bālak Dās ('Bālyogī'), Magnus Dennis, Ian Duncan (Bhagavānnāth), Finnian Moore Gerety, M. M. Gharote, Chris Gibbons, Hanumān Giri, Paraśurām Giri, Luis Gonzalez-Reimann, Marshall Govindan, Viswanatha Gupta, Jacqueline Hargreaves, Shankaranarayana Jois, Nirajan Kafle, Csaba Kiss, Ulrich Timme Kragh, Somānanda Kuyogin, Philipp Maas, Anne Monius, 'Yogī Bābā' Anup Nāth, Campā Nāth, Karen O'Brien-Kop, André Padoux, Seth Powell, Samaṇi Pratibhā Prajñā, Robin C. Rinehart, Kazuyo Sakaki, Deepak Sarma, Kurtis Schaeffer, Jason Schwartz, Vishal Sharma, Daniel Simpson, John Smith, Péter-Dániel Szántó, Vincent Tournier, Ganga White, Michael Witzel and Dominik Wujastyk (whose *Roots of Āyurveda* was an inspiration for this volume).

We would like to thank the staff of the Mehrangarh Fort Museum Trust, Jodhpur, for their continued generosity and collaboration: Dr Kr. Mahendra Singhji, Karni Singh Jasol, M. S. Tanwar, D. K. Nathani. Especial thanks to H. H. Gaj Singh, Maharaja of Jodhpur, for his support.

Mark would like to thank Karandip Singh and Navaz Sandhu for their hospitality and friendship during a writing retreat at Ballyhack Cottage in Shimla. Thanks also to the peerless Anita Roy.

James would like to thank his family, especially Claudia, Lily and Willa, for their unfailing support and understanding through this long and often demanding project.

We thank Josephine Greywoode, our editor, and Anna Hervé, our editorial manager at Penguin Classics, Ian Pindar, our copy-editor, Alex Bell, our indexer, Stephen Ryan and Alison Tulett, our proofreaders at Penguin, and David Godwin, our agent.

This project was partly funded through a Kickstarter online crowd-sourcing campaign. We would like to acknowledge the following patrons for their backing: Agama Yoga School, Tim

Allman, Lisa and Paul Angerame, Julien Balmer, George Barker, Georgina Bridges, David Cornell, Magnus Dennis, Rob Drummond, Steve Farmer, Tara Fraser, Jeff Goldring, Chris Handy, Kai Hitzer, Little River Yoga, Gillian MacCabe, Adam Murby, Dianna Oles, Anne O'Brien, Lubomír Ondračka, Sebastian Pole, Steven Richman, Elizabeth Ryerson, Eric Shaw, Zubin Shroff, J. Sherburne, Hilary Thornburn, Felicia Tomasko, Alan Walford, Randal Williams, Erica Rodefer Winters and Yogamatters. Thanks also to those who helped to promote and publicize the Kickstarter campaign: John B. Abbot, Bea Beatrice, Jennifer Davidson, Christina L. Desser, Elephant Journal, Phil Goldberg, Roseanne Harvey, Carol Horton, Autumn Jacobsen, Judith Hanson Lasater, Jill Miller, Danny Paradise, Jennifer Prugh, Matthew Redican at Signals.tv, Matthew Remski, Richard Rosen, Matthew Ryan, Matthew Sweeney, Priya Thomas, *Yoga Dork* and *Yoga Journal*. In particular we thank Scott Virden Anderson and the Yoga Science Foundation for their support of this project. We would also like to express our gratitude to the late Georg Feuerstein (1947–2012) for his enthusiastic support of this project at its inception.

Especial thanks to Elizabeth de Michelis for her support of this project, and for her continued contributions to the scholarly study of yoga

Index